T0226492

# Lipidology

*Editors*

EDWARD A. GILL
CHRISTIE M. BALLANTYNE
KATHLEEN L. WYNE

# CARDIOLOGY CLINICS

www.cardiology.theclinics.com

*Consulting Editors*
ROSARIO FREEMAN
JORDAN M. PRUTKIN
DAVID M. SHAVELLE
AUDREY H. WU

May 2015 • Volume 33 • Number 2

**ELSEVIER**

1600 John F. Kennedy Boulevard • Suite 1800 • Philadelphia, Pennsylvania, 19103-2899

http://www.theclinics.com

**CARDIOLOGY CLINICS Volume 33, Number 2**
**May 2015 ISSN 0733-8651, ISBN-13: 978-0-323-37592-4**

Editor: Adrianne Brigido
Developmental Editor: Susan Showalter

*Cardiology Clinics* (ISSN 0733-8651) is published quarterly by Elsevier Inc., 360 Park Avenue South, New York, NY 10010-1710. Months of issue are February, May, August, and November. Business and Editorial Offices: 1600 John F. Kennedy Blvd., Ste. 1800, Philadelphia, PA 19103-2899. Customer Service Office: 3251 Riverport Lane, Maryland Heights, MO 63043. Periodicals post-age paid at New York, NY and additional mailing offices. Subscription prices are $320.00 per year for US individuals, $530.00 per year for US institutions, $155.00 per year for US students and residents, $390.00 per year for Canadian individuals, $665.00 per year for Canadian institutions, $455.00 per year for international individuals, $665.00 per year for international institutions and $220.00 per year for Canadian and international students/residents. To receive student/resident rate, orders must be accompanied by name of affiliated institution, data of term, and the *signature* of program/residency coordinator on institution letterhead. Orders will be billed at individual rate until proof of status is received. Foreign air speed delivery is included in all *Clinics* subscription prices. All prices are subject to change without notice. **POSTMASTER:** Send address changes to *Cardiology Clinics*, Elsevier Health Sciences Division, Subscription Customer Service, 3251 Riverport Lane, Maryland Heights, MO 63043. **Customer Service: 1-800-654-2452 (U.S. and Canada); 314-447-8871 (outside U.S. and Canada). Fax: 314-447-8029. E-mail: journalscustomerservice-usa@ elsevier.com (for print support); journalsonlinesupport-usa@elsevier.com (for online support).**

*Reprints.* For copies of 100 or more, of articles in this publication, please contact the Commercial Reprints Department, Elsevier Inc., 360 Park Avenue South, New York, NY 10010-1710. Tel.: 212-633-3874; Fax: 212-633-3820; E-mail: reprints@elsevier.com.

*Cardiology Clinics* is also published in Spanish by McGraw-Hill Interamericana Editores S. A., P.O. Box 5-237, 06500, Mexico D. F., Mexico; in Portuguese by Reichmann and Alfonso Editores Rio de Janeiro, Brazil; and in Greek by Dimitrios P. Lagos, 8 Pondon Street, GR115-28 Ilissia, Greece.

*Cardiology Clinics* is covered in *MEDLINE/PubMed (Index Medicus), Excerpta Medica, The Cumulative Index to Nursing and Allied Health Literature* (CINAHL).

# Contributors

## EDITORIAL BOARD

**ROSARIO FREEMAN, MD, MS, FACC**
Associate Professor of Medicine; Director, Coronary Care Unit; Director, Echocardiography Laboratory, University of Washington Medical Center, Seattle, Washington

**JORDAN M. PRUTKIN, MD, MHS, FHRS**
Assistant Professor of Medicine, Division of Cardiology/Electrophysiology, University of Washington Medical Center, Seattle, Washington

**DAVID M. SHAVELLE, MD, FACC, FSCAI**
Associate Professor, Keck School of Medicine; Director, General Cardiovascular Fellowship Program; Director, Cardiac Catheterization Laboratory, Los Angeles County + USC Medical Center; Division of Cardiovascular Medicine, University of Southern California, Los Angeles, California

**AUDREY H. WU, MD**
Assistant Professor, Internal Medicine, University of Michigan, Ann Arbor, Michigan

## EDITORS

**EDWARD A. GILL, MD, FASE, FAHA, FACC, FACP, FNLA**
Professor of Medicine, Division of Cardiology; Adjunct Professor of Radiology, UW Department of Medicine; Director of Harborview Medical Center Echocardiography, University of Washington School of Medicine; Clinical Professor of Diagnostic Ultrasound, Seattle University, Seattle, Washington

**KATHLEEN L. WYNE, MD, PhD**
Associate Professor, Division of Endocrinology, The Ohio State University, Columbus, Ohio

**CHRISTIE M. BALLANTYNE, MD, FACC, FACP, FAHA, FNLA**
Chief, Sections of Cardiovascular Research and Cardiology; Professor of Medicine, Department of Medicine; Professor of Genetics, Baylor College of Medicine; Director of the Center for Cardiovascular Disease Prevention, Houston Methodist DeBakey Heart and Vascular Center, Houston, Texas

## AUTHORS

**BHAVIN B. ADHYARU, MS, MD**
Assistant Professor, Division of General Internal Medicine and Geriatrics, Department of Medicine, Emory University School of Medicine, Atlanta, Georgia

**KRISTEN M.J. AZAR, RN, MSN, MPH**
Palo Alto Medical Foundation Research Institute, Palo Alto, California

**SAMIRA BAHRAINY, MD**
Staff Physician, VA Medical Center, Puget Sound, Seattle, Washington

**CHRISTIE M. BALLANTYNE, MD, FACC, FACP, FAHA, FNLA**
Chief, Sections of Cardiovascular Research and Cardiology; Professor of Medicine, Department of Medicine; Professor of Genetics, Baylor College of Medicine; Director of the Center for Cardiovascular Disease Prevention, Houston Methodist DeBakey Heart and Vascular Center, Houston, Texas

**SETH J. BAUM, MD**
Division of Medicine, Charles E. Schmidt College of Biomedical Science, Florida Atlantic University, Boca Raton, Florida

**OZLEM BILEN, MD**
Medical Resident, Department of Medicine, Baylor College of Medicine, Houston, Texas

**VERA BITTNER, MD, MSPH, FNLA**
Division of Cardiovascular Disease, Department of Medicine, University of Alabama at Birmingham, Birmingham, Alabama

**VICTORIA ENCHIA BOUHAIRIE, MD**
Clinical Fellow in Endocrinology, Division of Endocrinology, Metabolism, and Lipid Research, Department of Medicine, Washington University School of Medicine, St Louis, Missouri

**ELIOT A. BRINTON, MD, FAHA, FNLA**
Director, Atherometabolic Research, Utah Foundation for Biomedical Research; President, Utah Lipid Center, Salt Lake City, Utah

**LISANDRO D. COLANTONIO, MD, MSc**
Department of Epidemiology, University of Alabama at Birmingham, Birmingham, Alabama

**MARY R. DICKLIN, PhD**
Metabolic Sciences, Midwest Center for Metabolic & Cardiovascular Research, Glen Ellyn, Illinois

**STEPHEN P. FORTMANN, MD**
Kaiser Permanente Center for Health Research, Portland, Oregon

**EDWARD A. GILL, MD, FASE, FAHA, FACC, FACP, FNLA**
Professor of Medicine, Division of Cardiology; Adjunct Professor of Radiology, UW Department of Medicine; Director of Harborview Medical Center Echocardiography, University of Washington School of Medicine; Clinical Professor of Diagnostic Ultrasound, Seattle University, Seattle, Washington

**ANNE CAROL GOLDBERG, MD**
Associate Professor of Medicine, Division of Endocrinology, Metabolism, and Lipid Research, Department of Medicine, Washington University School of Medicine, St Louis, Missouri

**KATHERINE G. HASTINGS, BA**
Stanford University School of Medicine, Stanford, California

**LINDA HEMPHILL, MD**
Assistant Physician, Massachusetts General Hospital; Instructor in Medicine, Harvard Medical School, Boston, Massachusetts

**CYNTHIA HERRICK, MD**
Instructor in Medicine, Division of Endocrinology, Metabolism and Lipid Research, Department of Medicine, Washington University School of Medicine, St Louis, Missouri

**ZAIN HUDANI, BPharm, MSc Candidate**
University of Waterloo School of Pharmacy, Waterloo, Ontario, Canada

**TERRY A. JACOBSON, MD**
Director, Lipid Clinic and Cardiovascular Risk Reduction Program; Professor, Department of Medicine, Emory University School of Medicine, Atlanta, Georgia

**KEVIN C. MAKI, PhD**
Metabolic Sciences, Midwest Center for Metabolic & Cardiovascular Research, Glen Ellyn, Illinois

**PATRICK M. MORIARTY, MD**
Professor of Medicine; Director of the Division of Clinical Pharmacology and Atherosclerosis/Lipoprotein-Apheresis Center, University of Kansas Medical Center, Kansas City, Kansas

**MERLE MYERSON, MD, EdD, FACC, FNLA**
Director, Cardiovascular Disease Prevention Program & Lipid Clinic, Cardiology Section, Institute for Advanced Medicine (HIV); Attending Cardiologist, Divisions of Cardiology and Infectious Diseases, Mount Sinai St. Luke's, Mount Sinai Roosevelt, New York, New York

**VANI NIMBAL, MPH**
Palo Alto Medical Foundation Research
Institute, Palo Alto, California

**LATHA P. PALANIAPPAN, MD, MS**
Stanford University School of Medicine,
Stanford, California

**YASHASHWI POKHAREL, MD, MSCR**
Clinical Postdoctoral Fellow, Section of
Cardiovascular Research, Department of
Medicine, Baylor College of Medicine; Center
for Cardiovascular Disease Prevention,
Methodist DeBakey Heart and Vascular
Center, Houston, Texas

**JIA PU, PhD**
Palo Alto Medical Foundation Research
Institute, Palo Alto, California

**CARLOS ROJAS-FERNANDEZ, BSc
(Pharm), PharmD**
Schlegel Research Chair in Geriatric
Pharmacotherapy, Schlegel-UW Research
Institute for Ageing & School of Pharmacy,
University of Waterloo; School of Public Health
and Health Systems, Faculty of Applied Health
Sciences, University of Waterloo, Waterloo,
Ontario, Canada; Michael G. DeGroote School
of Medicine, Department of Family Medicine,
McMaster University, Hamilton, Ontario,
Canada

**ROBERT ROMANELLI, PhD**
Palo Alto Medical Foundation
Research Institute, Palo Alto,
California

**ELIZABETH A. WEEDIN, DO**
Section of General Obstetrics
and Gynecology, Department of
Obstetrics and Gynecology,
University of Oklahoma Health
Sciences Center, Oklahoma City,
Oklahoma

**ROBERT WILD, MD, MPH, PhD**
Section of Reproductive Endocrinology
and Infertility, Department of Obstetrics
and Gynecology, University of Oklahoma
Health Sciences Center, Oklahoma City,
Oklahoma

**DON WILSON, MD, FNLA**
Department of Pediatric Endocrinology,
Cook Children's Medical Center,
Fort Worth, Texas

**BEINAN ZHAO, MS**
Palo Alto Medical Foundation
Research Institute, Palo Alto,
California

# Contents

> Familial hypercholesterolemia is a common, inherited disorder of cholesterol metabolism that leads to early cardiovascular morbidity and mortality. It is under-diagnosed and undertreated. Statins, ezetimibe, bile acid sequestrants, niacin, lomitapide, mipomersen, and low-density lipoprotein (LDL) apheresis are treatments that can lower LDL cholesterol levels. Early treatment can lead to substantial reduction of cardiovascular events and death in patients with familial hypercholesterolemia. It is important to increase awareness of this disorder in physicians and patients to reduce the burden of this disorder.

> This review discusses the 2013 American College of Cardiology (ACC)/American Heart Association (AHA) Guideline on the Treatment of Blood Cholesterol to Reduce Atherosclerotic Cardiovascular Risk in Adults and compares it with the 2014 National Lipid Association (NLA) Recommendations for Patient-Centered Management of Dyslipidemia. The review discusses some of the distinctions between the guidelines, including how to determine a patient's atherosclerotic cardiovascular disease risk, the role of lipoprotein treatment targets, the importance of moderate- and high-intensity statin therapy, and the use of nonstatin therapy in light of the IMProved Reduction of Outcomes: Vytorin Efficacy International Trial (IMPROVE-IT) trial.

> Patients with familial hypercholesterolemia (FH) have early development of atherosclerosis and cardiovascular disease (CVD). Lipid lowering medications are not always successful in reducing increased low-density lipoprotein C (LDL-C) levels. Lipoprotein apheresis (LA) therapy lowers LDL-C by more than 60%. LA has proven its clinical benefit in reducing CVD events for patients with FH and hypercholesterolemia. LA also reduces Lp(a) levels, inflammatory markers and blood viscosity.

> Recent studies have revealed evidence that poorly controlled cholesterol, triglycerides, and their metabolites during pregnancy may be associated with cardiometabolic dysfunction and have significant detrimental fetal and maternal vascular consequences. Cardiometabolic dysfunction during pregnancy may not only

contribute to long-term effects of the mother and child's vascular health but also potentially create cardiovascular risk for generational offspring. This article provides updates on this rapidly expanding and multifaceted topic and reviews new insight regarding why recognition of this disordered maternal cholesterol and triglyceride metabolism is likely to have long-term effect on the increasing atherosclerotic burden of the burgeoning population.

Understanding opportunities to reduce dyslipidemia before, during, and after pregnancy has major implications for cardiovascular disease risk prevention for the entire population. The best time to screen for dyslipidemia is before pregnancy or in the early antenatal period. The differential diagnosis of hypertriglyceridemia in pregnancy is the same as in nonpregnant women except that clinical lipidologists need to be aware of the potential obstetric complications associated with hypertriglyceridemia. Dyslipidemia discovered during pregnancy should be treated with diet and exercise intervention, as well as glycemic control if indicated. A complete lipid profile assessment during each trimester of pregnancy is recommended.

A statin is first-line drug therapy for dyslipidemia. Clinical trial data suggest there is an increase in the incidence of new-onset type 2 diabetes mellitus with statin use. The National Lipid Association (NLA) Statin Diabetes Safety Task Force concluded that the cardiovascular benefit of statin therapy outweighs the risk for developing diabetes. The NLA panel advocated following the standards of care from the American Diabetes Association for screening and diagnosis of diabetes, and emphasized the importance of lifestyle modification. This article summarizes NLA's review of the evidence, expanding it to include recent results, and outlines the clinical recommendations.

Statins are widely used in secondary and primary prevention of atherosclerotic cardiovascular disease. They reduce cardiovascular events and mortality, and have an excellent safety record. Recent case reports suggest a possible association between statins and adverse effects on cognition. This article reviews recent literature related to statins and cognition and provides recommendations to clinicians. Cognitive considerations should not play a role in decision making for most patients for whom statins are indicated. Future trials of statin, or any novel antilipemic agent should include systematic assessment of cognition.

Lipid lowering, particularly with 3-hydroxy-3-methylglutaryl-coenzyme A reductase inhibitors ("statins"), reduces the risk of cardiovascular disease. Patients with chronic liver disease present challenges to the use of lipid medications. In the case of most liver disorders, the concern has been one of safety. There is evidence that most lipid-lowering medications can be used safely in many situations, although large outcomes trials are lacking. This review examines lipid physiology and cardiovascular risk in specific liver diseases and reviews the evidence for lipid lowering and the use of statins in chronic liver disease.

Hereditary dyslipidemias are often underdiagnosed and undertreated, yet with significant health implications, most importantly causing preventable premature cardiovascular diseases. The commonly used clinical criteria to diagnose hereditary lipid disorders are specific but are not very sensitive. Genetic testing may be of value in making accurate diagnosis and improving cascade screening of family members, and potentially, in risk assessment and choice of therapy. This review focuses on using genetic testing in the clinical setting for lipid disorders, particularly familial hypercholesterolemia.

The development of antiretroviral medications to treat patients infected with HIV has changed this disease from one that was fatal to a chronic and more manageable condition. However, these patients are at increased risk for cardiovascular disease due to the HIV itself, use of antiretroviral medications, and because they are living to an age when cardiovascular disease is more prevalent. At present there are no specific guidelines for management of risk factors, in particular dyslipidemia, for this patient population. We present recommendations based on those for the general population and how these may be applied to patients living with HIV.

About one-half of individuals with an acute myocardial infarction have a low-density lipoprotein cholesterol level of less than 100 mg/dL at the time of occurrence, but remain at risk for recurrent events. This residual risk is likely mediated by multiple factors, including burden of atherosclerosis, residual dyslipidemia, nonlipid risk factors, and suboptimal implementation of lifestyle therapy and evidence-based pharmacologic therapy. This article reviews management options for this high-risk population.

Mendelian randomization data strongly suggest that hypertriglyceridemia (HTG) causes atherosclerotic cardiovascular disease (ASCVD), and so triglyceride (TG) level–lowering treatment in HTG is now more strongly recommended to address the residual ASCVD risk than has been the case in (generally earlier) published guidelines. Fibrates are the best-established agents for TG level lowering and are generally used as first-line treatment of TG levels greater than 500 mg/dL and prescription omega-3 and niacin are also useful. Statins are the best-established agents for ASCVD prevention, and so are usually used as first-line treatment of TG levels less than 500 mg/dL.

This article reviews racial/ethnic differences in dyslipidemia—prevalence of dyslipidemia, its relation to coronary heart disease (CHD) and stroke mortality rates, response to lipid-lowering agents, and lifestyle modification. Asian Indians, Filipinos, and Hispanics are at higher risk for dyslipidemia, which is consistent with the higher CHD mortality rates in these groups. Statins may have greater efficacy for Asians, but the data are mixed. Lifestyle modifications are recommended. Culturally-tailored prevention and intervention should be provided to the minority populations with elevated risk for dyslipidemia and considerably more research is needed to determine the best approaches to helping specific subgroups.

# CARDIOLOGY CLINICS

---

ISSUES OF RELATED INTEREST

*Endocrinology and Metabolism Clinics,* December 2014 (Vol. 43, No. 4)
**Lipids**
Donald A. Smith, *Editor*
Available at http://www.endo.theclinics.com/

---

**NOW AVAILABLE FOR YOUR iPhone and iPad**

# Preface
# The World and Lipidology as It Relates to Cardiology

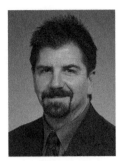

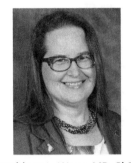

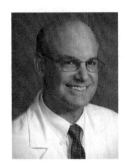

| | | |
|---|---|---|
| Edward A. Gill, MD, FASE, FAHA, FACC, FACP, FNLA | Kathleen L. Wyne, MD, PhD | Christie M. Ballantyne, MD, FACC, FACP, FAHA, FNLA |

*Editors*

What are hyperlipidemia and dyslipidemia? What is a Lipidologist? Is there a specialty dedicated to the diagnosis and treatment of lipid disorders? Should there be such a specialty? If so, how should it be recognized? What patients should be managed by Lipidologists? These are the questions that we hope the reader will be pondering as they peruse through the articles of this issue of *Cardiology Clinics* devoted to "Practical Lipidology for the Cardiovascular Specialist."

In order to define hyperlipidemia or dyslipidemia, on approach is to recognize this state as total I cholesterol, low density lipoprotein cholesterol (LDL-C), triglyceride, apolipoprotein (apo)-B, or Lp(a) levels above the 90th percentile. Also, high density lipoprotein-cholesterol (HDL-C) or apo A-I levels below the 10th percentile for the general population is another.

Cardiovascular disease continues to be the greatest killer of Americans despite remarkable progress in neutralizing its devastating effects. In fact, acute myocardial infarction decreased in prevalence throughout the 1990s and 2000s, especially ST elevation MI. In addition, mortality from acute MI decreased by as much as 50% in the 1990s and 2000s.[1] Cardiovascular disease is in fact growing in developing countries, and despite improvement in the United States, it is estimated that the global burden of coronary heart disease (CHD) increased by 29% between 1990 and 2010 due to increases in therapy and longevity along with global population growth.[1] There is significant regional variation in CHD mortality with the largest number of deaths seen in South Asia. Meanwhile, the highest death rate for CHD is seen in Eastern Europe and Central Asia.[1] The burden of cardiovascular disease in ethnic groups is hence emphasized and discussed in detail by Dr Palaniappan.

It cannot be emphasized enough that cardiovascular disease is largely preventable and, at the very least, can be delayed. Prevention has never been more possible today with the combination of tailored exercise, diet, and pharmacologic treatments, despite that our great pharmacologic therapies and lifestyle change are constantly being counterbalanced by an epidemic of obesity and type 2 diabetes.

The field of Lipidology experienced a dramatic turn of events in November 2013 when the ACC/AHA guidelines for treatment of cholesterol disorders were released and published simultaneously in *Circulation* and *JACC*.[2] These guidelines have been discussed hugely over the past 18 months and we continue to do so within this issue. Drs Jacobson and Adhyaru discuss the ACC/AHA guidelines and contrast them to recommendations recently released by the National Lipid Association. The two key issues have been the lack of recommendations of lipid level goals, specifically LDL goals, and the lack of recommended roles of lipid-lowering agents beyond the statins.

In addition, Drs Goldberg and Bouhairie discuss familial hypercholesterolemia from the

Cardiol Clin 33 (2015) xiii–xiv
http://dx.doi.org/10.1016/j.ccl.2015.03.001
0733-8651/15/$ – see front matter © 2015 Published by Elsevier Inc.

pathophysiology to treatment of these patients with strikingly high LDL cholesterol levels, and Drs Ballantyne, Bilen, and Pokharel take us through the newest breakthroughs in genetics and their role in diagnosing and treating lipid disorders.

This issue will take the reader on a journey of lipid recognition, appreciation of pathophysiology, and treatment of lipid disorders and will certainly recognize the difficulty we as caregivers face with the precise treatment of these disorders, particularly with regard to the need or lack thereof of LDL or other goals such as non-HDL, and with regard to which pharmacologic agents to prescribe. In the end, we believe the importance of lifestyle means of prevention, including weight loss, maintenance of ideal body weight, diet, and exercise, needs to be emphasized.

The guest editors would like to thank Dr Rosario Freeman for the invitation to put together this issue of *Cardiology Clinics*. It has been a pleasure to do so, and we have enjoyed working with all the contributors. A special thanks to the staff at Elsevier, particularly, Adrianne Brigido and Susan Showalter, for establishing goals and timelines, and for keeping us on track.

Edward A. Gill, MD, FASE, FAHA, FACC,
FACP, FNLA
Division of Cardiology
UW Department of Medicine
Harborview Medical Center Echocardiography
University of Washington School of Medicine
Seattle University
325 Ninth Avenue, Box 359748
Seattle, WA 98104-2499, USA

Kathleen L. Wyne, MD, PhD
Division of Endocrinology
The Ohio State University
566 McCampbell Hall
1581 Dodd Drive
Columbus, OH 43210, USA

Christie M. Ballantyne, MD, FACC, FACP,
FAHA, FNLA
Sections of Cardiovascular Research
and Cardiology
Baylor College of Medicine
Center for Cardiovascular Disease Prevention
Houston Methodist DeBakey Heart and
Vascular Center
6565 Fannin, M.S. A-601
Houston, TX 77030, USA

E-mail addresses:
eagill@u.washington.edu (E.A. Gill)
kittiewyne@hotmail.com (K.L. Wyne)
cmb@bcm.edu (C.M. Ballantyne)

## REFERENCES

1. Moran AE, Forouzanfar MH, Roth GA, et al. The global burden of ischemic heart disease in 1990 and 2010: the Global Burden of Disease 2010 study. Circulation 2014;129:1493–501.
2. Stone NJ, Robinson JG, Lichtenstein AH. 2013 ACC/AHA guideline on the treatment of blood cholesterol to reduce atherosclerotic cardiovascular risk in adults: a report of the American College of Cardiology/American Heart Association Task Force on Practice guidelines. Circulation 2014;129: S1–45.

# Familial Hypercholesterolemia

Victoria Enchia Bouhairie, MD, Anne Carol Goldberg, MD*

## KEYWORDS

- Familial hypercholesterolemia • Statins • Ezetimibe • Bile acid sequestrants • LDL apheresis
- Lomitapide • Mipomersen

## KEY POINTS

- Familial hypercholesterolemia (FH) is a common genetic disorder leading to high cholesterol levels from birth and increased risk of atherosclerotic cardiovascular disease.
- Heterozygous FH occurs in approximately 1 in 250 people in many populations.
- Homozygous FH can lead to coronary artery disease in childhood and adolescence.
- Early treatment can decrease the risk of premature atherosclerotic cardiovascular disease in FH patients.

## INTRODUCTION

Familial hypercholesterolemia (FH) is an inherited condition resulting in high levels of low-density lipoprotein cholesterol (LDL-C) and increased risk of premature cardiovascular disease in men and women. FH causes lifetime exposure to high LDL-C levels. It is not rare, but it is underdiagnosed. Although therapies for FH are available, it is commonly undertreated. Early diagnosis and treatment mitigate the excess risk of premature atherosclerotic cardiovascular disease that occurs with FH.[1–3]

### Pathophysiology

The pathophysiology of FH is due to decreased function of LDL receptors (LDLRs) (**Box 1**).

### Genetics of Familial Hypercholesterolemia

FH is an autosomal-dominant disorder with a gene dosage effect. Patients who are homozygotes (or compound heterozygotes) have much higher LDL-C levels and earlier coronary artery disease (CAD) onset than heterozygous patients.[1–4] The underlying defect in FH was initially thought to be due to increased synthesis of cholesterol, but it is now known that the fractional catabolic rate of LDL is decreased in heterozygous FH individuals compared with normal subjects.[5] The LDLR pathway was characterized by Brown and Goldstein and revealed receptor-mediated endocytosis.[6]

The most common form of FH is a monogenic, autosomal-dominant disorder, which causes defects in the gene that encodes the LDLR.[1–3]

More than 900 mutations of this gene have been identified,[1] most pathogenic, leading to the LDLR having decreased capacity to clear LDL from the circulation.

There are also defects in the LDLR binding region of apolipoprotein B (apoB)[1] and rare gain-of-function proprotein convertase subtilisin/kexin type 9 (PCSK9) gene mutations.[7] A rare

Conflict of Interest Statement: Dr V.E. Bouhairie receives support from Award Number T32DK007120 from the National Institute of Diabetes and Digestive and Kidney Diseases. The content is solely the responsibility of the authors and does not necessarily represent the official views of the National Institute of Diabetes and Digestive and Kidney Diseases or the National Institutes of Health; Dr A.C. Goldberg: Research Support: Research contracts to institution— Merck, Genzyme/ISIS/Sanofi-Aventis, GlaxoSmithKline, Amgen, Amarin, Regeneron/Sanofi-Aventis, Roche/Genentech, Pfizer; Consulting: Tekmira, Astra-Zeneca, uniQure; Editorial: Merck Manual.
Division of Endocrinology, Metabolism, and Lipid Research, Department of Medicine, Washington University School of Medicine, Campus Box 8127, 660 South Euclid, St Louis, MO 63110, USA
* Corresponding author.
E-mail address: agoldber@dom.wustl.edu

cardiology.theclinics.com

> **Box 1**
> **Pathophysiology of familial hypercholesterolemia**
>
> - Decreased LDLR function due to a genetic defect, typically one of the following classes[1]:
>   - LDLR is not synthesized
>   - LDLR is not properly transported from the endoplasmic reticulum to the Golgi apparatus for expression on the cell surface
>   - LDLR does not properly bind LDL on the cell surface
>   - LDLR does not properly cluster in clathrin-coated pits for receptor endocytosis
>   - LDLR is not recycled back to the cell surface
> - Therefore, LDLR-mediated endocytosis is decreased
> - Leading to markedly elevated LDL levels
> - Premature development of atherosclerotic plaque

autosomal-recessive form of FH caused by loss-of-function mutations in the LDL receptor adaptor protein 1 (LDLRAP1), which encodes a protein required for clathrin-mediated internalization of the LDLR, has also been described (**Table 1**).[3]

### Prevalence of Familial Hypercholesterolemia

Historically, the prevalence of heterozygous FH was 1 in 500 persons. Recent genetic studies suggest a prevalence of 1 in 200 to 250.[8,9] In populations such as French Canadians, Ashkenazi Jews, Lebanese, and several South African populations, the prevalence may be as high as 1 in 100.[10] Based on a prevalence of 1 in 500, there are an estimated 620,000 FH patients in the United States,[11] but this number may be as high as 1,500,000 based on a prevalence of 1 in 250. The historical prevalence estimate of homozygous (or compound heterozygous) patients is 1 in 1 million, and this would also change based on current studies. Recent data from the Netherlands suggest that the prevalence could be as low as 1 in 160,000 and is likely to be about 1 in 250,000.[9] Most patients with homozygous FH have extreme hypercholesterolemia with rapidly accelerated atherosclerosis when left untreated.[3,10]

Although single-gene disorders play a crucial role in the cause of FH, linkage studies suggest that some cases are caused by the presence of multiple single-nucleotide polymorphisms.[12] Heterozygotes arise when a mutation is inherited from one parent only, whereas homozygotes develop when the same mutated gene is inherited from both parents. Compound heterozygotes are due to inheritance of a different mutation from each parent. Untreated heterozygotes have LDL-C in the range of 155 to 500 mg/dL, whereas untreated homozygotes (or compound heterozygotes) typically have LDL-C greater than 500 mg/dL. Recent data suggest wide variation in LDL-C levels.[1–3,10]

## PATIENT EVALUATION
### Screening Strategies

Although the atherosclerotic manifestations of FH usually occur in adulthood, the clinical effects of the disease can start in the first decade of life in homozygous patients.[3] Unfortunately, FH is often diagnosed late and after the occurrence of a major coronary event. A combination of screening methods to identify at-risk individuals is needed[11,13,14] to prevent premature atherosclerosis.

There are many barriers to the diagnosis and treatment of FH. Many individuals and family members with FH who have CAD have other

**Table 1**
**Types of mutations causing familial hypercholesterolemia**

| Mutation | Gene | Mechanism | Numbers of Mutations (% of FH Cases) |
|---|---|---|---|
| LDLR | LDLR | LDLR is absent or has decreased capacity to clear LDL from circulation | >900 (85%–90%) |
| ApoB (also known as familial defective apoB) | ApoB | Impaired LDLR binding—mutation at binding site on LDL particle | Mutations around the 3500 residues—most common is Arg3500Gln (5%–10%) |
| PCSK9 gain of function | PCSK9 | Increased PCSK9 level leads to increased degradation of LDLRs | Rare |
| LDLR adaptor protein | LDLRAP1 | Protein needed for clathrin-mediated internalization of LDLR | Rare; autosomal-recessive hypercholesterolemia |

common CAD risk factors; thus, genetic hypercholesterolemia is not suspected and ultimately not diagnosed. Primary care physicians manage most patients with hypercholesterolemia, and there is often a lack of awareness of FH among physicians and the general public with only very severe cases being referred to specialists.[2,13]

Cascade screening, in which health care providers actively screen for disease among the first-degree and second-degree relatives of patients diagnosed with FH,[13] can increase detection rates but risks missing affected individuals. Several national and international guidelines recommend universal screening for elevated serum cholesterol by age 20 and cascade testing of first-degree relatives of all individuals with FH.[2,11,13,15,16] For children, cholesterol screening should be done at age 9 to 11 and considered beginning at age 2 in those with a family history of premature cardiovascular disease or elevated cholesterol.[11,17,18]

## Diagnosis

Diagnosis of FH is based on lipid levels, family history, physical findings (if present), and, if available, genetic analysis (**Box 2**). Physical examination findings of tendon xanthomas, arcus corneae (under the age of 45), and tuberous xanthomas or xanthelasma (under the age of 25) when present at an early age should also prompt suspicion for

FH. However, physical findings are not present in all patients with FH.[1]

There are 3 well-defined clinical diagnostic tools that are used to diagnose FH:

- The US Make Early Diagnoses Prevent Early Deaths Program Diagnostic Criteria,[19]
  - Uses total and LDL-C measurements and family history
- The Dutch Lipid Clinic Network Diagnostic Criteria[20]
  - Uses a point system of LDL-C levels, physical examination findings, and family and personal history of CAD; presence of genetic mutations
- The Simon Broome Register Diagnostic Criteria[15]
  - Uses LDL-C levels, family history, tendon xanthomas, presence of genetic mutations

The Dutch Lipid Clinic criteria are generally not useful in children. These sets of criteria are typically used to diagnose heterozygous FH.

The diagnosis of homozygous (or compound heterozygous) FH has been defined in several ways,[3,10] with one possible definition shown in **Box 3**. However, recent data on the heterogeneity and prevalence of genetically defined homozygous FH suggest that older criteria may not always apply.[9]

---

**Box 2**
**Clinical approach to diagnosis of familial hypercholesterolemia**

*Consider FH in the following*

- Presence of premature atherosclerotic cardiovascular disease
- Fasting LDL-C levels greater than 190 mg/dL in adults after exclusion of secondary causes of elevated LDL-C (hypothyroidism, nephrotic syndrome)
- Fasting untreated LDL-C levels that have an 80% probability of FH in the general population:
  - $\geq$250 mg/dL in adults $\geq$30 years
  - $\geq$220 mg/dL in adults aged 20 to 29
  - $\geq$190 mg/dL in patients under the age of 20
- Presence of full corneal arcus under the age of 40
- Presence of tendon xanthomas
- Family history of premature atherosclerotic cardiovascular disease
- Family history of high cholesterol levels

---

**Box 3**
**Diagnosis of homozygous familial hypercholesterolemia**

Genetic analysis showing mutations in 2 alleles at gene locus for *LDLR, APOB, PCKS9, LDLRAP1*

OR

Presence of untreated LDL greater than 500 mg/dL or treated LDL greater than 300 mg/dL plus:

Presence of cutaneous or tendon xanthomas before the age of 10 years

OR

Both parents with evidence of heterozygous FH (except for the rare LDLRAP1 mutations)

Note that the range of untreated LDL-C levels in homozygous FH can be lower, especially in children.
*Data from* Cuchel M, Bruckert E, Ginsberg H. Homozygous familial hypercholesterolaemia: new insights and guidance for clinicians to improve detection and clinical management. A position paper from the Consensus Panel on Familial Hypercholesterolaemia of the European Atherosclerosis Society. Eur Heart J 2014;35(32):2146–57; and Raal FJ, Santos RD. Homozygous familial hypercholesterolemia: current perspectives on diagnosis and treatment. Atherosclerosis 2012;223:262–8.

## Genetic Testing

Clinical criteria may not identify all patients with FH, and genetic testing is part of the screening strategies in many countries, with the costs covered by national health services.[2,3,13,15,16] In the United States, it is done infrequently, partly because of cost and lack of insurance coverage. Genetic testing in certain populations has changed the understanding of the frequency of both heterozygous and homozygous FH. However, a mutation is not always found in patients with clinical FH, and lack of a mutation should not change treatment.[1]

## Prognosis

Patients with heterozygous FH are generally asymptomatic in childhood and early adulthood. About 5% of heart attacks in patients under the age of 60 and as many as 20% under the age of 45 are due to FH.[1,2]

Homozygous or compound heterozygous FH has a severe and variable clinical presentation usually within the first decade of life. Most of these individuals have extreme hypercholesterolemia with rapidly accelerated atherosclerosis when left untreated. The variation depends on the amount of LDLR activity.[3,10] CAD is the most common cause of premature death in these patients, but other cardiovascular diseases, including aortic and supravalvular aortic stenosis and aortic root disease, are also common.[3,10]

### Risk assessment tools

Risk assessment tools do not adequately predict 10-year coronary heart disease (CHD) risk in FH patients, and the Framingham Risk Score is not recommended in FH patients.[4] Risk calculators underestimate risk in patients with FH because of the significant effect of exposure to high cholesterol levels from birth.

## TREATMENT

The lifetime risk of CHD and premature onset CHD is very high in individuals with FH. Early treatment is beneficial and long-term drug therapy can substantially reduce or eliminate the added lifetime risk of CHD from having FH and can lower the CHD event rate in heterozygous FH patients to levels similar to those of the general population.[2,21,22] The 2013 American College of Cardiology/American Heart Association (ACC/AHA) cholesterol treatment guideline recommends potent statin use in adult patients with LDL-C levels of 190 mg/dL or higher.[23] The National Lipid Association recommends that both children and adults with LDL-C of 190 mg/dL or higher (or

non-high-density lipoprotein [HDL] cholesterol ≥220 mg/dL) after lifestyle changes be started on drug therapy.[17,24]

## Lifestyle and Noncholesterol Risk Factor Modification

Lifestyle and noncholesterol risk factor modification is an important part of treatment (**Box 4**).[13,24]

Homozygous patients require treatment as soon as the diagnosis is made and need lifestyle, medication, and additional modalities. Treatment of homozygous FH patients can delay major cardiovascular events and early death.[3,25]

## Pharmacologic Therapy

Statins should be the initial drug for all adults with FH and in children with heterozygous FH starting at 8 to 10 years of age.[4,13,15–17,24] Patients with homozygous FH should be treated as soon as the diagnosis is made.[3,10,13] The US Food and Drug Administration (FDA) has approved lovastatin, atorvastatin, simvastatin, and rosuvastatin in children over the age of 10 years and pravastatin in those over 8 years of age.[26] Statins increase the expression of LDLRs by reducing HMG-CoA reductase, the rate-limiting step in cholesterol

---

**Box 4**
**Lifestyle and noncholesterol risk factor modification**

- Dietary modification contributes to improvement in lipid profiles
  - A heart-healthy diet including vegetables, fruit, nonfat dairy, beans, tree nuts, fish, and lean meats should be encouraged
  - Restrict intake of saturated fat to less than 7% of calories
  - Avoid trans fats
  - If alcohol is used, amount should be moderate
  - Addition of plant stanols (2 g/d) and insoluble fiber (10–20 g/d) can provide some LDL-C lowering
  - Dietitian counseling is beneficial
- Physical activity
- Avoidance of weight gain
- Avoidance and cessation of smoking is mandatory
  - Discourage exposure to passive smoking
- Treat diabetes and hypertension
- Consider low-dose aspirin

synthesis. Moderate-potency to high-potency statins should be used as first-line treatment (atorvastatin, rosuvastatin, simvastatin, pitavastatin) (**Table 2**). Low-potency statins are usually inadequate for FH patients.[13,24] Adult FH patients should have a treatment goal of 50% LDL-C reduction or better from baseline. Statin therapy is effective in heterozygous FH patients and may also benefit homozygous patients who have some LDLR activity (see **Table 2**).[3,10]

Long-term safety of statins in the pediatric population is still unknown, but the current benefits of therapy outweigh the risk of untreated pediatric populations.[17,26–28] Children and adolescents being treated with statins should have regular follow-up with close monitoring of creatinine kinase, aspartate aminotransferase (AST), and alanine aminotransferase levels (ALT). Baseline levels, then repeat testing, should be done at 1 to 3 months after drug initiation and then yearly. If **creatine kinase** levels reach 5 times the upper limit of normal and AST or ALT levels reach 3 times the upper limit of normal, a 3-month drug-free holiday should be initiated with reintroduction of the same drug at a lower dose or a different statin if levels return to baseline.[29]

Patients with FH who have a higher risk of CHD require more intensive drug therapy.[4,13]

High-risk patients include those with the following:

- Clinically evident CHD or other atherosclerotic cardiovascular disease
- Diabetes
- Family history of very early CHD (<45 years in men and <55 years in women)
- Current smoking
- Two or more CHD risk factors
- High lipoprotein (a) ($\geq$50 mg/dL)

In these patients, the LDL goal is less than 100 mg/dL and non-HDL goal is less than 130 mg/dL.

### Combination Therapy

Many patients with FH will require more than one medication to obtain optimal LDL-C lowering. Patients may require multiple medications depending on their baseline LDL-C levels and their responsiveness to therapy. Drugs that can be added to statins for LDL-C reduction include ezetimibe, bile-acid sequestrants, and niacin (**Table 3**).

The addition of ezetimibe to a statin is the preferred approach in the treatment of patients with FH.[2,3,13,16] Some patients may require 3 or more medications to lower LDL-C adequately.

Fibrates are most useful for triglyceride lowering but may have some LDL-C lowering effect.

Ezetimibe, niacin, and bile acid sequestrants are also treatment options for drug intensification or for those intolerant of a statin; this should also be considered in FH patients who are not at very high risk when LDL-C does not decrease by 50% with statin monotherapy. It is important to note that doubling the dose of statin only achieves an additional LDL reduction by 6% to 7%.[30] Therefore, if additional reduction is needed, other medications should be added. Other options for those intolerant of statins include every-other-day statin therapy or lowering the dose while adding other treatment medications.

Drug interactions with statins are primarily due to cytochrome P450 metabolism, drug transporters, and glucuronidation; thus, caution should

**Table 2**
**Lipid-lowering medications for use in familial hypercholesterolemia: statins**

| Statin | Dose Range (mg) | Mean Reduction LDL-C (%) | Pharmacologic and Safety Issues |
|---|---|---|---|
| Rosuvastatin | 5–40 | 46–55 | Dose reduction in renal insufficiency, Asian, and elderly patients |
| Atorvastatin | 10–80 | 37–51 | Minimal renal excretion CYP3A4 substrate |
| Simvastatin | 5–80[a] | 26–47 | CYP3A4 substrate, dose reduction in severe renal insufficiency |
| Lovastatin | 10–80 | 21–40 | CYP3A4 substrate |
| Pravastatin | 10–80 | 20–36 | Dose reduction in severe renal insufficiency |
| Fluvastatin | 20–80 | 22–35 | Minimal renal excretion |
| Pitavastatin | 1–4 | 32–43 | Dose reduction in severe renal insufficiency |

[a] Simvastatin 80-mg dosage should only be used in patients previously taking this dose for greater than 1 year and no other contraindications.

**Table 3**
**Low-density lipoprotein–lowering drugs for familial hypercholesterolemia: nonstatins**

| Medication | Dose Range | Mean Reduction LDL-C (%) | Pharmacologic and Safety Issues |
|---|---|---|---|
| Ezetimibe | 10 mg daily | 15–20 | Diarrhea, abdominal pain, myalgias |
| Bile acid sequestrants | | | |
|   Colesevelam | 3.75–4.375 g/d | 15–18 | Should be given with meals. |
|   Colestipol | 4–15 g bid | 12–30 | Side effects: constipation, abdominal pain, |
|   Cholestyramine | 4–12 g bid | 7–30 | bloating, nausea, flatulence |
| | | | Interference with absorption of other medications: warfarin, digoxin, thyroid hormone, thiazide diuretics, amiodarone, glipizide, statins (less with colesevelam) |
| Niacin | 500–2000 mg daily | 5–20 | Side effects: flushing, pruritus, nausea, bloating, elevation of liver transaminases, hyperuricemia, and hyperglycemia |
| Fenofibrate (multiple preparations) | 30–200 mg daily | 0–20 | Reduced dosage in renal insufficiency Side effects: abdominal pain, gastrointestinal, elevation of liver enzymes, myalgias, risk of rhabdomyolysis, increased creatinine |

be used with medications metabolized by cytochrome P450 isoenzyme CYP 3A4.[31]

Ezetimibe is localized to the brush border of the small intestine and inhibits the absorption of cholesterol. It reduces LDL-C by about 15% to 20% when used alone and provides 20% additional reduction in combination with a statin.[32]

Bile acid sequestrants inhibit the enterohepatic reuptake and increase fecal loss of bile salts. They decrease LDL-C by preventing the reabsorption of bile acids in the terminal ileum. Because they are not absorbed systemically, they are considered safer to use than other cholesterol-lowering medications.[33] Like ezetimibe, the effect on LDL-C reduction can be additive with statins and even ezetimibe.[34] The need for suspensions or large numbers of pills, gastrointestinal side effects, and multiple drug-drug interactions limits patient adherence and use. Colesevelam, as compared with other bile acid sequestrants, has fewer gastrointestinal side effects and drug-drug interactions. Colesevelam is also approved for treatment of diabetes and may help patients achieve both glycemic and lipid goals.[35] Colesevelam is the recommended bile acid sequestrant for FH patients.[24]

Niacin, a water-soluble B vitamin, lowers LDL-C and raises HDL. It comes in crystalline and extended release forms. Because of concerns for liver toxicity, most nonprescription sustained release forms are not recommended.[24] The maximum dose of 2 g daily of niacin when added to statin is effective in lowering LDL-C.[24] Fibrates lower triglycerides and raise HDL-C. Because of

the increased risk of fibrate-induced myositis (particularly with gemfibrozil) with statins, they need to be used with caution.[31]

Women with FH who are of child-bearing age should be advised to use contraception while on therapy and to stop any statin (category X), niacin (category C), or ezetimibe (category C) therapy at least 4 weeks before stopping contraception.[24] Those who become pregnant on therapy or are breastfeeding should be advised to discontinue therapy immediately. colesevelam is a category B drug and can used when clinically indicated.[24] For pregnant women with homozygous FH, or heterozygous FH and atherosclerotic disease, LDL apheresis should be considered.[13,24]

## Low-Density Lipoprotein Apheresis

LDL apheresis is an important treatment modality for homozygous FH patients and for heterozygous patients who have not met treatment goals despite optimal tolerated medical therapy (**Box 5**).[24,36] It is an extracorporeal treatment that uses various methods to remove LDL from the circulation. LDL apheresis is currently FDA approved and has been shown in clinical trials to prevent and slow the progression of CHD.[13,37,38]

Apheresis is generally done every 1 to 2 weeks, with each session taking about 3 hours and removing greater than 60% of Apo-B-containing lipoproteins.[38] The LDL reduction with LDL apheresis is temporary and associated with a rebound elevation in lipid levels after the procedure. The efficacy of LDL apheresis can be enhanced by the

**Box 5**
**Low-density lipoprotein apheresis recommendations (National Lipid Association and American College of Cardiology/American Heart Association cholesterol guideline)**

*LDL apheresis is recommended for the following patients*

- LDL goal reduction has not been achieved despite diet and maximum drug therapy (after 6 months)
- Adequate drug therapy is not tolerated or contraindicated
- Functional homozygous FH patients with LDL-C 300 mg/DL or higher (or non-HDL cholesterol ≥330 mg/dL)
- Functional heterozygous FH patients with LDL-C 300 mg/dL or higher (or non-HDL ≥330 mg/dL) and 0–1 risk factors
- Functional heterozygous FH patients with LDL-C 200 mg/dL or higher (or non-HDL cholesterol ≥230 mg/dL) and with risk characteristics such as 2 or more risk factors or high lipoprotein (a) 50 mg/dL or higher
- Functional heterozygotes with LDL-C 160 mg/dL or higher (or non-HDL cholesterol ≥190 mg/dL) and very high-risk characteristics (established CHD, other cardiovascular disease, or diabetes).

*Data from* Ito M, McGowan M, Moriarty P. National Lipid Association Expert Panel on Familial Hypercholesterolemia. Management of familial hypercholesterolemias in adult patients: recommendations from the National Lipid Association Expert Panel on Familial Hypercholesterolemia. J Clin Lipidol 2011;5:S38–45; and Stone NJ, Robinson JG, Lichtenstein AH, et al. Report on the treatment of blood cholesterol to reduce atherosclerotic cardiovascular disease in adults: full panel report supplement. 2013. Available at: http://circ.ahajournals.org/content/suppl/2013/11/07/01.cir.0000437738.63853.7a.DC1/Blood_Cholesterol_Full_Panel_Report.docx. Accessed January 21, 2015.

addition of statin therapy. LDL apheresis treatment in homozygous FH patients has improved their life expectancy to more than 50 years.[38] Cost and limited availability decrease widespread use of LDL apheresis.

### Homozygous Familial Hypercholesterolemia: Treatment Considerations

Treatment starts at the time of diagnosis and involves age-appropriate diet, statin, ezetimibe, and often apheresis.[3,13] The FDA has approved 2 novel treatments for homozygous FH individuals older than 18 years of age: lomitapide and mipomersen (**Table 4**).[39] Lomitapide also has European approval. Lomitapide is a microsomal triglyceride transfer (MTP) protein inhibitor available as a capsule and used as an adjunct to other cholesterol-lowering medications, lifestyle changes, and LDL apheresis if needed. The function of MTP, which resides in the lumen of endoplasmic reticulum of enterocytes and

**Table 4**
**Pharmacologic agents approved for homozygous familial hypercholesterolemia**

| Treatment | Dosage | Mean Reduction LDL-C (%) | Drug Interactions | Safety Issues | Side Effects |
|---|---|---|---|---|---|
| Mipomersen | 200 mg subcutaneously once per week | 24–28 | None | Increased hepatic transaminases Increased hepatic fat | Injection site reactions, pyrexia, malaise, fatigue, headache, nausea |
| Lomitapide | 5 to 60 mg orally per day | 38–50 | Cytochrome p450 3A4 (atorvastatin) | Increased hepatic enzymes Increased hepatic fat Cytochrome p450 3A4 interactions | Diarrhea, gastrointestinal side effects Requires low-fat diet and supplemental fat-soluble vitamins |

hepatocytes, is to assist in the transfer of triglycerides to apolipoprotein B to form very-low-density lipoprotein particles.[40] Lomitapide enabled some homozygous FH patients to discontinue or decrease the frequency of apheresis in some in a clinical trial.[41] Because of concerns about hepatotoxicity, prescription of lomitapide requires an FDA-approved Risk Evaluation and Mitigation Strategy (REMS) program.

Mipomersen is delivered by subcutaneous injection with weekly dosing. It is an antisense oligonucleotide that causes a reduction in LDL by binding to messenger RNA and inhibiting apolipoprotein B-100 synthesis.[42] LDL, apo B, and lipoprotein (a) concentrations are reduced.[43,44] Reported side effects include injection site reactions, flulike symptoms, increased ALT, and steatosis.[42–44] Thus, this medication also requires frequent monitoring of liver function tests and prescription approval via REMS.

## SURGICAL THERAPY

For patients who do not achieve sufficient lipid reduction by the above-mentioned modalities, other potential treatment options include partial ileal bypass and liver transplantation. Liver transplantation produces a significant lowering of LDL-C by providing normal LDLRs. Liver transplantation is now used primarily in children with homozygous FH when apheresis is not an option or with concurrent heart transplantation.[13,45] Its use, however, is limited due to the risk of transplant surgery and the limited number of donor livers.[13,24,29] Partial ileal bypass is rarely used and works by interrupting enterohepatic bile acid circulation.[13,24]

## TREATMENT RESISTANCE/COMPLICATIONS
### Side Effects of Medications

#### Statins and muscle problems

Statin side effects, particularly muscle complaints, are the limiting factors in their optimal usage. Muscle symptoms are the most common cause of statin discontinuation. They are typically dose dependent and can vary with the statin used. Statin-induced myopathy appears to be positively associated with the dose and potency of the statin.[23,46] Symptoms tend to occur more often with increasing age and number of medications, and decreasing renal function and body size. Management of statin-related myopathy can be difficult (**Box 6**).[23,46]

#### Statins and liver issues

Although liver toxicity from statins is often a concern for patients and physicians, it is not common, and serious hepatotoxicity is extremely rare. Hepatic aminotransferase elevation is usually mild and does not require discontinuation of the statin. It may be dose dependent.

Only about 1% of patients have aminotransferase increases to greater than 3 times the upper limit of normal, and the elevation often decreases even if patients continue on the statin. A common cause is hepatic steatosis, which responds to weight loss. Statins can be used cautiously in the presence of liver disease as long as it is not decompensated.[47] In particular, nonalcoholic fatty liver disease is not a contraindication. Hepatic transaminases should be obtained at baseline and during treatment if there is a clinical indication for their measurement.[23] Routine monitoring of hepatic transaminases was removed from product labeling

---

**Box 6**
**Approach to statin-related muscle problems**

- Discontinue statin in patients who develop muscle symptoms until they can be evaluated. For severe symptoms, evaluate for rhabdomyolysis.
- For mild to moderate symptoms, evaluate for conditions increasing the risk of muscle symptoms, including renal or hepatic impairment, hypothyroidism, vitamin D deficiency, rheumatologic disorders, and primary muscle disorders
- Statin-induced myalgias are likely to resolve within 2 months of discontinuing the drug.
- If symptoms resolve, the same or lower dose of the statin can be reintroduced.
- If symptoms recur, use a low dose of a different statin and increase as tolerated.
- If the cause of symptoms is determined to be unrelated, restart the original statin.

*Data from* Stone NJ, Robinson J, Lichtenstein AH, et al. 2013 ACC/AHA guideline on the treatment of blood cholesterol to reduce atherosclerotic cardiovascular risk in adults: a report of the American College of Cardiology/American Heart Association Task Force on Practice Guidelines. J Am Coll Cardiol 2014;63(25 Pt B):2889–934; and Rosenson RS, Baker SK, Jacobson TA. An assessment by the Statin Muscle Safety Task Force: 2014 update. J Clin Lipidol 2014;8:S58–71.

by the FDA in 2012. If aminotransferases remain greater than 3 times the upper limit of normal, change to a different statin and identifying other contributing conditions or drugs should be considered.[48] Irreversible liver damage resulting from statins is extremely rare, with a rate of liver failure of 1 case per 1 million person-years of use.[49]

Clinical trials and meta-analyses have shown a small increase in the risk of diabetes with statin use. In most cases of FH, the benefits of statin treatment far outweigh this risk.[23]

## DRUGS IN DEVELOPMENT

Drugs in development have the potential for additive effects with statins or other lipid-lowering medications to achieve further reduction of LDL-C.

The most promising new therapeutic approach for FH involves monoclonal antibodies to PCSK9. PCSK9 increases LDL-C by binding to the epidermal growth factor-like repeat A domain of the LDLR, causing LDL-receptor degradation, thus reducing the amount of LDL cleared from the plasma.[7] Gain-of-function mutations of PCSK9 result in elevation of LDL, whereas loss-of-function mutations lead to life-long low LDL levels and are associated with decreased risk of cardiovascular disease.[50] Given by subcutaneous injection once every 2 to 4 weeks, monoclonal antibodies that inhibit the binding of PCSK9 to LDLRs have produced 40% to 70% reductions of LDL-C in a variety of clinical situations, including FH.[51–55] Cardiovascular outcomes trials with several of these antibodies are in progress.

## SUMMARY

FH is a serious and treatable condition with a significantly increased risk of cardiovascular disease. Its onset is in early childhood with resultant premature death if not treated adequately. FH is underdiagnosed and undertreated, and more effort needs to be made to effectively screen and diagnose these patients because early treatment is necessary to decrease morbidity and mortality to the same level as in the general population. Lifestyle and diet changes are necessary but generally insufficient, and patients should be started on moderate-potency and high-potency statin therapy as initial treatment. Combination therapy is required in many patients. LDL apheresis should be considered in heterozygous and homozygous FH patients who have insufficient response to medical therapy. Recent medications for treatment of homozygous FH patients have been approved with other new treatment options currently undergoing clinical trials.

## REFERENCES

1. Hopkins P, Toth P, Ballantyne CM, et al. Familial hypercholesterolemias: prevalence, genetics, diagnosis and screening recommendations from the National Lipid Association Expert Panel on Familial Hypercholesterolemia. J Clin Lipidol 2011;5(3 Suppl): S9–17.
2. Nordestgaard B, Chapman M, Humphries S, et al. Familial hypercholesterolaemia is underdiagnosed and undertreated in the general population: guidance for clinicians to prevent coronary heart disease: consensus statement of the European Atherosclerosis Society. Eur Heart J 2013;34(45):3478–3490a.
3. Cuchel M, Bruckert E, Ginsberg H, et al. Homozygous familial hypercholesterolaemia: new insights and guidance for clinicians to improve detection and clinical management. A position paper from the Consensus Panel on Familial Hypercholesterolaemia of the European Atherosclerosis Society. Eur Heart J 2014;35(32):2146–57.
4. Robinson JG, Goldberg AC, National Lipid Association Expert Panel on Familial Hypercholesterolemia. Treatment of adults with familial hypercholesterolemia and evidence for treatment: recommendations from the National Lipid Association Expert Panel on Familial Hypercholesterolemia. J Clin Lipidol 2011;5(3 Suppl):S18–29.
5. Langer T, Strober W, Levy RI. The metabolism of low density lipoprotein in familial type II hyperlipoproteinemia. J Clin Invest 1972;51(6):1528–36.
6. Brown M, Goldstein J. A receptor-mediated pathway for cholesterol homeostasis. Science 1986;232(4746): 34–47.
7. Abifadel M, Elbitar S, El Khoury P, et al. Living the PCSK9 adventure: from the identification of a new gene in familial hypercholesterolemia towards a potential new class of anticholesterol drugs. Curr Atheroscler Rep 2014;16(9):439.
8. Benn M, Watts GF, Tybjaerg-Hansen A, et al. Familial hypercholesterolemia in the Danish general population: prevalence, coronary artery disease, and cholesterol-lowering medication. J Clin Endocrinol Metab 2012;97(11):3956–64.
9. Sjouke B, Kusters D, Kindt I, et al. Homozygous autosomal dominant hypercholesterolaemia in the Netherlands: prevalence, genotype–phenotype relationship, and clinical outcome. Eur Heart J 2014. http://dx.doi.org/10.1093/eurheartj/ehu058.
10. Raal FJ, Santos RD. Homozygous familial hypercholesterolemia: current perspectives on diagnosis and treatment. Atherosclerosis 2012;223:262–8.
11. Goldberg A, Hopkins P, Toth P, et al, National Lipid Association Expert Panel on Familial Hypercholesterolemia. Familial hypercholesterolemia: screening, diagnosis and management of pediatric and adult patients: clinical guidance from the National Lipid

Association Expert Panel on Familial Hypercholesterolemia. J Clin Lipidol 2011;5:S1–8.

12. Talmud PJ, Shah S, Whittall R, et al. Use of low-density lipoprotein cholesterol gene score to distinguish patients with polygenic and monogenic familial hypercholesterolaemia: a case-control study. Lancet 2013;381(9874):1293–301.

13. Watts GF, Gidding S, Wierzbicki AS, et al. Integrated guidance on the care of familial hypercholesterolemia from the International FH Foundation. J Clin Lipidol 2014;8:148–72.

14. Haase A, Goldberg A. Identification of people with heterozygous familial hypercholesterolemia. Curr Opin Lipidol 2012;23(4):282–9.

15. DeMott K, Nherera L, Shaw EJ, et al. Clinical guidelines and evidence review for familial hypercholesterolaemia: the identification and management of adults and children with familial hypercholesterolaemia. London: National Collaborating Centre for Primary Care and Royal College of General Practitioners; 2008.

16. Watts GF, Sullivan DR, Poplawski N, et al. Familial hypercholesterolaemia: a model of care for Australasia. Atheroscler Suppl 2011;12(2):221–63.

17. Daniels SR, Gidding SS, de Ferranti SD, National Lipid Association Expert Panel on Familial Hypercholesterolemia. Pediatric aspects of familial hypercholesterolemias: recommendations from the National Lipid Association Expert Panel on Familial Hypercholesterolemia. J Clin Lipidol 2011;5:S30–7.

18. Expert Panel on Integrated Guidelines for Cardiovascular Health and Risk Reduction in Children and Adolescents, National Heart, Lung, and Blood Institute. Expert panel on integrated guidelines for cardiovascular health and risk reduction in children and adolescents: summary report. Pediatrics 2011; 128(Suppl 5):S213–56.

19. Williams RR, Hunt SC, Schumacher MC. Diagnosing heterozygous familial hypercholesterolemia using new practical criteria validated by molecular genetics. Am J Cardiol 1993;72(2):171–6.

20. World Health organization. Familial hypercholesterolaemia. Report of a second WHO consultation. Geneva (Switzerland): World Health Organization; 1999.

21. Neil A, Cooper J, Betteridge J, et al. Reductions in all-cause, cancer, and coronary mortality in statin-treated patients with heterozygous familial hypercholesterolaemia: a prospective registry study. Eur Heart J 2008;29:2625–33.

22. Versmissen J, Oosterveer DM, Yazdanpanah M, et al. Efficacy of statins in familial hypercholesterolaemia: a long term cohort study. BMJ 2008;337: a2423.

23. Stone NJ, Robinson J, Lichtenstein AH, et al. 2013 ACC/AHA guideline on the treatment of blood cholesterol to reduce atherosclerotic cardiovascular risk in adults: a report of the American College of Cardiology/American Heart Association Task Force on Practice Guidelines. J Am Coll Cardiol 2014; 63(25 Pt B):2889–934.

24. Ito M, McGowan M, Moriarty P, National Lipid Association Expert Panel on Familial Hypercholesterolemia. Management of familial hypercholesterolemias in adult patients: recommendations from the National Lipid Association Expert Panel on Familial Hypercholesterolemia. J Clin Lipidol 2011;5:S38–45.

25. Raal FJ, Pilcher GJ, Panz VR, et al. Reduction in mortality in subjects with homozygous familial hypercholesterolemia associated with advances in lipid-lowering therapy. Circulation 2011;124:2202–7.

26. Forrester J. Redefining normal low-density lipoprotein cholesterol: a strategy to unseat coronary disease as the nation's leading killer. J Am Coll Cardiol 2010;56(8):630–6.

27. Wiegman A, Hutten BA, de Groot EE. Efficacy and safety of statin therapy in children with familial hypercholesterolemia: a randomized controlled trial. JAMA 2004;292(3):331–7.

28. McCrindle BW, Urbina EM, Dennison BA, et al. Drug therapy of high-risk lipid abnormalities in children and adolescents: a scientific statement from the American Heart Association Atherosclerosis, Hypertension, and Obesity in Youth Committee, Council of Cardiovascular Disease in the Young, with the Council on Cardiovascular Nursing. Circulation 2007;115:1948–67.

29. Varghese M. Familial hypercholesterolemia. A review. Ann Pediatr Cardiol 2014;7(2):107–17.

30. Jones P, Davidson M, Stein E, et al. Comparison of the efficacy and safety of rosuvastatin versus atorvastatin, simvastatin, and pravastatin across doses (STELLAR* Trial). Am J Cardiol 2003;92(2):152–60.

31. Kellick KA, Bottorff M, Toth PP. A clinician's guide to statin drug-drug interactions. J Clin Lipidol 2014;8: S30–46.

32. Gagne C, Gaudet D, Bruckert E, et al. Efficacy and safety of ezetimibe coadministered with atorvastatin or simvastatin in patients with homozygous familial hypercholesterolemia. Circulation 2002;105(21): 2469–75.

33. Insull W Jr. Clinical utility of bile acid sequestrants in the treatment of dyslipidemia: a scientific review. South Med J 2006;99:257–73.

34. Huijgen R, Abbink E, Bruckert E, et al. Colesevelam added to combination therapy with a statin and ezetimibe in patients with familial hypercholesterolemia: a 12-week, multicenter, randomized, double-blind, controlled trial. Clin Ther 2010;32(4):615–25.

35. Zieve F, Kalin M, Schwartz S, et al. Results of the glucose-lowering effect of WelChol study (GLOWS): a randomized, double-blind, placebo-controlled pilot study evaluating the effect of colesevelam hydrochloride on glycemic control in subjects with type 2 diabetes. Clin Ther 2007;29(1):74–83.

36. Stone, NJ, Robinson JG, Lichtenstein AH, et al. Report on the Treatment of blood cholesterol to reduce atherosclerotic cardiovascular disease in adults: full panel report supplement. 2013. Available at: http://circ.ahajournals.org/content/suppl/2013/11/07/01.cir.0000437738.63853.7a.DC1/Blood_Cholesterol_Full_Panel_Report.docx. Accessed January 21, 2015.

37. Thompson G. LDL apheresis. Atherosclerosis 2003; 167(1):1–13.

38. Thompson GR, Catapano A, Saheb S, et al. Severe hypercholesterolaemia: therapeutic goals and eligibility criteria for LDL apheresis in Europe. Curr Opin Lipidol 2010;21(6):492–8.

39. Rader D, Kastelein J. Lomitapide and mipomersen: two first-in-class drugs for reducing low-density lipoprotein cholesterol in patients with homozygous familial hypercholesterolemia. Circulation 2014;129(9): 1022–32.

40. Cuchel M, Bloedon L, Szapary P, et al. Inhibition of microsomal triglyceride transfer protein in familial hypercholesterolemia. N Engl J Med 2007;356:148–56.

41. Cuchel M, Meagher EA, du Toit Theron H, et al. Efficacy and safety of a microsomal triglyceride transfer protein inhibitor in patients with homozygous familial hypercholesterolaemia: a single-arm, open-label, phase 3 study. Lancet 2013;381:40–6.

42. Stein E, Dufour R, Gagne C, et al. Apolipoprotein B synthesis inhibition with mipomersen in heterozygous familial hypercholesterolemia: results of a randomized, double-blind, placebo-controlled trial to assess efficacy and safety as add-on therapy in patients with coronary artery disease. Circulation 2012; 126(19):2283–92.

43. Raal FJ, Santos RD, Blom DJ, et al. Mipomersen, an apolipoprotein B synthesis inhibitor, for lowering of LDL cholesterol concentrations in patients with homozygous familial hypercholesterolaemia: a randomized, double-blind, placebo-controlled trial. Lancet 2010;375(9719):998–1006.

44. McGowan M, Tardif J, Ceska R, et al. Randomized, placebo-controlled trial of mipomersen in patients with severe hypercholesterolemia receiving maximally tolerated lipid-lowering therapy. PloS ONE 2012;7:e49006.

45. Palacio CH, Harring TR, Nguyen NT, et al. Homozygous familial hypercholesterolemia: case series and review of the literature. Case Rep Transplant 2011; 2011:154908.

46. Rosenson RS, Baker SK, Jacobson TA. An assessment by the statin muscle safety task force: 2014 update. J Clin Lipidol 2014;8:S58–71.

47. Herrick C, Litvin M, Goldberg AC. Lipid lowering in liver and chronic kidney disease. Best Pract Res Clin Endocrinol Metab 2014;28:339–52.

48. Bays H, Cohen DE, Chalasani N, et al. An assessment by the statin liver safety task force: 2014 update. J Clin Lipidol 2014;8:S47–57.

49. Cohen DE, Anania FA, Chalasani N. An assessment of statin safety by hepatologists. Am J Cardiol 2006; 97:77C–81C.

50. Cohen JC, Boerwinkle E, Mosley TH Jr, et al. Sequence variations in PCSK9, low LDL, and protection against coronary heart disease. N Engl J Med 2006;354:1264–72.

51. Stein EA, Raal F. Reduction of low-density lipoprotein cholesterol by monoclonal antibody inhibition of PCSK9. Annu Rev Med 2014;65:417–31.

52. Stein EA, Honarpour N, Wasserman SM, et al. Effect of the proprotein convertase subtilisin/kexin 9 monoclonal antibody, AMG 145, in homozygous familial hypercholesterolemia. Circulation 2013;128(19): 2113–20.

53. Stein E, Mellis S, Yancopoulos G, et al. Effect of a monoclonal antibody to PCSK9 on LDL cholesterol. N Engl J Med 2012;366:1108–18.

54. Raal F, Scott R, Somaratne R, et al. Low-density lipoprotein cholesterol-lowering effects of AMG 145, a monoclonal antibody to proprotein convertase subtilisin/kexin type 9 serine protease in patients with heterozygous familial hypercholesterolemia: the Reduction of LDL-C with PCSK9 Inhibition in Heterozygous Familial Hypercholesterolemia Disorder (RUTHERFORD) randomized trial. Circulation 2012; 126(20):2408–17.

55. Stein EA, Gipe D, Bergeron J, et al. Effect of a monoclonal antibody to PCSK9, REGN727/SAR236553, to reduce low-density lipoprotein cholesterol in patients with heterozygous familial hypercholesterolaemia on stable statin dose with or without ezetimibe therapy: a phase 2 randomised controlled trial. Lancet 2012;380(9836): 29–36.

# New Cholesterol Guidelines for the Management of Atherosclerotic Cardiovascular Disease Risk

## A Comparison of the 2013 American College of Cardiology/American Heart Association Cholesterol Guidelines with the 2014 National Lipid Association Recommendations for Patient-Centered Management of Dyslipidemia

Bhavin B. Adhyaru, MS, MD[a], Terry A. Jacobson, MD[b],*

## KEYWORDS

- Clinical recommendations • Guidelines • Low-density lipoprotein cholesterol (LDL-C)
- Atherosclerotic cardiovascular disease (ASCVD) • Dyslipidemia • Atherogenic cholesterol

## KEY POINTS

- The 2013 American College of Cardiology (ACC)/American Heart Association (AHA) guideline proposes a pooled risk calculator as an improved method to assess quantitative atherosclerotic cardiovascular disease (ASCVD) risk in primary prevention.
- The 2013 ACC/AHA Guideline recommends shifting away from low-density lipoprotein cholesterol (LDL-C) targets and goals and focuses in on the intensity of statin therapy.
- The 2014 National Lipid Association (NLA) recommendations provides a more comprehensive, patient-centered approach to identifying ASCVD risk.
- The NLA recommendations emphasizes the use of statins as first-line therapy, and advocate the use of non–high-density lipoprotein cholesterol (HDL-C) and LDL-C as markers of the atherogenic risk.
- The NLA recommendations emphasize the importance of using evidence-based nonstatin therapy to achieve non–HDL-C and LDL-C goals.

Conflicts of Interest & Financial Disclosures: Dr T.A. Jacobson is a consultant for Amarin, Amgen, Astra-Zeneca, Merck, and Regeneron/Sanofi.
[a] Division of General Internal Medicine & Geriatrics, Department of Medicine, Emory University School of Medicine, 49 Jesse Hill Jr Drive, Atlanta, GA 30303, USA; [b] Lipid Clinic and Cardiovascular Risk Reduction Program, Department of Medicine, Emory University School of Medicine, 49 Jesse Hill Jr Drive, Atlanta, GA 30303, USA
* Corresponding author.
*E-mail address:* tjaco02@emory.edu

Cardiol Clin 33 (2015) 181–196
http://dx.doi.org/10.1016/j.ccl.2015.02.001
0733-8651/15/$ – see front matter © 2015 Elsevier Inc. All rights reserved.

cardiology.theclinics.com

## THE 2013 AMERICAN COLLEGE OF CARDIOLOGY/AMERICAN HEART ASSOCIATION GUIDELINE ON THE TREATMENT OF BLOOD CHOLESTEROL
### Scope and Methodology

Almost one-third of the population in the United States will die as a result of heart attack and stroke associated with atherosclerotic cardiovascular disease (ASCVD), which is currently the leading cause of death in the United States.[1–3]

To provide an update to the 2004 Adult Treatment Panel (ATP) III guidelines,[4,5] the National Heart Lung Blood Institute (NHLBI) formulated a multidisciplinary expert panel consisting of cardiologists, medical subspecialists, and experts in clinical lipidology in 2008.[1] The panel elected to include only randomized controlled trials (RCTs) involving statins, systematic reviews, and metaanalyses for the treatment of blood cholesterol to reduce ASCVD. In the guideline, clinical ASCVD included coronary heart disease (acute coronary syndromes, history of myocardial infarction [MI], stable or unstable angina, coronary or other arterial revascularization), stroke or transient ischemic attack, and peripheral arterial disease presumed to be of atherosclerotic origin. The panel constructed 3 critical questions, and an independent contractor helped search for evidence for each of these critical questions based on inclusion and exclusion criteria. The search included data from 1995 to 2009; however, major RCTs and metaanalyses through July 2013 were included in the discussions of their final recommendations. The RCTs were graded from good to poor quality, with only good or fair quality RCTs included for consideration. The final recommendations were approved by at least a majority of the voting members of the expert panel. In 2013, the NHLBI turned over its recommendations to the American College of Cardiology (ACC) and the American Heart Association (AHA), who were charged with further review and guideline dissemination to the broader provider community. The synthesis of the evidence is based on the NHLBI grading of recommendations (**Table 1**) as well as the ACC/AHA (**Table 2**) classification system.

---

**Table 1**
**NHLBI grading of recommendations**

| Grade | Strength of Recommendation |
|-------|----------------------------|
| A | Strong recommendation <br> There is high certainty based on evidence that the net benefit (benefits minus risk/harm of service/intervention) is substantial. |
| B | Moderate recommendation <br> There is moderate certainty based on evidence that the net benefit is moderate to substantial, or there is high certainty that the net benefit is moderate. |
| C | Weak recommendation <br> There is at least moderate certainty based on evidence that there is small net benefit. |
| D | Recommendation against <br> There is at least moderate certainty based on evidence that it has no net benefit or that risks/harms outweigh benefits. |
| E | Expert opinion ("There is insufficient evidence or evidence is unclear or conflicting, but this is what the work group recommends.") <br> Net benefit is unclear. Balance of benefits and harms cannot be determined because of no evidence, insufficient evidence, unclear evidence, or conflicting evidence, but the work group thought it was important to provide clinical guidance and make a recommendation. Further research is recommended in this area. |
| N | No recommendation for or against ("There is insufficient evidence or evidence is unclear or conflicting.") <br> Net benefit is unclear. Balance of benefits and harms cannot be determined because of no evidence, insufficient evidence, unclear evidence, or conflicting evidence, and the work group thought no recommendation should be made. Further research is recommended in this area. |

*Abbreviation:* NHLBI, National Heart Lung Blood Institute.
*From* Stone NJ, Robinson JG, Lichtenstein AH, et al. 2013 ACC/AHA guideline on the treatment of blood cholesterol to reduce atherosclerotic cardiovascular risk in adults: a report of the American College of Cardiology/American Heart Association Task Force on Practice Guidelines. Circulation 2014;129(25 Suppl 2):S6; with permission.

**Table 2**
**ACC/AHA recommendation classification and level of evidence**

| | | Size of Treatment Effect | | | |
|---|---|---|---|---|---|
| | **Level** | **Class I**<br>*Benefit >>> Risk*<br>Procedure/Treatment Should Be Performed/Administered | **Class IIa**<br>*Benefit >> Risk*<br>*Additional Studies With Focused Objectives Needed*<br>It Is Reasonable to Perform Procedure/Administer Treatment | **Class IIb**<br>*Benefit ≥ Risk*<br>*Additional Studies With Broad Objectives Needed; Additional Registry Data Would Be Helpful*<br>Procedure/Treatment May Be Considered | **Class III No Benefit or CLASS III Harm**<br><br> | | |
| | | | | | Procedure/Test<br>COR III: No benefit — Not Helpful<br>COR III: Harm — Excess Cost W/O Benefit or Harmful | Treatment<br>No Proven Benefit<br>Harmful to Patients |
| Estimate of certainty (precision) of treatment effect | **Level A**<br>Multiple populations evaluated<br>Data derived from multiple randomized clinical trials or metaanalyses | Recommendation that procedure or treatment is useful/effective<br>Sufficient evidence from multiple randomized trials or metaanalyses | Recommendation in favor of treatment or procedure being useful/effective<br>Some conflicting evidence from multiple randomized trials or metaanalyses | Recommendation's usefulness/efficacy less well established<br>Greater conflicting evidence from multiple randomized trials or meta-analyses | Recommendation that procedure or treatment is useful/effective and may be harmful<br>Sufficient evidence from multiple randomized trials or meta-analyses | |
| | **Level B**<br>Limited populations evaluated<br>Data derived from a single randomized trial or nonrandomized studies | Recommendation that procedure or treatment is useful/effective<br>Evidence from single randomized trial or nonrandomized studies | Recommendation in favor of treatment or procedure being useful/effective<br>Some conflicting evidence from single randomized trial or nonrandomized studies | Recommendation's usefulness/efficacy less well established<br>Greater conflicting evidence from single randomized trial or nonrandomized studies | Recommendation that procedure or treatment is not useful/effective and may be harmful<br>Evidence from single randomized trial or nonrandomized studies | |
| | **Level C**<br>Very limited populations evaluated<br>Only consensus opinion of experts, case studies, or standard of care | Recommendation that procedure or treatment is useful/effective<br>Only expert opinion, case studies, or standard of care | Recommendation in favor of treatment or procedure being useful/effective<br>Only diverging expert opinion, case studies, or standard of care | Recommendation's usefulness/efficacy less well established<br>Only diverging expert opinion, case studies, or standard of care | Recommendation that procedure or treatment is not useful/effective and may be harmful<br>Only expert opinion, case studies, or standard of care | |

*Abbreviations:* COR, class of recommendation; W/O, without.
*From* Stone NJ, Robinson JG, Lichtenstein AH, et al. 2013 ACC/AHA guideline on the treatment of blood cholesterol to reduce atherosclerotic cardiovascular risk in adults: a report of the American College of Cardiology/American Heart Association task force on practice guidelines. Circulation 2014;129(25 Suppl 2):S5; with permission.

## Groups Benefiting from Statin Therapy ("Statin Benefit Groups")

The ACC/AHA panel found in its review of statin RCTs that there was a consistent reduction in ASCVD events from statin therapy in both secondary and primary prevention. The intensity of statin therapy was defined based on the average expected LDL-C response. As shown in **Table 3**, the 3 types of statin therapy include high intensity (≥50% reduction in LDL-C), moderate intensity (30 to <50% reduction), and low intensity (<30% reduction).

The guideline found 4 major groups where the benefit of a statin on ASCVD risk reduction outweighed the risk of adverse events (**Fig. 1**)[1]:

1. Patients with clinical ASCVD (eg, acute coronary syndromes, history of MI, stable or unstable angina, stroke, transient ischemic attack, or peripheral arterial disease).
2. Patients with primary elevation of LDL-C of 190 mg/dL or higher.
3. Patients with diabetes (type 1 and 2) aged 40 to 75 years with LDL-C of 70 to 189 mg/dL and without clinical ASCVD.
4. Patients without diabetes or clinical ASCVD and estimated 10-year ASCVD risk of 7.5% or greater.

For primary prevention, in patients age 40 to 75 years with LDL-C of 70 to 189 mg/dL without diabetes or clinical ASCVD, the decision to initiate statin is based on 10-year ASCVD risk using new pooled risk equations (discussed in more detail elsewhere in this article). The data used to identify who would benefit from a statin was based on 3 trials (Air force/Texas coronary atherosclerosis prevention study [AFCAPS-TexCAPS], Primary Prevention of Cardiovascular Disease With Pravastatin in Japan [MEGA], and Justification for the Use of Statins in Primary Prevention: An Intervention Trial Evaluating Rosuvastatin Trial [JUPITER]) that included patients with LDL-C of greater than 70 mg/dL and less than 190 mg/dL in primary prevention. It was determined that patients with a ASCVD risk of 7.5% or higher benefited most from moderate- to high-intensity statin therapy. This value is not an absolute threshold to start statin therapy, but this is when physicians and patients should engage in discussion of the risks and benefits of statin therapy.[6–8]

In patients with a 10-year ASCVD risk of 5.0% to 7.4%, a similar amount of evidence supports moderate- to high-intensity statin therapy, although there is evidence that the benefit of a moderate intensity statin outweighs the risk of adverse events in this group. For patients with an ASCVD risk of less than 5% or those not in a statin benefit group (ie, age <40 or age >75), it is important to consider the risks and benefits of statin therapy as well as considering other risk factors that may better inform treatment decisions such as:

- LDL-C of 160 mg/dL or greater
- Family history of premature ASCVD with onset less than 55 years old in first degree male relatives or less than 65 years old in first-degree female relative

**Table 3**
**Intensity of statin therapy according to the 2013 American College of Cardiology/American Heart Association Guideline**

| High-Intensity Statin Therapy | Moderate-Intensity Statin Therapy | Low-Intensity Statin Therapy |
|---|---|---|
| Daily dose lowers LDL-C on average, by approximately ≥50% | Daily dose lowers LDL-C on average, by approximately 30% to <50% | Daily dose lowers LDL-C on average, by <30% |
| Atorvastatin 40–80 mg<br>Rosuvastatin 20–40 mg | Atorvastatin 10–20 mg<br>Rosuvastatin 5–10 mg<br>Simvastatin 20–40 mg<br>Pravastatin 40–80 mg<br>Lovastatin 40 mg<br>Fluvastatin XL 80 mg<br>Fluvastatin 40 mg twice daily<br>Pitavastatin 2–4 mg | Simvastatin 10 mg<br>Pravastatin 10–20 mg<br>Lovastatin 20 mg<br>Fluvastatin 20–40 mg<br>Pitavastatin 1 mg |

*Abbreviation:* LDL-C, low-density lipoprotein cholesterol.

*Adapted from* Stone NJ, Robinson JG, Lichtenstein AH, et al. 2013 ACC/AHA guideline on the treatment of blood cholesterol to reduce atherosclerotic cardiovascular risk in adults: a report of the American College of Cardiology/American Heart Association task force on practice guidelines. Circulation 2014;129(25 Suppl 2):S25; with permission.

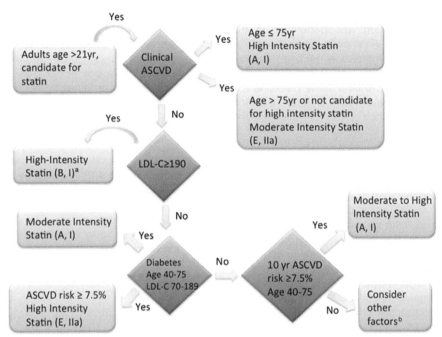

**Fig. 1.** The major recommendations based on the 2013 American College of Cardiology/American Heart Association (ACC/AHA) guidelines for atherosclerotic cardiovascular disease (ASCVD) prevention. Recommendations are given with the National Heart Lung Blood Institute (NHLBI) grade and ACC/AHA classification (eg, A, I). [a] Note. For patients >21 years with untreated primary LDL-C >190 mg/dL after maximum intensity of statin, addition of nonstatin drug can be considered (E, IIbC). [b] Consider for additional assessment of ASCVD risk in patients who do not fall within 1 of the 4 statin benefit groups: LDL-C ≥160 mg/dL, family history of premature ASCVD, coronary artery calcium score (CAC) ≥300 Agatston units of 75th percentile, high-sensitivity C-reactive protein ≥2 mg/L, ankle–brachial index <0.9, and high lifetime risk at age 20 to 59. LDL-C, low-density lipoprotein cholesterol. (*Adapted from* Stone NJ, Robinson JG, Lichtenstein AH, et al. 2013 ACC/AHA guideline on the treatment of blood cholesterol to reduce atherosclerotic cardiovascular risk in adults: a report of the American College of Cardiology/American Heart Association Task Force on Practice Guidelines. Circulation 2014;129(25 Suppl 2):S15; with permission.)

- Coronary artery calcium score of 300 Agatston units or more, or greater than 75th percentile
- Highly sensitive C-reactive protein of 2 mg/L or greater
- Ankle-brachial index of less than 0.9
- High lifetime risk at age 20 to 59 years.

## Pooled Cohort Risk Equations for Atherosclerotic Cardiovascular Disease Risk Assessment

To determine an individual's risk, the guideline recommends the estimation of a 10-year risk for ASCVD events (CHD and stroke). This differs from the 10-year risk score from the previous National Cholesterol Education Program (NCEP)/ATP III guideline, which only included hard CHD events (nonfatal MI and CHD death).[9] The risk assessment is based on pooled cohort risk assessment and can be calculated by many online calculators and risk prediction apps.[10]

The Framingham 10-year general CVD risk was used as the basis for the development of the pooled cohort risk. However, to make it more generalizable, data from large, racially and geographically diverse cohort studies were included (Atherosclerosis Risk in Communities [ARIC] study, Cardiovascular Health Study, Coronary Artery Risk Development in Young Adults [CARDIA]) combined with the Framingham original and offspring cohorts.[1] The cohort included 11,240 white women, 9098 white men, 2641 African-American women, and 1647 African-American men. These data were used to develop sex- and race-specific equations to predict the 10-year risk of a first hard ASCVD event. The ATP III panel considered diabetes to be a CHD risk equivalent and for this reason did not include diabetes in their multivariable risk equations. Because a recent metaanalysis did not show that diabetes is a CHD risk equivalent, diabetes was included as an independent predictor variable in the new pooled cohort risk equations.[11]

The pooled cohort had good internal validation, and external validation was performed in the Whites and African-Americans from the Multi-Ethnic Study of Atherosclerosis (MESA)[12] and the Reasons for Geographic And Racial Differences in Stroke Study (REGARDS).[13] The guideline authors did note that even in their external validation there was overprediction of ASCVD risk in all of the groups.[1]

### Low-Density Lipoprotein Cholesterol Treatment Targets

The evidence included in the ACC/AHA guideline was based on RCTs that compared a fixed dose or compared high-intensity versus moderate-intensity statins. Based on this, they did not find evidence to support titrating therapy to achieve a specific LDL-C or non–HDL-C goal as recommended by the ATP III. The panel gave no recommendation for or against specific LDL-C or non–HDL-C targets for primary prevention of ASCVD. The panel also argued that, given the lack of evidence to treat to a specific target or that even if lower lipid levels were better (vs the statin dose), the use of multidrug therapy may be harmful and not evidence based.

The guideline provides an approach to monitor statin therapy. They recommend an initial lipid panel followed by a second lipid panel 4 to 12 weeks after initiation of statin therapy to determine adherence and appropriate LDL-C response to therapy (**Fig. 2**). If a patient is already on a statin where the baseline LDL-C is unknown, an LDL-C less than of 100 mg/dL was observed in individuals receiving high-intensity statin therapy in RCTs. If a patient with ASCVD is on a moderate- or low-intensity statin with an LDL-C of less than 100 mg/d, then based on current evidence, that patient would have a greater reduction in ASCVD events if a high-intensity statin was given and tolerated. Therefore, we could conclude based on the ACC/AHA guidelines that, if a patient with ASCVD is on a moderate-intensity statin with LDL-C of less than 100 mg/dL, they still should be switched to a high-intensity statin.

### THE 2014 NATIONAL LIPID ASSOCIATION RECOMMENDATIONS FOR PATIENT-CENTERED MANAGEMENT OF DYSLIPIDEMIA
#### Scope and Methodology

The National Lipid Association (NLA) convened their expert panel to develop a patient-centered approach to the management of dyslipidemia.[2] The guideline was developed with 2 parts, the first discussing the screening and classification of lipoprotein lipid levels, targets for intervention in dyslipidemia, ASCVD risk assessment, atherogenic cholesterol (non-HDL, LDL-C) as targets for therapy, and lifestyle/drug therapies to reduce ASCVD events. The second part addressed lifestyle therapies, special populations including the elderly, children, women, other ethnic groups (Hispanics, Asian Americans, African Americans), patients with HIV, high-risk inflammatory conditions (rheumatoid arthritis), and those with high residual risk on statin therapy.

The guideline was developed to provide an update to the revised ATP III guideline published in 2004 and to consider new evidence from RCT trials involving statin and nonstatin therapy, as well as combination statin therapy. The evidence that was evaluated not only included RCTs, but also metaanalyses, epidemiologic and observational studies, metabolic and genetic studies, and mechanistic investigations. The following core principles were used to develop the guideline:

1. Elevated levels of cholesterol carried by apolipoprotein (Apo) B-containing lipoproteins (non–HDL-C and LDL-C, called atherogenic cholesterol) are a root cause of atherosclerosis, the major underlying process contributing to ASCVD events.
2. Reducing elevated levels of atherogenic cholesterol will lower ASCVD risk in proportion to the extent that atherogenic cholesterol is lowered.
3. The intensity of risk reduction therapy should be adjusted to the patient's absolute risk for an ASCVD event.
4. Both intermediate- and long-term (or lifetime) risk should be considered when assessing potential benefits and hazards of risk reduction therapies.
5. Statin treatment is the primary and most evidence-based modality for reducing ASCVD risk.
6. Lipid targets and goals are important clinical and motivational tools for patients and providers, and LDL-C monitoring is important in assessing adherence to therapy, adequacy of response to therapy, and determining lipid-related residual risk.

### Atherogenic Cholesterol (Non–High-Density Lipoprotein Cholesterol and Low-Density Lipoprotein Cholesterol)

Although LDL-C has typically been the primary target of therapy, the NLA consensus was that non–HDL-C is a better primary target than LDL-C. The non–HDL-C comprises cholesterol carried by all potentially atherogenic particles that include LDL, intermediate density lipoproteins, very

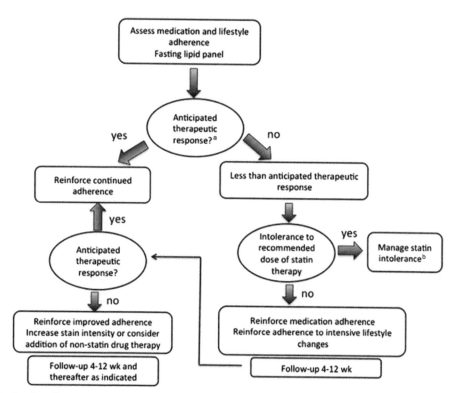

**Fig. 2.** Monitoring therapeutic response and adherence to statin therapy by the 2013 American College of Cardiology/American Heart Association (ACC/AHA) guidelines. [a] Indicators of anticipated therapeutic response and adherence to selected statin intensity: high-intensity statin therapy reduces LDL-C by approximately ≥50% from the untreated baseline and moderate-intensity statin therapy reduces LDL-C by approximately 30% to <50% from the untreated baseline. [b] Management of statin intolerance: (1) To avoid unnecessary discontinuation of statins, obtain history of prior or current muscle symptoms to establish a baseline before statin therapy; (2) If unexplained severe muscle symptoms, discontinue statin and address possibility of rhabdomyolysis by evaluating a creatine kinase (CK), creatinine, and urinalysis; (3) If mild to moderate muscle symptoms develop during statin therapy, discontinue statin until symptoms can be evaluated, consider other conditions that might increase risk for muscle symptoms (ie, hypothyroidism, reduced renal/hepatic function, vitamin D deficiency), if symptoms resolve give the patient original or lower dose of the same statin to establish a causal relationship, increase dose as tolerated; if persistent muscle symptoms are unrelated to statin therapy, resume statin therapy at the original dose. (*Adapted from* Stone NJ, Robinson JG, Lichtenstein AH, et al. 2013 ACC/AHA guideline on the treatment of blood cholesterol to reduce atherosclerotic cardiovascular risk in adults: a report of the American College of Cardiology/American Heart Association task force on practice guidelines. Circulation 2014;129(25 Suppl 2):S43; with permission.)

low-density lipoproteins, and very low-density lipoproteins remnants, chylomicron remnants, and lipoprotein (a). In several metaanalyses of statin[14,15] and nonstatin trials,[16] it was found that non–HDL-C correlated more closely with ASCVD risk than LDL-C both at baseline and during therapy. This may be owing to several factors, including that (1) some triglyceride-rich lipoprotein remnants enter the arterial wall similar to LDL-C, contributing to the initiation and progression of atherosclerosis, (2) non–HDL-C correlates more closely with all Apo-B–containing lipoproteins and with the total burden of all atherogenic particles, and (3) elevated levels of triglycerides and very low-density lipoprotein-C reflect hepatic production of particles with greater atherogenic potential resulting in longer residence time in circulation. Apo-B is an optional secondary target for treatment because it is also a very robust predictor of ASCVD risk during statin therapy.[17,18] Based on population studies, desirable levels for secondary prevention are non–HDL-C of less than 100 mg/dL, LDL-C of less than 70 mg/dL, and Apo B of less than 80 mg/dL.

## Assessment of Atherosclerotic Cardiovascular Disease Risk

According to the NLA, risk assessment is based on the identification of high-risk and very high-risk groups, the counting of individual ASCVD risk factors, and the classification of individual risk status as very high risk, high risk, moderate risk, and low risk. These classifications help to determine when to consider drug therapy, what treatment goals to select, and how to match the intensity of therapy to the patient's absolute risk of an ASCVD event. **Table 4** shows the major ASCVD risk factors and **Tables 5** and **6** show treatment goals in relation to risk categories. **Fig. 3** shows a sequential method for identifying a patient's risk.

Individuals with clinical ASCVD and patients with diabetes with 2 or more ASCVD risk factors are at "very high risk" and should have the most aggressive goals for atherogenic cholesterol (non–HDL-C <100 mg/dL, LDL-C <70 mg/dL). Interestingly, chronic kidney disease stage 5 represents a group at very high risk of ASCVD; however, data from RCTs have not shown consistent benefits and clinical judgment should be used when deciding treatment for this group.

For patients with 2 major ASCVD risk factors, other major ASCVD risk indicators can be considered (**Box 1**) in clinical decision making, or quantitative risk assessment can be performed to identify those at high risk. The thresholds recommended for commonly used risk scores are shown below. These risk cutpoints differ than the cutpoints in both the 2013 AHA/ACC guidelines and the ATP III guidelines using the Framingham risk calculator. Of note, these cutpoints are not the same as the "statin benefit groups" as outlined in the 2013 AHA/ACC cholesterol guideline. These cutpoints are intended to inform clinical judgment by placing patients into their different risk categories.

1. ATP III Framingham risk calculator: 10% or greater 10-year risk for a hard CHD event.
2. Pooled cohort equations: 15% or greater 10-year risk for a hard ASCVD event.

**Table 5**
**Treatment goals for non–HDL-C, LDL-C, and Apo B according to the National Lipid Association Recommendations**

| | Treatment Goals | | |
|---|---|---|---|
| Risk Category | Non–HDL-C (mg/dL) | LDL-C (mg/dL) | Apo B[a] (mg/dL) |
| Low | <130 | <100 | <90 |
| Moderate | <130 | <100 | <90 |
| High | <130 | <100 | <90 |
| Very high | <100 | <70 | <80 |

*Abbreviations:* Apo B, apolipoprotein B; HDL-C, high-density lipoprotein cholesterol; LDL-C, low-density lipoprotein cholesterol.
[a] Apo B is a secondary, optional target of treatment.
*From* Jacobson TA, Ito MK, Maki KC, et al. National Lipid Association recommendations for patient-centered management of dyslipidemia: part 1 - executive summary. J Clin Lipidol 2014;8(5):476; with permission.

3. Framingham long-term (30-year to age 80) risk calculator: 45% or greater risk for CVD (MI, CHD death, or stroke).

## Treatment Algorithm

First-line pharmacologic treatment for elevated atherogenic cholesterol levels is a moderate- or high-intensity statin (discussed in the ACC/AHA guideline section). For patients with contraindication or intolerance to statin therapy, nonstatin drug therapy may be considered. The nonstatin drug classes for LDL-C reduction include the cholesterol absorption inhibitors, bile acid sequesterants, and nicotinic acid, and the nonstatin drugs for triglyceride reduction include the fibrates, nicotinic acid, and the long-chain omega-3 fatty acids.

**Table 4**
**Major risk factors for atherosclerotic cardiovascular disease according to the National Lipid Association recommendations**

| Risk Factor | Parameter |
|---|---|
| Age | Male ≥45 y<br>Female ≥55 y |
| Family history of early coronary heart disease | <55 y of age in a male first-degree relative<br><65 y of age in a female first-degree relative |
| Current cigarette smoking | |
| High blood pressure | ≥140/≥90 mm Hg or on blood pressure medication |
| Low high-density lipoprotein cholesterol | Male <40 mg/dL<br>Female <50 mg/dL |

*From* Jacobson TA, Ito MK, Maki KC, et al. National Lipid Association recommendations for patient-centered management of dyslipidemia: part 1 - executive summary. J Clin Lipidol 2014;8(5):479; with permission.

**Table 6**
**Criteria for ASCVD risk assessment, treatment goals, and levels at which to consider drug therapy according to the National Lipid Association recommendations**

| Risk Category | Criteria | Treatment Goal | | Consider Drug Therapy | |
|---|---|---|---|---|---|
| | | Non–HDL-C (mg/dL) | LDL-C (mg/dL) | Non–HDL-C (mg/dL) | LDL-C (mg/dL) |
| Low | 0–1 major ASCVD risk factors Consider other risk indicators, if known | <130 | <100 | ≥190 | ≥160 |
| Moderate | 2 major ASCVD risk factors Consider quantitative risk scoring Consider other risk indictors[a] | <130 | <100 | ≥160 | ≥130 |
| High | ≥3 major ASCVD risk factors Diabetes   0–1 other major ASCVD risk factor   No evidence of end organ damage CKD stage 3B or 4 LDL-C >190 mg/dL Quantitative risk score reaching the   high risk threshold | <130 | <100 | ≥130 | ≥100 |
| Very high | ASCVD Diabetes   ≥2 major risk factors or   Evidence of end-organ damage[a] | <100 | <70 | ≥100 | ≥70 |

For patients with ASCVD or diabetes mellitus, consideration should be given to use of moderate- or high-intensity statin therapy, irrespective of baseline atherogenic cholesterol levels.

*Note:* End-organ damage is indicated by increased albumin/creatinine ratio (≥30 mg/g), CKD, or retinopathy.

*Abbreviations:* ASCVD, atherosclerotic cardiovascular disease; CKD, chronic kidney disease; HDL-C, high-density lipoprotein cholesterol; LDL-C, low-density lipoprotein cholesterol.

[a] For those at moderate risk, additional testing may be considered for some patients to assist with decisions about risk stratification. These include metabolic syndrome and risk indicators such as (1) severe disturbance in a major ASCVD risk factor such as multipack per day smoking or strong family history of premature coronary heart disease, (2) coronary calcium score of ≥300 Agatston units, (3) LDL-C ≥ 160 mg/dL or non–HDL-C ≥190 mg/dL, (4) high-sensitivity C-reactive protein of ≥2.0 mg/L, (5) lipoprotein (a) ≥50 mg/dL, (6) urine albumin/creatinine ratio ≥30 mg/g.

*From* Jacobson TA, Ito MK, Maki KC, et al. National Lipid Association recommendations for patient-centered management of dyslipidemia: part 1 - executive summary. J Clin Lipidol 2014;8(5):477; with permission.

If the goal levels of atherogenic cholesterol have not been achieved, the statin dosage may be increased or switched to a more efficacious agent. If, after a trial of the highest tolerable dose of a high-intensity statin, goal levels have not been achieved, the clinician can consider addition of a second cholesterol-lowering agent or referral to a lipid specialist. Once goals have been achieved, response to therapy should be monitored periodically.

There are several adverse events related to statin therapy that have been reported. The most common adverse effects are muscle-related complaints (ie, myalgias, muscle aches, or muscle discomfort) that are related mostly to the dose of the statin than the degree of LDL reduction. Musculoskeletal complaints are common in older patients and in those who are more physically active; therefore, it is important to assess for these causes before attributing symptoms to statin therapy. It is also important to consider other medications and conditions (hypothyroidism), which may interact with statins thus increasing the risk of muscle symptoms.[19,20] There has been a modest increase in the risk of type 2 diabetes observed with statin therapy, and higher intensity statin therapy increases this risk to a greater extent than less intensive regimens. It is recommended to check a hemoglobin A1c level before initiation of a statin and within a year afterward in those with risk factors for the metabolic syndrome or diabetes.[21–24] Short-term memory impairment has been reported; however, observational studies have failed to find significant evidence for memory loss with those on long-term statin therapy.[23,25] See the articles elsewhere in this issue for a more in-depth discussion about statins and their effects on diabetes risk and cognition.

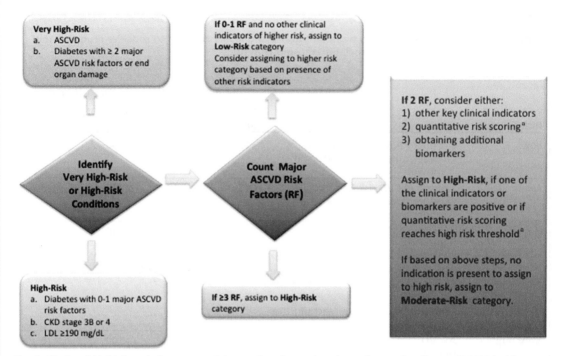

**Fig. 3.** National Lipid Association sequential steps in atherosclerotic cardiovascular disease (ASCVD) risk assessment. [a] The 10-year Framingham risk is ≥10%; American College of Cardiology/American Heart Association pooled cohort equations 10-year risk is ≥15%; Framingham long-term (30-year to age 80) risk is ≥45%.

---

**Box 1**
**National Lipid Association risk indicators considered for risk refinement**

1. A severe disturbance in a major ASCVD risk factor, such as multipack per day smoking, or strong family history of premature CHD.

2. Indicators of subclinical disease, including coronary artery calcium.

   a. ≥300 Agatston units is considered high risk.

3. LDL-C ≥160 and/or non–HDL-C ≥190 mg/dL.

4. High-sensitivity C-reactive protein ≥2.0 mg/L.

5. Lipoprotein (a) ≥50 mg/dL (protein) using an isoform insensitive assay.

6. Urine albumin/creatinine ratio ≥30 mg/g.

*Abbreviations:* ASCVD, atherosclerotic cardiovascular disease; CHD, coronary heart disease; HDL-C, high-density lipoprotein cholesterol; LDL-C, low-density lipoprotein cholesterol.

*From* Jacobson TA, Ito MK, Maki KC, et al. National Lipid Association recommendations for patient-centered management of dyslipidemia: part 1 - executive summary. J Clin Lipidol 2014;8(5):481; with permission.

There are observational data as well as some RCTs comparing lower and higher dosages of statin therapy that suggest that ASCVD event risk reduction is associated with lower levels of atherogenic cholesterol and that greater reductions in atherogenic cholesterol levels are associated with greater ASCVD benefits. The associations between on-treatment levels of LDL-C (and non–HDL-C) follow a log–linear relationship, supporting the view that the primary mechanism of action of statins is through reductions in levels of atherogenic lipoproteins. Until there are further data from RCTs for add-on therapies, the NLA recommends that consideration be given to combination therapy with the highest tolerated statin dose to further lower atherogenic cholesterol (non–HDL-C and LDL-C) to goal levels.

## COMPARISON AND CONTRASTS OF THE NEW GUIDELINES

Since its inception, several aspects of the new 2013 ACC/AHA guidelines have been controversial, including the absence of treatment goals, the role of combination therapy on top of statin therapy, and the utility of the pooled cohort equations to assess ASCVD risk.

A recent article reviewing various clinical practice guidelines for lipid management shows major differences in the assessment of risk and treatment targets.[26] Most national and international practice guidelines use LDL-C or non–HDL-C as targets of therapy whereas the 2013 ACC/AHA cholesterol guidelines use LDL-C more as a means of assessing adherence to therapy. The risk assessments vary from using the pooled cohort ASCVD risk equations to the Framingham risk score. This does pose significant challenges to the practicing clinician on how to manage and evaluate a patient's ASCVD risk. Prior studies have shown that few clinicians were actually using the risk prediction engines in primary prevention under the ATP III guidelines and that giving risk prediction scores to clinicians did not improve patient outcomes necessarily.[27–29] Therefore, the NLA guidelines chose not to put a heavy emphasis on quantitative risk scoring, but chose to emphasize the identification of high-risk conditions, the simple counting of cardiovascular risk factors, and the selective use of other risk factor indicators

when there is doubt about the necessity for treatment. The NLA guidelines were created to provide a more comprehensive and patient-centered approach to determining an individual's risk and management. Specifically, the NLA recommendations were designed to offer expert advice in where RCT evidence was lacking.

There are some similarities between the guidelines in that both recommend lipid screening for primary prevention at 5-year intervals and lifestyle therapy is advocated as a first step in all treatment algorithms. The goal of therapy for both guidelines is ASCVD risk reduction and moderate- to high-intensity statin is the central focus of pharmacotherapy. Both recommend patient–provider discussion of risk and benefit regarding drug treatment and regular lipid follow-up is warranted to assess adherence to therapy.

There are several other important differences between the guidelines (**Table 7**). One includes the evidence base that was used in forming recommendations. Whereas the ACC/AHA includes only statin RCTs and metaanalyses, the NLA incorporates statin and nonstatin RCTs and metaanalysis, along with observational studies,

**Table 7**
**A comparison of the 2013 ACC/AHA and the 2014 NLA guidelines**

|  | 2013 ACC/AHA Guideline | 2014 NLA Recommendations |
|---|---|---|
| Evidence base | RCTs of statin therapy Metaanalyses and systematic review of RCTs | RCT of statin therapy and nonstatin therapies Meta analyses and systematic review of RCTs Observational and epidemiologic studies Genetic studies Metabolic and mechanistic studies |
| ASCVD risk assessment | 4 major statin benefit groups CV risk calculator based on pooled cohort risk equations (10-year risk and lifetime risk) | Identification of patients with "very high-risk" or "high-risk" conditions Counting of ASCVD risk factors to determine risk factor category If 2 major ASCVD risk factors, consider either: other key clinical criteria, quantitative risk scoring, or obtaining additional biomarkers |
| Treatment goals and lipid monitoring | No specific LDL-C target or goal of therapy Monitor LDL-C to assess adherence to therapy | Target non–HDL-C and LDL-C based on risk category Use non–HDL-C and LDL-C goals to assess adherence to therapy, adequacy of treatment response, and residual risk related to lipids |
| Nonstatin therapy | No recommendation for nonstatin therapy except for patients with LDL-C >190 mg/dL on maximum dose statin therapy, or patients with statin intolerance | If non–HDL-C and LDL-C goals are not met with statin therapy, addition of evidence based nonstatin therapy should be considered |

*Abbreviations:* ACC, American College of Cardiology; AHA, American Heart Association; ASCVD, atherosclerotic cardiovascular disease; CHD, coronary heart disease; CV, cardiovascular; HDL-C, high-density lipoprotein cholesterol; LDL-C, low-density lipoprotein cholesterol; NLA, National Lipid Association; RCT, randomized, controlled trial.

genetic studies, and mechanistic studies in formulating its recommendations. Although RCTs represent a high quality of evidence, there may be important insights from observational studies, such as assessing ASCVD risk across populations or determining safety signals in large observational cohorts. Finally, for many of the important questions in clinical medicine, there is an absence of RCTs to inform clinical judgment. Therefore, it is important that guidelines give recommendations, even in cases where RCTs are lacking.

## Low-Density Lipoprotein Cholesterol Treatment Goals

Other areas of controversy are the importance of treatment targets, whether non–HDL-C is a better target of therapy than LDL-C, and what are the additional benefits of adding nonstatin therapy. The 2013 ACC/AHA guidelines emphasize that RCTs used fixed doses of statins and it therefore should not be assumed that dosage titration is correct. They stress that the evidence suggests that it is the dose of the statin that is more important than either the degree of LDL-C reduction or the obtainment of lipid goals. However, the Treating to New Targets (TNT) trial did show that atorvastatin 80 mg compared with atorvastatin 10 mg did achieve LDL levels (77 vs 100 mg/dL) quite similar to the ATP III goals of therapy (<70 and 100 mg/dL, respectively). This difference in LDL-C was associated with a relative risk reduction in major cardiovascular events of 22% (hazard ratio, 0.78; 95% CI, 0.69–0.89; $P<0.001$; absolute risk reduction, 3.2%).[30]

## Combination Statin Therapy

The AHA/ACC guideline refer to several trials wherein the addition of an additional lipid-lowering agent on top of statin therapy did not further lower ASCVD risk. The AIM-HIGH and HPS-2-THRIVE trials studied niacin in combination with statin therapy, but failed to show additional ASCVD risk reduction despite additional LDL-C and non–HDL-C reduction.[31,32] Not discussed in the AHA/ACC guidelines was the fact that both of these high-risk populations studied were already at or near their LDL goals (70 and 63 mg/dL, respectively), despite the additional fact that this limitation of both of these trials has been discussed elsewhere in considerable detail.[33] Similarly, the Action to Control Cardiovascular Risk in Diabetes (ACCORD-Lipid) trial did not find additional risk reduction in patients with diabetes mellitus when fenofibrate was added to statin therapy.[34] Again also of note, the patients were already close to their LDL goal (mean of 100.6 mg/dL) before fenofibrate was added and their final LDL values (mean LDL of 81 mg/dL) were no different between placebo and fenofibrate by study end. Despite these results, there is some evidence that fibrates can be considered in select patients with high triglycerides and low HDL-C based on individual trial subgroup analysis and from a metaanalysis that has shown ASCVD risk reduction. However, these findings of benefit in subgroups with high triglycerides and low HDL need to be confirmed prospectively. Finally, it cannot be refuted that, in the prestatin era, clinical trials involving monotherapy with either cholestyramine in the Lipid Research Clinics Coronary Primary Prevention trial, niacin in the Coronary Drug Project, and ileal bypass surgery in the POSCH study all reduced ASCVD risk significantly.[35–38]

## Implications of the IMProved Reduction of Outcomes: Vytorin Efficacy International Trial

Excitingly, the recent IMProved Reduction of Outcomes: Vytorin Efficacy International Trial (IMPROVE-IT) study suggests that the addition of ezetimibe to simvastatin is safe and more efficacious than statin therapy alone. This trial was an RCT of 18,144 post-acute coronary syndrome patients with baseline LDL-C of 50 to 125 mg/dL randomized to either simvastatin 40 mg or simvastatin 40 mg plus ezetimibe 10 mg. The primary endpoint was cardiovascular death, MI, hospital admission for unstable angina, stroke, or coronary revascularization 30 days or more after randomization. The absolute risk reduction for the primary endpoint at the end of 5.7 years was 2.0% with a number needed to treat of 50. In addition, the benefit was demonstrated with the achievement of lower LDL-C levels of 50 versus 65 mg/dL, respectively.[39] This is consistent with the Cholesterol Treatment Trialists' metaanalysis of 27 statin trials,[40,41] which showed a greater reduction in risk with larger LDL reductions and no evidence of a threshold level of LDL-C wherein there was no longer a benefit. These new data suggest clearly that there may be additional benefit by further targeting LDL-C and non–HDL-C to lower levels, and that nonstatin therapy can reduce effectively ASCVD risk in combination with-high dose statins. Whether lower doses of statins can be used with ezetimibe in patients who are intolerant to statins needs to be determined.

## Atherosclerotic Cardiovascular Disease Risk Assessment

The ASCVD pooled cohort equations remains an important area of controversy. Although a strength of the ACC/AHA guideline is their incorporation of more recent epidemiologic cohorts with greater ethnic diversity, there remain several issues with its validation. A general concern is whether any type of global risk prediction score is needed, given that no trial has ever randomized patients by their absolute risk or tried to tailor or match the intensity of therapy to their absolute risk. For example, the Controlled Rosuvastatin Multinational Trial in Heart Failure (CORONA; heart failure)[42] and A Study to Evaluate the Use of Rosuvastatin in Subjects on Regular Hemodialysis: An Assessment of Survival and Cardiovascular Events (AURORA; hemodialysis)[43] trials included high-risk vascular patients and found no event reduction despite significant reductions in LDL-C. Although the AHA/ACC guidelines appropriately point out that patients with congestive heart failure or on dialysis have not been shown to benefit from statin therapy, it raises some questions about the utility of the equations in certain comorbid patient populations and in populations in where there are few outcomes data, such as Americans of Hispanic or Asian origin. A study by Ridker and Cook[44] showed that the event rate predicted by the ASCVD prediction score systematically overestimated observed risks in external cohorts. Additionally, family history was not included as a part of the ASCVD pooled cohort equations, although it has been shown to be an important risk factor behind smoking and diabetes.[45] The guideline authors also state that even in their external validation in REGARDS and MESA, the pooled cohort equations overestimated 10-year ASCVD risk. The authors of the REGARDS study argue that the overestimation of risk in the REGARDS study may be owing to short follow-up periods, increased use of statin therapy and revascularization, and methodologic issues in identifying ASCVD events.[46,47] Although the REGARDS study is reported by the guideline authors to be confirmatory of the new risk prediction tool, the reliance on patient and family self-report of events, the generalizability of extrapolating 5-year data to 10-year event rates, and the reliance on the Medicare claims database to be a surrogate for active surveillance limits the use and generalizability of this database.

In addition, a recent study evaluated several ASVD risk assessment models from the ACC/AHA and ATP III on a European cohort (Rotterdam study).[48] They found that all 3 models had poor calibration and all 3 models overestimated ASCVD risk in the Rotterdam cohort. Overall, the study demonstrates that the pooled cohort risk equations may not be generalizable to other populations.

## Importance of Shared Decision Making and a Patient-Centered Approach

Ultimately, both guidelines point out that the decision to start statin therapy should be a shared decision between the patient and physician. As noted by Montori and colleagues,[49] the 10-year risk threshold of 7.5% is a value judgment and that the use of shared decision-making tools may help to translate the guidelines into practice.

It is important to recognize that clinical practice guidelines are a tool to help guide a physician in making decisions for his or her patients. They should not be followed uncritically or blindly. A patient-centered approach should be used when applying guidelines. Of note, the 2013 ACC/AHA guideline provided an important paradigm shift by looking at ASCVD risk and focusing in on "statin benefit" groups. They have simplified greatly clinical practice by just focusing clinicians on statin dose and statin intensity. Their focus on starting higher dose statins may seem appropriate based on the lack of statin titration by health care providers. However, the assumption that side effects would be similar with high-intensity versus moderate-intensity statins is not borne out by observational or clinical studies.[22,50,51] Patients enrolled in statin trials tend to be healthier generally than the general population and those with previous side effects to statin therapy, such as those with myalgia, are generally not included in RCTs. The clinical reality for practicing providers is that many patients cannot tolerate a high-intensity statin as initial therapy or need to be titrated slowly based on age or frailty. As in many disease states, titration of therapy to maximally tolerated doses should be an important alternative.

## Lipid Targets and Low-Density Lipoprotein Cholesterol Monitoring

The abandonment of target lipid goals takes away an important clinical and motivational tool that providers can use with their patients. Goal setting is an important behavioral tool that providers have used successfully in many disease states, including lifestyle counseling, blood pressure control, and diabetes management. Finally, by indirectly deemphasizing frequent LDL-C monitoring, a major concern is that this might have a significant adverse effect on adherence to lipid-lowering therapy. The recent move by 2015 National Committee for Quality Assurance (NCQA) Healthcare Effectiveness Data and Information Set (HEDIS) to remove baseline LDL-C levels and LDL-C monitoring in patients with CHD or diabetes mellitus, along with similar moves by the ACC/AHA Taskforce on Lipid Performance Measurement, may have unanticipated effects. Such adverse effects include a possible drop in statin adherence and the loss of an important quality indicator, in monitoring the change in a population's LDL-C levels.[52,53]

The NLA provides some alternative perspectives based on evidence that (1) there is utility in treating to LDL-C and non–HDL-C targets; (2) non–HDL-C is a better overall predictor of ASCVD risk than LDL-C both before and on statin therapy; (3) titration of statin therapy may be desirable in certain patient groups, such as those with statin intolerance or those who are frail, elderly, or have significant comorbidities; (4) clinicians and patients may benefit by setting specific lipid goals of therapy based on principles of shared decision making and evidence from behavioral medicine; and (5) frequent lipid monitoring is encouraged to identify patient barriers to statin adherence, encourage patient–provider communication, reward patients for positive changes in compliance to lifestyle and drug therapy, ensure adequate patient response to therapy, and treat lipid-related residual risk. In light of the recent IMPROVE-IT trial, combination nonstatin therapy should be considered in patients not reaching their LDL-C and non–HDL-C goals and the emphasis should be placed back on lipids and not just statin benefit groups.

### The Way Forward

Overall, both sets of guidelines complement each other and try to move the needle forward in ASCVD prevention. Given the stakes involved and the growing burden of ASCVD in the United States, it is even more important that all stakeholders including large medical subspecialty organizations (ACC, AHA, NLA, American Diabetes Association, American Association of Clinical Endocrinologists) government and regulatory agencies (Centers for Medicare and Medicaid Services, Medicare, Medicaid, Veteran's Administration, Centers for Disease Control and Prevention), private insurers, primary care (American Academy of Family Physicians, American College of Physicians) and medical subspecialty groups, allied health professionals (nursing, nurse practitioners, pharmacists, dieticians, physician assistants, health educators, public health workers, exercise physiologists, etc), and the general public (consumers, patients, patient advocacy groups) come together to better understand guideline commonalities and remain united in working together to implement the necessary clinical and public health measures needed to reduce ASCVD.

Although one can debate the evidence base, disagree on the importance of clinical or expert judgment, or make different decisions based on different biases, preferences, or values, a guideline at its best must be acceptable to major stakeholders and implementable to be effective. An inclusive and transparent process among various stakeholders will ensure broad guideline endorsement, uptake, and adoption. Now is the time for all stakeholders to work together to devise an improved and actionable plan that will center the focus back to the prevention of the leading cause of death and disability in the United States from the ravages of ASCVD.

### REFERENCES

1. Stone NJ, Robinson JG, Lichtenstein AH, et al. 2013 ACC/AHA guideline on the treatment of blood cholesterol to reduce atherosclerotic cardiovascular risk in adults: a report of the American College of Cardiology/American Heart Association task force on practice guidelines. Circulation 2014;129(25 Suppl 2):S1–45.
2. Jacobson TA, Ito MK, Maki KC, et al. National Lipid Association recommendations for patient-centered management of dyslipidemia: part 1-executive summary. J Clin Lipidol 2014;8(5):473–88.
3. Go AS, Mozaffarian D, Roger VL, et al. Heart disease and stroke statistics–2014 update: a report from the American Heart Association. Circulation 2014;129(3):e28–292.
4. Grundy SM, Cleeman JI, Merz CN, et al. Implications of recent clinical trials for the national cholesterol education program Adult Treatment Panel III guidelines. Circulation 2004;110(2):227–39.
5. National Cholesterol Education Program Expert Panel on Detection E. Treatment of high blood cholesterol in A. Third report of the National Cholesterol Education Program (NCEP) Expert Panel on Detection, Evaluation, and Treatment of High Blood Cholesterol in Adults (Adult Treatment Panel III) final report. Circulation 2002;106(25):3143–421.
6. Ridker PM, Danielson E, Fonseca FA, et al. Rosuvastatin to prevent vascular events in men and women with elevated C-reactive protein. N Engl J Med 2008;359(21):2195–207.
7. Downs JR, Clearfield M, Weis S, et al. Primary prevention of acute coronary events with lovastatin in men and women with average cholesterol levels: results of AFCAPS/TexCAPS. Air force/Texas Coronary Atherosclerosis Prevention Study. JAMA 1998;279(20):1615–22.
8. Nakamura H, Arakawa K, Itakura H, et al. Primary prevention of cardiovascular disease with pravastatin in Japan (MEGA Study): a prospective randomised controlled trial. Lancet 2006;368(9542):1155–63.

9. Expert Panel on Detection E. Treatment of high blood cholesterol in a. Executive summary of the third report of the national cholesterol education program (NCEP) expert panel on detection, evaluation, and treatment of high blood cholesterol in adults (Adult Treatment Panel III). JAMA 2001; 285(19):2486–97.

10. Association AH. 2013 Prevention guidelines tools. CV risk calculator. 2013. Available at: http://my.american heart.org/cvriskcalculator. Accessed January 19, 2015.

11. Bulugahapitiya U, Siyambalapitiya S, Sithole J, et al. Is diabetes a coronary risk equivalent? systematic review and meta-analysis. Diabet Med 2009;26(2): 142–8.

12. Bild DE, Bluemke DA, Burke GL, et al. Multi-Ethnic Study of Atherosclerosis: objectives and design. Am J Epidemiol 2002;156(9):871–81.

13. Howard VJ, Cushman M, Pulley L, et al. The Reasons for Geographic And Racial Differences in Stroke Study: objectives and design. Neuroepidemiology 2005;25(3):135–43.

14. Robinson JG, Wang S, Smith BJ, et al. Meta-analysis of the relationship between non-high-density lipoprotein cholesterol reduction and coronary heart disease risk. J Am Coll Cardiol 2009;53(4):316–22.

15. Boekholdt SM, Arsenault BJ, Mora S, et al. Association of LDL cholesterol, non-HDL cholesterol, and apolipoprotein B levels with risk of cardiovascular events among patients treated with statins: a meta-analysis. JAMA 2012;307(12):1302–9.

16. Robinson JG. Are you targeting non-high-density lipoprotein cholesterol? J Am Coll Cardiol 2009; 55(1):42–4.

17. Harper CR, Jacobson TA. Using apolipoprotein B to manage dyslipidemic patients: time for a change? Mayo Clin Proc 2010;85(5):440–5.

18. Robinson JG, Wang S, Jacobson TA. Meta-analysis of comparison of effectiveness of lowering apolipoprotein B versus low-density lipoprotein cholesterol and nonhigh-density lipoprotein cholesterol for cardiovascular risk reduction in randomized trials. Am J Cardiol 2012;110(10):1468–76.

19. Abd TT, Jacobson TA. Statin-induced myopathy: a review and update. Expert Opin Drug Saf 2011; 10(3):373–87.

20. Toth PP, Thanassoulis G, Williams K, et al. The risk-benefit paradigm vs the causal exposure paradigm: LDL as a primary cause of vascular disease. J Clin Lipidol 2014;8(6):594–605.

21. Harper CR, Jacobson TA. Avoiding statin myopathy: understanding key drug interactions. Clin Lipidol 2011;6(6):665–74.

22. Rosenson RS, Baker SK, Jacobson TA, et al. An assessment by the statin muscle safety task force: 2014 update. J Clin Lipidol 2014;8(Suppl 3): S58–71.

23. Guyton JR, Bays HE, Grundy SM, et al. An assessment by the statin intolerance panel: 2014 update. J Clin Lipidol 2014;8(Suppl 3):S72–81.

24. Cohen JD, Brinton EA, Ito MK, et al. Understanding statin use in America and gaps in patient education (USAGE): an internet-based survey of 10,138 current and former statin users. J Clin Lipidol 2012;6(3):208–15.

25. Rojas-Fernandez CH, Goldstein LB, Levey AI, et al. An assessment by the statin cognitive safety task force: 2014 update. J Clin Lipidol 2014;8(Suppl 3): S5–16.

26. Morris PB, Ballantyne CM, Birtcher KK, et al. Review of clinical practice guidelines for the management of LDL-related risk. J Am Coll Cardiol 2014;64(2): 196–206.

27. Jacobson TA, Gutkin SW, Harper CR. Effects of a global risk educational tool on primary coronary prevention: the atherosclerosis assessment via total risk (AVIATOR) study. Curr Med Res Opin 2006; 22(6):1065–73.

28. Sheridan SL, Viera AJ, Krantz MJ, et al. The effect of giving global coronary risk information to adults: a systematic review. Arch Intern Med 2010;170(3): 230–9.

29. Shillinglaw B, Viera AJ, Edwards T, et al. Use of global coronary heart disease risk assessment in practice: a cross-sectional survey of a sample of U.S. physicians. BMC Health Serv Res 2012;12:20.

30. LaRosa JC, Grundy SM, Waters DD, et al. Intensive lipid lowering with atorvastatin in patients with stable coronary disease. N Engl J Med 2005;352(14): 1425–35.

31. AIM-HIGH Investigators, Boden WE, Probstfield JL, et al. Niacin in patients with low HDL cholesterol levels receiving intensive statin therapy. N Engl J Med 2011;365(24):2255–67.

32. The HPS2-THRIVE Collaborative Group, Landray MJ, Haynes R, et al. Effects of extended-release niacin with laropiprant in high-risk patients. N Engl J Med 2014;371(3):203–12.

33. Ginsberg HN, Reyes-Soffer G. Niacin: a long history, but a questionable future. Curr Opin Lipidol 2013; 24(6):475–9.

34. The ACCORD Study Group, Ginsberg HN, Elam MB, et al. Effects of combination lipid therapy in type 2 diabetes mellitus. N Engl J Med 2010;362(17): 1563–74.

35. Canner PL, Berge KG, Wenger NK, et al. Fifteen year mortality in coronary drug project patients: long-term benefit with niacin. J Am Coll Cardiol 1986;8(6):1245–55.

36. Buchwald H. Risk reduction and the program on the surgical control of the hyperlipidemias. Circulation 2001;104(9):E47.

37. The lipid research clinics coronary primary prevention trial results. II. The relationship of reduction in

incidence of coronary heart disease to cholesterol lowering. JAMA 1984;251(3):365–74.

38. The lipid research clinics coronary primary prevention trial results. I. Reduction in incidence of coronary heart disease. JAMA 1984;251(3):351–64.

39. Kohno T. Report of the American Heart Association (AHA) scientific sessions 2014, Chicago. Circ J 2015;79:34–40.

40. Cholesterol Treatment Trialists' (CTT) Collaboration, Baigent C, Blackwell L, et al. Efficacy and safety of more intensive lowering of LDL cholesterol: a meta-analysis of data from 170,000 participants in 26 randomised trials. Lancet 2010;376(9753):1670–81.

41. Mihaylova B, Emberson J, Blackwell L, et al. The effects of lowering LDL cholesterol with statin therapy in people at low risk of vascular disease: meta-analysis of individual data from 27 randomised trials. Lancet 2012;380(9841):581–90.

42. Rogers JK, Jhund PS, Perez AC, et al. Effect of rosuvastatin on repeat heart failure hospitalizations: the CORONA trial (Controlled Rosuvastatin Multinational Trial in Heart Failure). JACC Heart Fail 2014; 2(3):289–97.

43. Fellstrom BC, Jardine AG, Schmieder RE, et al. Rosuvastatin and cardiovascular events in patients undergoing hemodialysis. N Engl J Med 2009; 360(14):1395–407.

44. Ridker PM, Cook NR. Statins: new American guidelines for prevention of cardiovascular disease. Lancet 2013;382(9907):1762–5.

45. Qureshi N, Armstrong S, Dhiman P, et al. Effect of adding systematic family history enquiry to cardiovascular disease risk assessment in primary care: a matched-pair, cluster randomized trial. Ann Intern Med 2012;156(4):253–62.

46. Muntner P, Safford MM, Cushman M, et al. Comment on the reports of over-estimation of ASCVD risk using the 2013 AHA/ACC risk equation. Circulation 2014;129(2):266–7.

47. Cook NR, Ridker PM. Response to comment on the reports of over-estimation of ASCVD risk using the 2013 AHA/ACC risk equation. Circulation 2014; 129(2):268–9.

48. Kavousi M, Leening MJ, Nanchen D, et al. Comparison of application of the ACC/AHA guidelines, Adult Treatment Panel III guidelines, and European Society of Cardiology guidelines for cardiovascular disease prevention in a European cohort. JAMA 2014;311(14):1416–23.

49. Montori VM, Brito JP, Ting HH. Patient-centered and practical application of new high cholesterol guidelines to prevent cardiovascular disease. JAMA 2014;311(5):465–6.

50. Bruckert E, Hayem G, Dejager S, et al. Mild to moderate muscular symptoms with high-dosage statin therapy in hyperlipidemic patients–the PRIMO study. Cardiovasc Drugs Ther 2005;19(6):403–14.

51. Jacobson TA. Statin safety: lessons from new drug applications for marketed statins. Am J Cardiol 2006;97(8A):44C–51C.

52. NCQA updates HEDIS Quality Measure. Available at: http://www.ncqa.org/Newsroom/NewsArchive/2014 NewsArchive/NewsReleaseJuly12014.aspx. Accessed January 19, 2015.

53. Drozda JJ, Ferguson TB Jr, Jneid H, et al. 2014 ACC/AHA update of secondary prevention lipid measures: a report of the American College of Cardiology/American Heart Association Task Force on Performance Measures. J Am Coll Cardiol, in press.

# Lipoprotein Apheresis

Patrick M. Moriarty, MD[a,*], Linda Hemphill, MD[b]

## KEYWORDS

- Lipoprotein apheresis • Familial hypercholesterolemia • LDL-C • CVD • Atherosclerosis • Lp(a)

## KEY POINTS

- Patients with familial hypercholesterolemia (FH) have early development of atherosclerosis and cardiovascular disease (CVD).
- Lipid level–lowering medications are not always successful in reducing increased low-density lipoprotein C (LDL-C) levels.
- Lipoprotein apheresis (LA) reduces LDL-C levels by more than 60% in patients with FH and reduces CVD events.
- LA also reduces lipoprotein (a) (Lp(a)) levels and CVD events.
- LA reduces inflammatory markers and blood viscosity.

## INTRODUCTION

Apheresis, derived from the Greek word aphairein, meaning to take away, is applied to patients with familial hypercholesterolemia (FH) who are resistant to standard lipid level–lowering medications. Apheresis devices used for the reduction of plasma cholesterol levels can be separated into 3 general groups:

1. Nonselective plasma exchange, which simply removes all of the plasma volume through centrifugation, and was first introduced in 1967 by de Gennes and colleagues.[1]
2. Semiselective ultrafiltration, developed by Agishi and colleagues[2] in 1980, which uses a double-membrane filtration and involves elimination of atherogenic lipoproteins based on particle size and geometric properties.
3. Selective lipoprotein apheresis (LA), which was developed in 1981 by Stoffel and colleagues[3] using a device containing 2 columns of sapharose gel coupled with polyclonal sheep apolipoprotein B (apoB)-100 antibodies. Newer selective

LA devices have been developed involving not only antibodies to lipoproteins but negative charged environments to capture the positive charged apoB. The devices approved for use in the United States and Canada are based on the removal of charged lipoprotein particles.

## CRITERIA FOR LIPOPROTEIN APHERESIS

The US Food and Drug Administration (FDA) set the criteria for LA in 1997, when the Kaneka Liposorber and B Braun HELP (heparin-induced extracorporeal low-density lipoprotein precipitation) systems were approved in the United States based on the following criteria.

Patients must show that, after 6 months of the maximum tolerated lipid level–lowering therapy and compliance with a low-saturated-fat, low-cholesterol diet, one of the following is still met:

1. Functional homozygous FH with low-density lipoprotein cholesterol (LDL-C) level greater than or equal to 500 mg/dL

Disclosures: Dr P.M. Moriarty, Research for Amgen, Kowa, Lilly, Novartis, Sanofi, Regeneron, Genzyme, Pfizer, Catabasis, Espirion, B. Braun, and Kaneka; Consultant for Regeneron, Duke Clinical research Institute, Lilly, Catabasis, B Braun, Kaneka, and Genzyme; Honoraria from Esperion.
Dr L. Hemphill, Research: Regeneron, Sanofi and ISIS.
[a] Division of Clinical Pharmacology and Atherosclerosis/Lipoprotein-Apheresis Center, University of Kansas Medical Center, 3901 Rainbow Boulevard, Mail Stop 3008, Kansas City, KS 66160, USA; [b] Massachusetts General Hospital, Harvard Medical School, Boston, MA 02115, USA
* Corresponding author. Atherosclerosis/Lipoprotein-Apheresis Center, University of Kansas Medical Center, 3901 Rainbow Boulevard, Mail Stop 3008, Kansas City, KS 66160.
E-mail address: pmoriart@kumc.edu

2. Functional heterozygous FH with LDL-C level greater than or equal to 200 mg/dL in the presence of documented coronary artery disease (CAD)
3. Functional heterozygous FH with LDL-C level greater than or equal to 300 mg/dL in the absence of documented CAD

These requirements for therapy are much sterner than those of other countries that perform LA. In Germany, treatments are allowed for patients with CAD and LDL-C levels greater than 130 mg/dL, whereas Japan approves LA therapy for patients with CAD with a total cholesterol level greater than 250 mg/dL. To deal with this gap in treatment, some LA sites have negotiated with health care providers in allowing some high-risk patients with LDL-C levels greater than 160 mg/dL to receive LA.

Panels from the National Lipid Association (NLA) and the American Society for Apheresis (ASFA) recently recommended modifying the criterion for initiating LA therapy to include patients with any atherosclerotic cardiovascular disease (CVD), not just CAD, and lowering the LDL-C threshold in these patients to greater than or equal to 160 mg/dL.[4]

## POTENTIAL PATIENT POPULATION WHO QUALIFY FOR LIPOPROTEIN APHERESIS

An estimate of the LA eligible population in the United States by the strict FDA criteria, assuming a prevalence of heterozygous FH of 1 in 500, is approximately 15,000 patients eligible for LA.[5] From the population of individuals intolerant of 3-hydroxy-3-methylglutaryl-coenzyme A reductase inhibitors (statins) (prevalence 10%–25%), another 10,000 patients could be added to the number who would qualify for LA.[6,7] Despite these estimates the current census in the United States of patients receiving LA is only 550. Potential explanations for the low number of patients receiving LA therapy include a lack of awareness; insufficient numbers of LA centers (fewer than 50 in the United States), resulting in patients traveling long distances for treatments; complexity of initiating an LA center; and the likelihood that patients with poor venous access will require a shunt/fistula or the belief by physicians that future lipid level–lowering drugs such as proprotein convertase subtilisin/kexin type 9 (PCSK9) inhibitors will provide adequate treatment of these extremely high-risk patients. In contrast, to achieve a successful LA program requires a team effort by the patients, medical staff, and health care providers.

## BILLING AND CODING INFORMATION

LA therapy is covered by most private health insurers and government payers (eg, Medicare, Department of Veterans' Affairs). Coverage policies are typically based on the FDA indications but exceptions have been allowed (ongoing CVD and increased Lp(a) or LDL-C level more than 160 mg/dL). These exceptions are made on a case-by-case basis and may also depend on the health care provider and the state residency of the patient. Reimbursement for LA in the hospital or outpatient setting can be highly variable ($2000–$4000 per session) according to the insurer and the location in the United States.

In 2005, relative value units (RVUs) were specified for current procedural terminology (CPT) 36516. This specification applies exclusively to LA. In 2005 and 2006, about 85 RVUs were designated for this procedure and associated services under the direct supervision of physicians. Under the applicable ambulatory payment classification (APC 0112), Medicare payments are usually less than reimbursement under contracts negotiated between hospital providers and private insurers. It is recommended that all cases separately bill the insurer for professional services and again under CPT 36516.

## APPROVED LIPOPROTEIN APHERESIS MACHINES IN THE UNITED STATES
### Futura, B Braun, Melsungen, Germany

#### Heparin-induced extracorporeal low-density lipoprotein precipitation
In 1983, Wieland and Seidel[8] introduced the HELP system (**Fig. 1**). Following separation, the plasma is mixed 1:1 with a 0.3-M acetate buffer (pH 4.8) solution containing heparin at a concentration of 100 U/mL. Precipitation of heparin and low-density lipoprotein (LDL) occurs when the plasma buffer solution reaches an approximate pH of 5.2. The mechanism for the selective removal of lipoproteins is attributed to the negatively charged heparin precipitating with the positively charged apoB of LDL-C, very-low-density lipoproteins (VLDLs), and Lp(a). High-density lipoprotein cholesterol (HDL-C), which has a negatively charged membrane,[9] is normally spared from the precipitation process. A diethylaminoethyl cellulose filter adsorbs the residual heparin in the LDL-free plasma. Physiologic pH of the plasma and removal of excess fluid are achieved by dialysis and ultrafiltration.[10]

### MA03 Liposorber, Kaneka, Osaka, Japan

#### Dextran sulfate low-density lipoprotein adsorption
In 1987, Mabuchi and colleagues[11] reported on the dextran sulfate LDL adsorption (DSA) system (LA-15, Kaneka, Osaka, Japan) (**Fig. 2**). Plasma is exposed to a column of cellulose beads coated

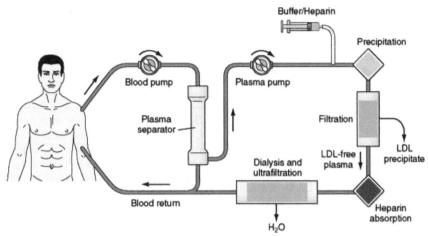

**Fig. 1.** HELP (Futura). (*From* Moriarty PM. Low-density lipoprotein apheresis. In: Ballantyne CM, editor. Clinical lipidology: a companion to Braunwald's heart disease. Philadelphia: Saunders Elsevier; 2009. p. 365; with permission.)

with dextran sulfate cellulose. Similar to the HELP system, selective removal of LDL, VLDL, and Lp(a) occurs through an electrostatic interaction of the polyanionic dextran sulfate ligands and the positively charged apoB lipoproteins. The machine contains 2 dextran sulfate columns. After the first column is exposed to 500 mL of plasma, it is then cleansed and regenerated with a solution containing 4.1% sodium chloride. During the first column's rinsing process, plasma flow is redirected to the second column. As with the HELP system, the DSA system retains most of the HDL in the plasma.

### Further lipoprotein apheresis information

A heparin bolus (2000–4000 IU) is used to achieve anticoagulation, followed by a continuous infusion of heparin at 1500 IU/h. Both treatments are performed through a peripheral antecubital venous access (needles of 16–18 gauge) or an

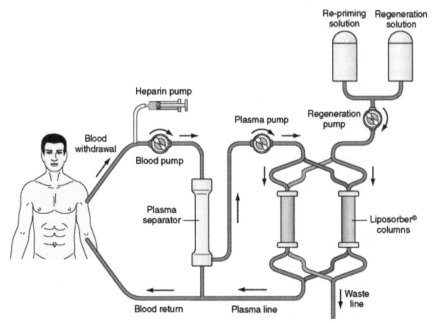

**Fig. 2.** DSA (MAO3). (*From* Moriarty PM. Low-density lipoprotein apheresis. In: Ballantyne CM, editor. Clinical lipidology: a companion to Braunwald's heart disease. Philadelphia: Saunders Elsevier; 2009. p. 366; with permission.)

arteriovenous fistula. At flow rates between 40 and 100 mL/min, treated plasma volume varies between the two machines. The HELP system treats 3000 mL of plasma and additional volume would overtax the collecting capability of its precipitating filter or increase bleeding risk because of lower fibrinogen levels. For the DSA system, each of the 2 dextran sulfate filters are cleansed after exposure to 500 mL of plasma, allowing an unlimited amount of plasma volume treated as long as its plasma separator remains patent. Plasma volume treated with the DSA system is based on the patient's body mass and hematocrit. During therapy, only a maximum of 300 to 600 mL of plasma/blood are extracorporeal at any time. Treatments last 2 to 4 hours (1.5–3 hours patient time and 1 hour nursing time for before and after the session) and are scheduled weekly, biweekly, or even less frequently, depending on baseline lipid levels and response to therapy. The biweekly treatments are most common.

### Contraindications/Complications/Adverse Events

The HELP and DSA systems are contraindicated for patients with hypersensitivity to heparin. In cases of sensitivity to heparin, the broad-spectrum synthetic protease inhibitor nafamostat mesilate has sometimes been used with the DSA system as an alternative anticoagulant. The occurrence of adverse events (AEs) is low and typically involves the blood circulating outside the body.[12] Hypotension is the most common AE (<2%) and the incidence of all other AEs (flushing, blotching, chest pain, anemia, abdominal discomfort, hemolysis, and arrhythmia) is less than 1%.[13,14] Unlike HELP, the DSA system increases plasma bradykinin (BK) levels by 900-fold. BK is a potent vasodilator and increase of plasma levels may cause an anaphylactoidlike reaction for patients also receiving angiotensin-converting enzyme inhibitors (ACEIs), which are blockers of BK degradation. To prevent this reaction, patients should discontinue the use of ACEI or switch to an angiotensin receptor blocker.

### Special Points of Interest

The DSA system is recommended for children with FH if they weigh more than 15 kg (33 lb) and are older than 5 years of age, whereas with the HELP system it is suggested that a patient's weight should be more than 37 kg (80 lb) before initiating therapy. Although not recommended, case studies have shown LA safety and effectiveness for women with FH throughout their pregnancies.[15] Plasma fibrinogen, a multifaceted protein involved in the vascular process of inflammation, coagulation, and viscosity, is acutely lowered by 65% with the HELP system compared with 30% or less with the DSA system.

### Clinical Benefit

Because of the small number of patients receiving LA therapy and the unethical practice of sham therapy, there is a lack of large, multicenter, placebo-controlled trials. One of the largest non-randomized trials followed the safety and efficacy of LA therapy (DSA) over a 6-year period. The study compared FH heterozygotes (n = 43) with CVD receiving LA plus combination lipid level–lowering therapy (low-dose statin plus probucol and resin or fibrate) with a similar group of FH heterozygotes (n = 87) receiving only lipid level–lowering therapy. Kaplan-Meier analysis of the primary end points (nonfatal myocardial infarction, coronary angioplasty, coronary artery bypass, and death from coronary heart disease [CHD]) found that the rate of events was 72% lower in the LA group (10%) compared with the drug-only group (36%) (P = .008).[16] **Fig. 3** shows the relative risk reduction found in multiple studies.

### LIPOPROTEINS AND OTHER PROTEINS ALTERED BY LIPOPROTEIN APHERESIS
### Low-density Lipoprotein (Apolipoprotein B–containing Particles)

LA acutely reduces apoB-containing particles by approximately 60% (see **Table 1**). Typically, the greater the baseline LDL-C level, the greater the reduction of apoB lipoproteins. The rebound of LDL-C and Lp(a) to approximately baseline levels ranges from 8 to 13 days.[20] Using multiple therapies along with LA, such as statins, increases the efficacy of LA and increases the probability of

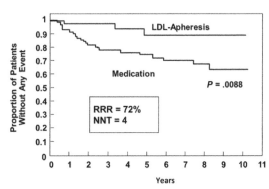

**Fig. 3.** LA and the reduction of CV events. NNT, numbers needed to treat; RRR, relative risk reduction. (*Data from* Refs.[17–19]).

**Table 1**
**Acute percentage lipid changes reductions following LA**

|  | HELP[47–50] (%) | DSA[11,24,48,51–53] (%) |
|---|---|---|
| Total cholesterol | 42–54 | 48–68 |
| LDL-C | 55–61 | 49–85 |
| HDL-C | 0–19 | 4–32 |
| Lp(a) | 55–68 | 19–70 |
| Triglycerides | 20–61 | 26–64 |

*From* Moriarty PM. Low-density lipoprotein apheresis. In: Ballantyne CM, editor. Clinical lipidology: a companion to Braunwald's heart disease. Philadelphia: Saunders Elsevier; 2009. p. 367; with permission.

treatment success, even in patients homozygous for FH.[21] Further, after chronic LA therapy, the pretreatment levels of apoB lipoproteins, such as LDL-C, are reduced by 20% to 40%.[13,22]

Along with the reduction of apoB lipoproteins, LA also modifies the composition of plasma LDL. Increased circulating levels of oxidized LDL (ox-LDL)[23] and small dense LDL[24] have been associated with an increased risk of CVD. LA significantly reduces ox-LDL levels[25] and decreases small dense LDL levels, whereas the total percentage of large buoyant LDL increases after treatment.[26] Despite the quantitative and qualitative changes to LDL, regular apheresis therapy does not seem to alter kinetic parameters of apoB metabolism.[27]

### High-density Lipoprotein Cholesterol

HDL-C levels are reduced and its functionality (reverse cholesterol transport activity) may be impaired in patients with FH.[28] The mechanism

by which LA acutely lowers HDL-C (10%–20%) is not fully understood because, unlike apoB lipoproteins, the HDL-C is negative charged. Some explanations involve filtration, hemodilution, activation of hepatic triglyceride lipase (HTGL), or the decreased activity of lecithin-cholesterol acyltransferase.[29] Several studies[30,31] of LA therapy have revealed a greater acute reduction of total HDL than apolipoprotein A-I, the primary HDL lipoprotein involved in reverse cholesterol transport, and that most of the HDL-C removed following LA is a proinflammatory type, as measured by the inability of HDL to inhibit LDL-induced monocyte chemotactic activity.[32,33]

Apolipoprotein E4 (ApoE4), a risk factor for CVD and Alzheimer disease, is a component of HDL-C that increases its binding affinity to the LDL receptor more than LDL-C.[34] Patients with FH seem to have a greater amount of ApoE4-bound HDL-C and LA therapy acutely removes this protein complex by more than 40%.[35,36] Acutely, total HDL-C returns to pretreatment levels in 24 hours, whereas long-term therapy preserves or enhances baseline levels.[20,37] LA significantly reduces LDL/HDL ratios and reduces more HDL (2.5 times) than apolipoprotein A1 (ApoA1), whereas nonselective plasma exchange increases LDL/HDL ratios and reduces equal amounts of HDL and ApoA1.[30] This difference is one of the significant distinctions between nonselective and selective apheresis.

HDL particle (HDL-P) number has been shown to be inversely associated with CHD, independent of total HDL-C levels and/or other atherogenic lipoproteins.[38] LA therapy acutely increases HDL-P by 16% and reduces total HDL-C levels.[39]

### Triglycerides and Other Apolipoproteins

Triglycerides (TGs) are acutely reduced by 18% to 64% (**Table 1**)[16,40] following LA. Similar to HDL-C,

**Table 2**
**LA therapy for increased Lp(a) levels**

| Apheresis | Jaeger et al,[45] 2009 Before | After | Rosada et al,[46] 2014 Before | After | Leebmann et al,[44] 2013 Before | After |
|---|---|---|---|---|---|---|
| Patients (n) | 120 | 120 | 37 | 37 | 170 | 166 |
| Duration (y) | 5.5 | 5.0 | 5.2 | 6.8 | 2 | 2 |
| LDL-C (mg/dL) | 125 | 45 (−65%) | 84 | 34 (−60%) | 100 | 33 (−60%) |
| Lp(a) (mg/dL) | 118 | 33 (−72%) | 112 | 36 (−68%) | 87 | 26 (−70%) |
| MACE total | 297 | 57 (−81%) | 67 | 20 (−70%) | 142 | 31 (−78%) |
| MACE per year | 1.05 | 0.14 (−86%) | 2.80 | 0.08 (−97%) | 0.41 | 0.09 (−78%) |

Percentages are mean percent change.
*Abbreviation:* MACE, major adverse cardiac events.

**Table 3**
**Acute changes to vascular markers following LA**

| Marker | Acute Changes (%)[30,54–67] |
|---|---|
| Proinflammatory | |
| MCP-1 | −15 to −18 |
| MMP-9 | −20 |
| TIMP-1 | −30 |
| LBP | −27 |
| Lp-PLA2 | −22 |
| VCAM-1 | −10 to −20 |
| ICAM-1 | −10 to −16 |
| E-selectin | −6 to −31 |
| Fibrinogen | −11 to −65 |
| Oxidized LDL | −65 |
| CRP | −10 to −80 |
| SAA | −21 to −35 |
| Pentraxin 3 | −20 |
| Vascular Function | |
| Nitric oxide | 25 to 45 |
| VEGF | 15 |
| IGF-I | −37 |
| Bradykinin | 0>2000 |
| ET-1 | −15 to −75 |
| PGI2 | 300 |
| Thrombotic | |
| Tissue factor | −26 |
| Von Willebrand factor | −29 to −56 |
| Thrombin | −55 |
| Factor V | −57 to −74 |
| Factor VII | −4 to −36 |
| Factor XI | −27 to 82 |
| Factor XII | −32 to 73 |
| sCD40L | −16 |
| Homocysteine | −15 to −25 |
| Fibrinogen | −10 to −65 |
| Fibrinolytic | |
| Plasminogen | −23 to −50 |
| Protein S | −11 to −35 |
| Protein C | −32 to −48 |
| Antithrombin | −11 to −25 |

High variation of values may be partially caused by differences in treated plasma and blood volumes.

*Abbreviations:* CRP, C-reactive protein; ET-1, endothelin-1; ICAM-1, intercellular adhesion molecule-1; IGF-I, insulinlike growth factor-I, LBP, lipopolysaccharide binding protein; Lp-PLA2, lipoprotein-associated phospholipase A2; MCP-1, monocyte chemoattractant protein-1; MMP-9, matrix metalloproteinase-9; PGI2, prostaglandin I2; SAA, serum amyloid A; sCD40L, soluble CD40 ligand; TIMP-1, tissue inhibitor of metalloproteinase-1; VCAM-1, vascular cellular adhesion molecule-1; VEGF, vascular endothelial growth factor.

*Adapted from* Moriarty PM. Low-density lipoprotein apheresis. In: Ballantyne CM, editor. Clinical lipidology: a companion to Braunwald's heart disease. Philadelphia: Saunders Elsevier; 2009. p. 369; with permission.

TG levels rebound to near pretreatment levels in 24 hours.[20] Reduction in TG levels have been attributed to the removal of the apoB portion of VLDL, HTGL activation, and heparin's ability to increase lipoprotein lipase activity.[40] LA therapy also reduces apolipoprotein C-III and apoE levels by 40% to 50%.[41]

## Lp(a)

The treatment of increased Lp(a) levels is not an FDA-approved indication in the absence of meeting the LDL-C criterion. However, the latest data reveal an increased atherogenicity and risk of CVD associated with Lp(a) regardless of LDL-C levels.[42,43] In 2010 the German government approved LA treatments for patients with ongoing CAD and Lp(a) levels greater than 60 mg/dL (Normal<30 mg/dL), irrespective of LDL-C levels. Since initiating LA for increased Lp(a) levels, 3 retrospective/prospective trials[44–46] have discovered a 70% to 81% reduction of major adverse cardiovascular events (**Table 2**). In the United States a few patients with isolated increased Lp(a) levels and ongoing CVD are receiving biweekly LA therapy.

### Inflammatory and Other Markers Affected

In addition to lipoproteins, LA modifies other markers associated with vascular disease, in particularly inflammatory proteins. **Table 3** lists immediate changes to certain plasma proteins following LA.

Vascular cells in response to injury secrete pentraxin 3, a member of the humoral arm of innate immunity. Pentraxin 3 levels are also increased in patients with FH and its level is strongly associated with vascular disease. Zanetti and colleagues[68] found that LA therapy acutely and chronically reduced plasma levels of pentraxin 3.

The reduction of these inflammatory and lipoproteins seems to markedly reduce plaque inflammation, as shown by van Wijk and colleagues[69] when they used F-fluorodeoxyglucose PET before and after LA (**Fig. 4**).

## RHEOLOGY

Hemorheology, or blood rheology, is the study of flow properties of blood and its elements. Blood viscosity is a measure of the resistance of blood to flow. Unlike plasma, blood behaves as a non-newtonian fluid, such that its viscosity varies with shear forces (rate or stress). The variation in viscosity is directly related to vascular resistance, which can profoundly influence CVD and atherosclerosis.[70] Mediators of blood viscosity (in addition to hematocrit, shear forces, and temperature) include red blood cell (RBC) deformability, RBC aggregation, and plasma viscosity. A single LA treatment reduces blood viscosity by more than 20%[71] and maintains this reduction for at least 7 days.[72] The improvement of blood rheology by LA is related to changes in RBC aggregation/deformability and plasma viscosity.[73,74] Fibrinogen is responsible for 20% of

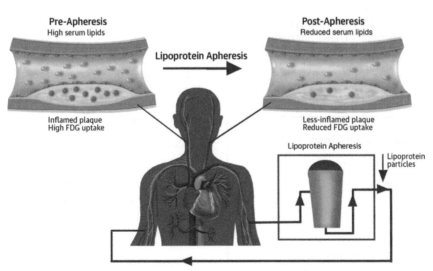

**Fig. 4.** Reduction of plaque inflammation as shown by F-fluorodeoxyglucose (FDG) PET scan. (*From* Zanetti M, Zenti M, Barazzoni R, et al. HELP LDL apheresis reduces plasma pentraxin 3 in familial hypercholesterolemia. PLoS One 2014;9(7):e101290.)

### Table 4
### Hemorheology markers: percentage changes following LA

| Markers | HELP | Liposorber |
|---|---|---|
| Plasma viscosity[a] | −15 | −11 |
| Blood viscosity[a] | −15 | −5 |
| RBC aggregation[a] | −52 | −31 |
| RBC deformability | 45 | 45 |
| Fibrinogen[a] | −62 | −11 |

Comparison from head-to-head study between HELP and Liposorber.
[a] P less than .05.
Data from Refs.[70–74]

plasma viscosity, which explains why the Futura HELP system LA improves rheology factors more effectively than the Liposorber DSA system (**Table 4**).[73]

## ALTERNATIVE USES

When standard therapy has failed, LA can be used for complex vascular diseases in which pathologic components of the blood or plasma need to be removed (**Box 1**). As mentioned previously, LA is performed in Germany for patients with increased plasma levels of Lp(a) and ongoing CVD, whereas clinicians in Japan treat more patients who have advanced (Fontaine classification ≥II) peripheral arterial disease than patients with FH. In 2013 the FDA approved LA therapy (DSA) for pediatric patients with primary focal segmental glomerulosclerosis (FSG) either before or after renal transplant. These alternative uses, and others, are listed in **Box 1**. Besides FSG, the FDA has approved none.

### Box 1
### Possible alternative applications of LA

Increased Lp(a) and ongoing CVD[43,44,75]

Peripheral arterial disease[17,56,59,76–79]

FSG[80–82]

Cardiac transplant[83–87]

Cerebral vascular events[88,89]

Age-related macular degeneration[50,90,91]

Sudden idiopathic hearing loss[92–94]

Preeclampsia[95]

## SUMMARY

LA therapy has proved its clinical benefit in reducing CVD events for patients with FH with hypercholesterolemia. Present FDA guidelines for the use of LA are based on 25-year-old data and more recent studies have shown that lower levels of plasma cholesterol, even in combination with a statin, further reduce CVD risk. Although lacking in multicenter randomized control studies, for the past 40 years LA therapy has extended the lives of the FH population, in particular homozygote patients.

The reduction of Lp(a) levels, improved rheology, and improved quality of HDL-C may be independent mechanisms by which LA reduces CVD. It seems that the removal of plasma inflammatory markers along with atherogenic lipoproteins might play a role in the immediate reduction of arterial wall inflammation. These potential benefits of LA would be further appreciated and implemented as therapy if more randomized clinical trials were performed using this technology in patients with other categories of vascular disease not necessarily associated with FH.

Despite the success of reducing LDL-C levels and almost universal coverage, only 2% of potential candidates are presently receiving LA therapy in the United States. Recently, the NLA, ASFA, and FH Foundation publically voiced their support for LA therapy and the need for patients to be offered this technology if they qualify. The future for most patients with FH may be aligned with newer lipid level–lowering medications such as PCSK9 inhibitors, but until that time LA is the most effective treatment available for this high-risk patient population.

## ACKNOWLEDGMENTS

The authors thank Audrey McCalley and Julie-Ann Dutton for their work in completing this article.

## REFERENCES

1. de Gennes JL, Touraine R, Maunand B, et al. Homozygous cutaneo-tendinous forms of hypercholesteremic xanthomatosis in an exemplary familial case. Trial of plasmapheresis and heroic treatment. Bull Mem Soc Med Hop Paris 1967;118(15):1377–402.
2. Agishi T, Kaneko I, Hasuo Y, et al. Double filtration plasmapheresis. Trans Am Soc Artif Intern Organs 1980;26:406–11.
3. Stoffel W, Borberg H, Greve V. Application of specific extracorporeal removal of low density lipoprotein in familial hypercholesterolaemia. Lancet 1981; 2(8254):1005–7.

4. Ito MK, McGowan MP, Moriarty PM, et al. Management of familial hypercholesterolemias in adult patients: recommendations from the national lipid association expert panel on familial hypercholesterolemia. J Clin Lipidol 2011;5(3 Suppl):S38–45.

5. Vishwanath R, Hemphill LC. Familial hypercholesterolemia and estimation of US patients eligible for low-density lipoprotein apheresis after maximally tolerated lipid-lowering therapy. J Clin Lipidol 2014;8:18–28.

6. Bruckert E, Hayem G, Dejager S, et al. Mild to moderate muscular symptoms with high-dosage statin therapy in hyperlipidemic patients–the PRIMO study. Cardiovasc Drugs Ther 2005;19(6):403–14.

7. Cohen JD, Brinton EA, Ito MK, et al. Understanding Statin Use in America and Gaps in Patient Education (USAGE): an internet-based survey of 10,138 current and former statin users. J Clin Lipidol 2012; 6(3):208–15.

8. Wieland H, Seidel D. A simple specific method for precipitation of low density lipoproteins. J Lipid Res 1983;24(7):904–9.

9. Davidson WS, Sparks DL, Lund-Katz S, et al. The molecular basis for the difference in charge between pre-beta- and alpha-migrating high density lipoproteins. J Biol Chem 1994;269(12):8959–65.

10. Susca M. Heparin-induced extracorporeal low-density lipoprotein precipitation futura, a new modification of HELP apheresis: technique and first clinical results. Ther Apher 2001;5(5):387–93.

11. Mabuchi H, Michishita I, Takeda M, et al. A new low density lipoprotein apheresis system using two dextran sulfate cellulose columns in an automated column regenerating unit (LDL continuous apheresis). Atherosclerosis 1987;68(1–2):19–25.

12. Schuff-Werner P. Clinical long-term results of H.E.L.P.-apheresis. Z Kardiol 2003;92(Suppl 3):III28–9 [in German].

13. Gordon BR, Kelsey SF, Dau PC, et al. Long-term effects of low-density lipoprotein apheresis using an automated dextran sulfate cellulose adsorption system. Liposorber study group. Am J Cardiol 1998;81(4):407–11.

14. Bosch T, Gahr S, Belschner U, et al. Direct adsorption of low-density lipoprotein by DALI-LDL-apheresis: results of a prospective long-term multicenter follow-up covering 12,291 sessions. Ther Apher Dial 2006; 10(3):210–8.

15. Klingel R, Göhlen B, Schwarting A, et al. Differential indication of lipoprotein apheresis during pregnancy. Ther Apher Dial 2003;7(3):359–64.

16. Mabuchi H, Koizumi J, Shimizu M, et al. Long-term efficacy of low-density lipoprotein apheresis on coronary heart disease in familial hypercholesterolemia. Hokuriku-FH-LDL-apheresis study group. Am J Cardiol 1998;82(12):1489–95.

17. Kroon AA, van Asten WN, Stalenhoef AF. Effect of apheresis of low-density lipoprotein on peripheral vascular disease in hypercholesterolemic patients with coronary artery disease. Ann Intern Med 1996;125(12):945–54.

18. Kroon AA, Aengevaeren WR, van der Werf T, et al. LDL-Apheresis Atherosclerosis Regression Study (LAARS). Effect of aggressive versus conventional lipid lowering treatment on coronary atherosclerosis. Circulation 1996;93(10):1826–35.

19. Aengevaeren WR, Kroon AA, Stalenhoef AF, et al. Low density lipoprotein apheresis improves regional myocardial perfusion in patients with hypercholesterolemia and extensive coronary artery disease. LDL-apheresis atherosclerosis regression study (LAARS). J Am Coll Cardiol 1996;28(7):1696–704.

20. Kroon AA, van't Hof MA, Demacker PN, et al. The rebound of lipoproteins after LDL-apheresis. Kinetics and estimation of mean lipoprotein levels. Atherosclerosis 2000;152(2):519–26.

21. Marais AD, Naoumova RP, Firth JC, et al. Decreased production of low density lipoprotein by atorvastatin after apheresis in homozygous familial hypercholesterolemia. J Lipid Res 1997;38(10):2071–8.

22. Pfohl M, Naoumova RP, Klass C, et al. Acute and chronic effects on cholesterol biosynthesis of LDL-apheresis with or without concomitant HMG-CoA reductase inhibitor therapy. J Lipid Res 1994; 35(11):1946–55.

23. Holvoet P, Mertens A, Verhamme P, et al. Circulating oxidized LDL is a useful marker for identifying patients with coronary artery disease. Arterioscler Thromb Vasc Biol 2001;21(5):844–8.

24. St-Pierre AC, Ruel IL, Cantin B, et al. Comparison of various electrophoretic characteristics of LDL particles and their relationship to the risk of ischemic heart disease. Circulation 2001;104(19):2295–9.

25. Napoli C, Ambrosio G, Scarpato N, et al. Decreased low-density lipoprotein oxidation after repeated selective apheresis in homozygous familial hypercholesterolemia. Am Heart J 1997;133(5):585–95.

26. Schamberger BM, Geiss HC, Ritter MM, et al. Influence of LDL apheresis on LDL subtypes in patients with coronary heart disease and severe hyperlipoproteinemia. J Lipid Res 2000;41(5):727–33.

27. Parhofer KG, Barrett PH, Demant T, et al. Effects of weekly LDL-apheresis on metabolic parameters of apolipoprotein B in heterozygous familial hypercholesterolemia. J Lipid Res 1996;37(11):2383–93.

28. Guerin M. Reverse cholesterol transport in familial hypercholesterolemia. Curr Opin Lipidol 2012; 23(4):377–85.

29. Richter WO, Jacob BG, Ritter MM, et al. Three-year treatment of familial heterozygous hypercholesterolemia by extracorporeal low-density lipoprotein immunoadsorption with polyclonal apolipoprotein B antibodies. Metabolism 1993;42(7):888–94.

30. Hershcovici T, Schechner V, Orlin J, et al. Effect of different LDL-apheresis methods on parameters

involved in atherosclerosis. J Clin Apher 2004;19(2): 90–7.

31. Schechner V, Berliner S, Shapira I, et al. Comparative analysis between dextran sulfate adsorption and direct adsorption of lipoproteins in their capability to reduce erythrocyte adhesiveness/aggregation in the peripheral blood. Ther Apher Dial 2004;8(1):39–44.

32. Opole IO, Belmont JM, Kumar A, et al. Effect of low-density lipoprotein apheresis on inflammatory and noninflammatory high-density lipoprotein cholesterol. Am J Cardiol 2007;100(9):1416–8.

33. Navab M, Ananthramaiah GM, Reddy ST, et al. The double jeopardy of HDL. Ann Med 2005;37(3):173–8.

34. Matsuura F, Wang N, Chen W, et al. HDL from CETP-deficient subjects shows enhanced ability to promote cholesterol efflux from macrophages in an apoE- and ABCG1-dependent pathway. J Clin Invest 2006;116(5):1435–42.

35. Orsoni A, Saheb S, Levels JH, et al. LDL-apheresis depletes apoE-HDL and pre-beta1-HDL in familial hypercholesterolemia: relevance to atheroprotection. J Lipid Res 2011;52(12):2304–13.

36. Moriarty PM. Association of ApoE and HDL-C with cardiovascular and cerebrovascular disease: potential benefits of LDL-apheresis therapy. J Clin Lipidol 2009;4(3):311–29.

37. Schmaldienst S, Banyai S, Stulnig TM, et al. Prospective randomised cross-over comparison of three LDL-apheresis systems in statin pretreated patients with familial hypercholesterolaemia. Atherosclerosis 2000;151(2):493–9.

38. Mackey RH, Greenland P, Goff DC Jr, et al. High-density lipoprotein cholesterol and particle concentrations, carotid atherosclerosis, and coronary events: MESA (Multi-ethnic Study of Atherosclerosis). J Am Coll Cardiol 2012;60(6):508–16.

39. Castillo SM, Tye S, Moriarty PM. Effect of lipid-apheresis on HDL-C functionality. Journal of American Cardiology 2013.

40. Richter WO, Donner MG, Schwandt P. Short- and long-term effects on serum lipoproteins by three different techniques of apheresis. Artif Organs 1996;20(4):311–7.

41. Le NA, Julie-Ann D, Moriarty P, et al. Acute changes in oxidative and inflammatory markers with LDL apheresis. Circulation 2006;114:II-111 [abstract].

42. Clarke R, Peden JF, Hopewell JC, et al. Genetic variants associated with Lp(a) lipoprotein level and coronary disease. N Engl J Med 2009;361(26): 2518–28.

43. Willeit P, Kiechl S, Kronenberg F, et al. Discrimination and net reclassification of cardiovascular risk with lipoprotein(a): prospective 15-year outcomes in the Bruneck Study. J Am Coll Cardiol 2014;64(9):851–60.

44. Leebmann J, Roeseler E, Julius U, et al. Lipoprotein apheresis in patients with maximally tolerated lipid-lowering therapy, lipoprotein(a)-hyperlipoproteinemia, and progressive cardiovascular disease: prospective observational multicenter study. Circulation 2013; 128(24):2567–76.

45. Jaeger BR, Richter Y, Nagel D, et al. Longitudinal cohort study on the effectiveness of lipid apheresis treatment to reduce high lipoprotein(a) levels and prevent major adverse coronary events. Nat Clin Pract Cardiovasc Med 2009;6(3):229–39.

46. Rosada A, Kassner U, Vogt A, et al. Does regular lipid apheresis in patients with isolated elevated lipoprotein (a) levels reduce the incidence of cardiovascular events? Artif Organs 2014;38:135–41 [Erratum appears in Artif Organs 2014;38(2): 177].

47. Geiss HC, Bremer S, Barrett PH, et al. In vivo metabolism of LDL subfractions in patients with heterozygous FH on statin therapy: rebound analysis of LDL subfractions after LDL apheresis. J Lipid Res 2004; 45(8):1459–67.

48. Bosch T, Keller C. Clinical effects of direct adsorption of lipoprotein apheresis: beyond cholesterol reduction. Ther Apher Dial 2003;7(3):341–4.

49. Nakamura T, Kawagoe Y, Ogawa H, et al. Effect of low-density lipoprotein apheresis on urinary protein and podocyte excretion in patients with nephrotic syndrome due to diabetic nephropathy. Am J Kidney Dis 2005;45(1):48–53.

50. Ramunni A, Giancipoli G, Guerriero S, et al. LDL-apheresis accelerates the recovery of nonarteritic acute anterior ischemic optic neuropathy. Ther Apher Dial 2005;9(1):53–8.

51. Bosch T, Schmidt B, Blumenstein M, et al. Lipid apheresis by hemoperfusion: in vitro efficacy and ex vivo biocompatibility of a new low-density lipoprotein adsorber compatible with human whole blood. Artif Organs 1993;17(7):640–52.

52. Rosamond W, Flegal K, Friday G, et al. Heart disease and stroke statistics–2007 update: a report from the American Heart Association Statistics Committee and Stroke Statistics Subcommittee. Circulation 2007;115(5):e69–171.

53. Stone PH. Triggering myocardial infarction. N Engl J Med 2004;351(17):1716–8.

54. Grutzmacher P, Landgraf H, Esser R, et al. In vivo rheologic effects of lipid apheresis techniques: comparison of dextran sulfate LDL adsorption and heparin-induced LDL precipitation. ASAIO Trans 1990;36:M327–30.

55. Thompson GR. LDL apheresis. Atherosclerosis 2003;167(1):1–13.

56. Mii S, Mori A, Sakata H, et al. LDL apheresis for arteriosclerosis obliterans with occluded bypass graft: change in prostacyclin and effect on ischemic symptoms. Angiology 1998;49(3):175–80.

57. Nakamura T, Ushiyama C, Osada S, et al. Effect of low-density lipoprotein apheresis on plasma endothelin-1 levels in diabetic hemodialysis patients

with arteriosclerosis obliterans. J Diabetes Complications 2003;17(6):349–54.

58. Kojima S, Ogi M, Sugi T, et al. Changes in plasma levels of nitric oxide derivative during low-density lipoprotein apheresis. Ther Apher 1997;1(4):356–61.

59. Kobayashi S, Moriya H, Negishi K, et al. LDL-apheresis up-regulates VEGF and IGF-I in patients with ischemic limb. J Clin Apher 2003;18(3):115–9.

60. Schaumann D, Welch-Wichary M, Voss A, et al. Prospective cross-over comparisons of three low-density lipoprotein (LDL)-apheresis methods in patients with familial hypercholesterolaemia [see comment]. Eur J Clin Invest 1996;26(11):1033–8.

61. Wang Y, Blessing F, Walli AK, et al. Effects of heparin-mediated extracorporeal low-density lipoprotein precipitation beyond lowering proatherogenic lipoproteins–reduction of circulating proinflammatory and procoagulatory markers. Atherosclerosis 2004; 175(1):145–50.

62. Julius U, Metzler W, Pietzsch J, et al. Intraindividual comparison of two extracorporeal LDL apheresis methods: lipidfiltration and HELP. Int J Artif Organs 2002;25(12):1180–8.

63. Geiss HC, Parhofer KG, Donner MG, et al. Low density lipoprotein apheresis by membrane differential filtration (cascade filtration). Ther Apher 1999;3(3): 199–202.

64. Blaha M. Adhesive selectin molecules MCP-1 and endothelin-1 during long-lasting LDL-apheresis in familial hyperlipoproteinemia. Ther Apher 2005; 9(3):A29.

65. Spieker LE, Ruschitzka F, Badimon JJ, et al. Shear stress-dependent platelet function after LDL cholesterol apheresis. Thromb Res 2004;113(6):395–8.

66. Empen K, Otto C, Brödl UC, et al. The effects of three different LDL-apheresis methods on the plasma concentrations of E-selectin, VCAM-1, and ICAM-1. J Clin Apher 2002;17(1):38–43.

67. Palumbo B, Cardinali L, Sinzinger H. LDL-Apheresis removes serum amyloid P and A in hypercholesterolemic patients. Thromb Res 2000;97(6):491–4.

68. Zanetti M, Zenti M, Barazzoni R, et al. HELP LDL apheresis reduces plasma pentraxin 3 in familial hypercholesterolemia. PLoS One 2014;9(7): e101290.

69. van Wijk DF, Sjouke B, Figueroa A, et al. Nonpharmacological lipoprotein apheresis reduces arterial inflammation in familial hypercholesterolemia. J Am Coll Cardiol 2014;64(14):1418–26.

70. Angelkort B, Amann B, Lawall H. Hemorheology and hemostatis in vascular disease. A pathophysiological review. Clin Hemorheol Microcirc 2002;26: 145–54.

71. Moriarty PM, Gibson CA, Kensey KR, et al. Effect of low-density lipoprotein cholesterol apheresis on blood viscosity. Am J Cardiol 2004;93(8):1044–6.

72. Rubba P, Iannuzzi A, Postiglione A, et al. Hemodynamic changes in the peripheral circulation after repeat low density lipoprotein apheresis in familial hypercholesterolemia. Circulation 1990;81:610–6.

73. Schuff-Werner P, Schütz E, Seyde WC, et al. Improved haemorheology associated with a reduction in plasma fibrinogen and LDL in patients being treated by heparin-induced extracorporeal LDL precipitation (HELP). Eur J Clin Invest 1989;19(1):30–7.

74. Iannuzzi A, Bianciardi G, Faccenda F, et al. Correction of erythrocyte shape abnormalities in familial hypercholesterolemia after LDL-apheresis: does it influence cerebral hemodynamics? Heart Vessels 1997;12:234–40.

75. Alonso R, Andres E, Mata N, et al. Lipoprotein(a) levels in familial hypercholesterolemia: an important predictor of cardiovascular disease independent of the type of LDL receptor mutation. J Am Coll Cardiol 2014;63(19):1982–9.

76. Tsuchida H, Shigematsu H, Ishimaru S, et al. Effect of low-density lipoprotein apheresis on patients with peripheral arterial disease. Peripheral Arterial Disease LDL Apheresis Multicenter Study (P-LAS). Int Angiol 2006;25(3):287–92.

77. Kobayashi S, Moriya H, Maesato K, et al. LDL-apheresis improves peripheral arterial occlusive disease with an implication for anti-inflammatory effects. J Clin Apher 2005;20(4):239–43.

78. Takagi M, Yamada T, Yamaguchi H, et al. The role of low-density lipoprotein apheresis as postoperative care of bypass grafting for chronic arterial occlusion. Cardiovasc Surg 1996;4(4):459–65.

79. Walzl B, Walzl M, Lechner P, et al. Heparin-induced extracorporeal LDL precipitation (HELP): a new therapeutic intervention in cerebrovascular diseases and peripheral arterial occlusive disease. Wien Med Wochenschr 1993;143(22):563–70 [in Germany].

80. Hattori M, Chikamoto H, Akioka Y, et al. A combined low-density lipoprotein apheresis and prednisone therapy for steroid-resistant primary focal segmental glomerulosclerosis in children. Am J Kidney Dis 2003;42(6):1121–30.

81. Iwagami M, Negishi K. Kidney diseases. In: HN, Noiri E, editors. The concise manual of apheresis therapy. Tokyo, Japan: Springer; 2014. p. 259–69.

82. Muso E, Mune M, Fujii Y, et al. Significantly rapid relief from steroid-resistant nephrotic syndrome by LDL apheresis compared with steroid monotherapy. Nephron 2001;89(4):408–15.

83. Sosland RP, Gollub SB, Wilson DB, et al. The first case report of the treatment of transplant coronary artery disease with dextran sulfate adsorption lipid apheresis. Ther Apher Dial 2010;14(2):218–21.

84. Julius U, Tselmin S, Fischer S, et al. Lipid apheresis after heart transplantation – the Dresden experience. Tx Med 2010;22:355–62.

85. Park JW, Merz M, Braun P. Regression of transplant coronary artery disease during chronic low-density lipoprotein-apheresis. J Heart Lung Transplant 1997;16(3):290–7.

86. Matschke K, Mrowietz C, Sternitzky R, et al. Effect of LDL apheresis on oxygen tension in skeletal muscle in patients with cardiac allograft vasculopathy and severe lipid disorder. Clin Hemorheol Microcirc 2004;30(3–4):263–71.

87. Jaeger BR, Meiser B, Nagel D, et al. Aggressive lowering of fibrinogen and cholesterol in the prevention of graft vessel disease after heart transplantation. Circulation 1997;96(9 Suppl):II-154–8.

88. Pfefferkorn TK, Knüppel HP, Jaeger BR, et al. Increased cerebral $CO_2$ reactivity after heparin-mediated extracorporal LDL precipitation (HELP) in patients with coronary heart disease and hyperlipidemia. Stroke 1999;30(9):1802–6.

89. Walzl M, Lechner H, Walzl B, et al. Improved neurological recovery of cerebral infarctions after plasmapheretic reduction of lipids and fibrinogen. Stroke 1993;24(10):1447–51.

90. Moriarty PM, Whittaker TJ. Treatment of acute occlusion of the retinal artery by LDL-apheresis. J Clin Apher 2005;20(2):88–92.

91. Pulido JS, Multicenter Investigation of Rheopheresis for AMD (MIRA-1) Study Group. Multicenter prospective, randomized, double-masked, placebo-controlled study of rheopheresis to treat nonexudative age-related macular degeneration: interim analysis. Trans Am Ophthalmol Soc 2002;100:85–106 [discussion: 106–7].

92. Ullrich H, Kleinjung T, Steffens T, et al. Improved treatment of sudden hearing loss by specific fibrinogen aphaeresis. J Clin Apher 2004;19(2):71–8.

93. Balletshofer BM, Stock J, Rittig K, et al. Acute effect of rheopheresis on peripheral endothelial dysfunction in patients suffering from sudden hearing loss. Ther Apher Dial 2005;9(5):385–90.

94. Suckfull M, Hearing Loss Study Group. Fibrinogen and LDL apheresis in treatment of sudden hearing loss: a randomised multicentre trial. Lancet 2002;360(9348):1811–7.

95. Wang Y, Walli AK, Schulze A, et al. Heparin-mediated extracorporeal low density lipoprotein precipitation as a possible therapeutic approach in preeclampsia. Transfus Apher Sci 2006;35(2):103–10.

# Dyslipidemia in Pregnancy

Robert Wild, MD[a], Elizabeth A. Weedin, DO[a],*, Don Wilson, MD, FNLA[b]

## KEYWORDS

- Dyslipidemia • Hyperlipidemia • Pregnancy • Fetal metabolism • Metabolic syndrome

## KEY POINTS

- Exposure of the fetus to elevated levels of cholesterol and oxidative byproducts of cholesterol metabolism has been shown to result in programming of fetal arterial cells with a predisposition to atherosclerosis later in life.
- For many women, the reproductive years span 2 decades, representing an optimal time to reduce cardiovascular disease risk factors before conception.
- Recent discoveries highlight the importance of preventing or optimizing maternal dyslipidemia for the benefit of the mother and the child.
- Currently no reference standards are defined for lipid parameters during pregnancy, although it is well-known that pregnancy is a state of insulin resistance and that lipoprotein lipid profiles reflect this process.
- Overweight and obese women are significantly more likely to exceed the pregnancy-related weight gain recommendations.

## INTRODUCTION

Historically dyslipidemia in pregnancy has been considered physiologic with little clinical relevance. Lipids and lipoproteins have not been routinely measured at any time point during pregnancy, irrespective of their role in cardiovascular disease (CVD) or pregnancy outcomes. Recent evidence describing fatty streaks in the aortas of 6-month-old fetuses of mothers who were hypercholesterolemic[1] and studies in animal models have challenged the assumption that maternal cholesterol does not cross the placental barrier. Poorly controlled cholesterol, triglycerides, and their metabolites associated with cardiometabolic dysfunction seem to have significant detrimental maternal and fetal vascular consequences. Maternal cardiometabolic dysfunction may not only contribute to long-term effects of the mother and child's vascular health but also potentially create CVD risk for generational offspring.

In providing an update on this rapidly expanding and multifaceted topic, this article first outlines the basic understanding of the importance of cholesterol in fetal development. New insight is then reviewed regarding why this new recognition of disordered maternal cholesterol and triglyceride metabolism is likely to have a long-term effect for future generations. Diagnosing and treating dyslipidemia before, during, and after pregnancy in an effort to provide the best opportunity to reduce the increasing atherosclerotic burden of the rapidly expanding population.

## CHOLESTEROL AND FETAL DEVELOPMENT

Cholesterol is required for normal fetal development. It plays a key role in the formation of cell

Financial Disclosures: None.
[a] Section of Reproductive Endocrinology and Infertility, Department of Obstetrics and Gynecology, University of Oklahoma Health Sciences Center, 1100 N Lindsay Ave, Oklahoma City, OK 73104, USA; [b] Department of Pediatric Endocrinology, Cook Children's Medical Center, 1500 Cooper Street, Fort Worth, TX 76104, USA
* Corresponding author. 920 S.L. Young Boulevard, WP2410, Oklahoma City, OK 73104.
*E-mail address:* Elizabeth-weedin@ouhsc.edu

membranes, membrane integrity, and maintaining cholesterol-rich domains that are essential for most membrane-associated signaling cascades, including sonic hedgehog signaling.[2] Cholesterol is also a precursor of hormones, such as steroids, vitamin D, and bile acids. Sources of fetal cholesterol seem to include endogenous production, the maternal circulation, and synthesis within the yolk sac or placenta.

Because of its critical role in fetal development, it was previously thought that most cholesterol is synthesized de novo by the fetus. Emerging evidence, however, suggests that maternal cholesterol and the placenta may also play a meaningful role. For exogenous cholesterol to be available for fetal use, the yoke sac and placenta must take up maternal cholesterol via receptor-mediated or receptor-independent transport processes, transport lipids across cellular barriers, and/or secrete the maternally derived or newly synthesized cholesterol into the fetal circulation.[3,4] Cultured trophoblast cells have been shown to express low-density lipoprotein (LDL) receptors (LDLRs), LDLR-related proteins, scavenger receptors A, and high-density lipoprotein (HDL)–binding scavenger receptors B1 (SR-B1s) on their apical side. Cholesterol taken up by internalization of receptor-bound ApoB- or ApoE-carrying lipoproteins and oxidized LDL, and from SR-B1–bound HDL, is then released on the basolateral side.[4] Although the uptake of cholesterol by endothelial cells is well understood, knowledge about the mechanisms through which placental endothelial cells transport cholesterol to the fetal microcirculation, the regulation of efflux, and their ability to deliver substantial quantities of cholesterol is incomplete.

Maternal cholesterol has been shown to cross the placental and enter the fetal circulation, contributing substantially to the fetal cholesterol pool in animals and humans.[4,5] Vuorio and colleagues[6] found that plant stanol concentrations in cord blood of healthy newborns were 40% to 50% of maternal levels, demonstrating active maternal-fetal sterol transport. Compared with the umbilical arteries, the umbilical vein has been found to have a greater concentration of cholesterol.[7]

Maternal hypercholesterolemia, as seen in a woman with familial hypercholesterolemia (FH), may pose a significant risk to the fetus.[8] A substantial increase in maternal cholesterol has been shown to significantly increase cholesterol transfer from the mother to the fetus, without upregulation of liver X receptors.[9] Fetal cholesterol levels in mid-pregnancy are much higher than they are at term, and these levels correlate with maternal cholesterol before the sixth month of gestation.[9] This finding suggests maternal hypercholesterolemia does not, a priori, result in upregulation of cholesterol transport. However, exposure of the fetus to very high levels of cholesterol and oxidative products of cholesterol has been shown to result in programming of arterial cells with a predisposition to atherosclerosis later in life.[1] Similar findings have been observed in pregnant women who are obese, have the metabolic syndrome, and/or have diabetes.[10] Napoli and colleagues[1] have shown a direct correlation between the concentration of maternal cholesterol and the presence of fatty streaks in the fetus; effects more strongly correlated earlier in gestation.

Studies have also shown adverse fetal effects as a consequence of decreased exogenous cholesterol. Women with lower plasma cholesterol levels, for example, were found to have smaller newborns; a correlation has been reported between low plasma cholesterol and microcephaly.[11] Ultimately, however, the mechanisms underlying fetal effects related to maternal hypercholesterolemia remain incompletely understood.[9]

## PREVALENCE OF CARDIOVASCULAR DISEASE RISK FACTORS

According to the National Health and Nutrition Examination Survey 1999–2008 data, among women aged 18 to 44 years in the United States, 2.4% have diabetes, 7.7% are estimated to have hypertension, 25.4% use tobacco, 2.9% have chronic kidney disease, and 57.6% are either overweight or obese. Prepregnancy cardiometabolic and inflammatory risk factors predict the risk of hypertensive disorders of pregnancy. An increased risk of hypertension is seen in women who are obese. The odds of hypertension during pregnancy are 1.8 times greater for individuals who are normotensive yet obese before pregnancy. The odds of a hypertension-related complication during pregnancy are 3.5 times higher in women who are overweight and hypertensive before pregnancy.[12]

Approximately 50% of pregnancies are unplanned, limiting the ability to identify women with CVD risk factors before pregnancy. A Kaiser Family Foundation national survey recently noted that the rate of CVD screening for women aged 18 to 44 years was 58%, compared with 78% for women aged 45 to 64 years.[13] This proportion is even lower compared with blood pressure screening in 18- to 44-year olds. Another national survey found that among women aged 18 to 64 years, 15% were seen by general medicine physicians, 62% by gynecologists alone, and 23% by both. Those seen by gynecologists received more counseling and preventive services.[14] In an evaluation of 2 different health care plans servicing nearly 3.6 million members, hypertension was recognized in fewer than one-third of women during the course of their care. Furthermore, irrespective of which specialty provided the care, less than 70% of women received lipid screening, nutrition, or weight counseling. The survey also illustrated that limited knowledge about preeclampsia and future risk in reproductive age women was common among all specialties.

The most recent National Vital Statistics report illustrates that pregnancy rates for women aged 25 to 29 years have changed very little since 1990.[15] Rates for women in their 30s and 40s, however, have increased. Additionally, in the past 45 years, women aged 35 to 44 years in the United States have experienced the greatest increase in prevalence of obesity. With the known association between obesity and dyslipidemia, the implications of this trend are profound. Currently, 45% of women begin pregnancy either overweight or obese, a statistic that has almost doubled in the past 30 years. Furthermore, approximately 43% of pregnant women gain more weight than recommended during the course of their pregnancy. It is well understood that maternal obesity contributes to other high-risk conditions, such as gestational diabetes, hypertensive disorders, newborn macrosomia, and perinatal complications.[16] For many women, the reproductive years can span 2 decades, representing an optimal time to reduce CVD risk factors before conception, for the benefit of both the mother and her future offspring.

## FETAL CONSIDERATIONS

Because gestational dyslipidemia has historically been considered physiologic, with little clinical significance, lipid and lipoproteins have not been measured routinely during pregnancy. However, the recent discoveries of fatty streaks in the aortas of 6-month-old fetuses of mothers with hypercholesterolemia, and the identification of aortic atherosclerosis at autopsy of deceased children with normal levels cholesterol born to mothers with hypercholesterolemia, highlight the importance of correcting maternal dyslipidemia.[1,17] In New Zealand white rabbits, diet-induced maternal dyslipidemia causes a dose-dependent fetal and postnatal atherogenesis, which was reduced by lowering maternal cholesterol with cholestyramine.[18] Similar data have been obtained in a murine model.[19]

A large body of literature suggests that an unhealthy uterine environment can lead to maladaptations in postuterine life, many of which are suspected to be the origin of chronic, noncommunicable diseases. Atherosclerosis is among the first of several conditions for which a role of developmental programming was described.[20] Several factors have been suggested that may play a role in developmental programming of the fetus.[21] Genetic factors, metabolic or environmental disturbances of the mother, and the father's lifestyle and genetics are important prepregnancy components that may contribute to fetal programming. During pregnancy, maternal malnutrition (either underfeeding or overfeeding), maternal stress, chemical exposure, preeclampsia, hypertension, gestational diabetes, maternal smoking, second-hand smoke exposure, metabolic syndrome, hyperlipidemia, obesity, intrauterine growth retardation, placental function, and hypoxia may be important influences. At the cellular level, adaptation occurs through DNA methylation, genetics, lifestyle choices during childhood, and altered immune responses, ultimately contributing to childhood atherosclerosis. Recent animal studies have revealed that changes in DNA methylation and chromatin modification may be responsible for the epigenetic programming and increased atherosclerotic susceptibility.[22] However, the exact mechanisms underlying the effects of maternal hypercholesterolemia in the offspring are still unclear.

Despite this lack of clarity, increasing evidence shows that epigenetic programming of metabolism during embryonic or fetal development might be involved.[23] Epigenetic phenomena occur at the interface between the genome and the environment. The environment can influence epigenetic information that is superimposed on the DNA, which may have long-term consequences for the transcription of specific regions of the genome. Results of animal studies show that permanent changes in either DNA methylation or chromatin modification, or both, may be responsible for the epigenetic programming of increased atherosclerotic susceptibility.[24] For instance, maternal hypercholesterolemia in ApoE-deficient mice leads to the activation of genes involved in cholesterol synthesis and LDLR activity in adult offspring.[17,24] Other animal studies have shown that the genes involved in immune pathways and fatty acid metabolism are upregulated in the offspring of hypercholesterolemic dams.[25] These findings indicate that an adverse maternal environment may alter basic cellular programming of the fetus.[24] Further research is needed to unravel the exact mechanisms through which maternal hypercholesterolemia influences this process.

Depending on what deleterious influences occur in utero and during childhood, the adult phenotype of insulin resistance and obesity that results in car-diometabolic disease is expressed at different genetic set points.[19]

In utero, the fetus handles lipid metabolism in a dynamic fashion. Pregnancy is associated with increased permeability of the vascular endothelium by small molecules, which can lead to vascular inflammation. This permeability is further increased in the presences of diabetes. Additionally, it is now known that there is active transport of lipids to the fetus. This transport seems to vary at different stages of pregnancy. Early in gestation, the fetus seems to preferentially use lipids for the purposes of adequate membrane development and possibly for protection. Excess fat may, thereafter, be deposited in the liver, depending on gestational age and hepatic maturity. Additionally, fetal epicardial fat can be identified early in gestation. Presumably these mechanisms occur in an attempt to protect the fetal brain.[9]

The offspring of obese mothers have an increased risk of mortality in later life.[26] Minimal mortality is found in offspring of mothers with a normal body mass index (BMI).[26] Long-term studies have shown that offspring of mothers with a greater BMI and waist circumference have higher triglycerides and increased blood pressure and insulin resistance.[27]

## MATERNAL CONSIDERATIONS

Lipid and lipoprotein levels have been tracked throughout pregnancy in groups of women with uncomplicated and complicated pregnancies. Nonetheless, no reference standards for lipid or lipoproteins during pregnancy currently exist.[9] Pregnancy is a state of insulin resistance reflected by the lipid and lipoprotein profiles of the mother. Within 6 weeks of gestation, lipid levels drop slightly, followed by an increase during each trimester of pregnancy. Triglyceride levels increase sharply during pregnancy, as do cholesterol levels. LDL increases in a similar pattern as that of total cholesterol. On average, cholesterol and triglyceride levels do not exceed 250 mg/dL. However, when abnormal pregnancies are included, levels can exceed 300 mg/dL.[28] Abnormally high triglyceride levels in the first trimester are significantly associated with gestational hypertension, preeclampsia, induced preterm birth, and fetuses considered large for gestational age.[29] Estrogens increase triglyceride levels through stimulating hepatic production of very-low-density lipoprotein (VLDL) and inhibiting hepatic and adipose lipoprotein lipase. Progesterone opposes these actions, whereas cytokines and inflammatory factors are important contributors of insulin resistance. However, this physiologic increase in lipids and lipoproteins is a mechanism aimed at accommodating fetal demands for normal growth and development.[23]

Preeclampsia is characterized by endothelial dysfunction prompted by an increase in triglyceride and free fatty acid levels. Triglyceride levels and ApoB and small LDL particles are all increased in preeclampsia, vascular cell adhesion molecule specifically is increased and serves as an indicator of endothelial dysfunction. Whether ApoB or small LDL particles cause this endothelial disruption is currently unclear.[30] Additionally, some indication exists that endothelial dysfunction may be caused partly by oxidative stress and decreased prostacyclin. Metabolic syndrome and gestational diabetes are conditions that predispose women to preeclampsia and overt diabetes.[29] Women with polycystic ovarian syndrome, for example, are more likely to have adverse pregnancy outcomes even if they are not obese.[31] This finding is particularly important because these women have insulin resistance and are prone to metabolic syndrome and diabetes.

Medical conditions that cause abnormal lipids and lipoproteins should be investigated and, if present, treated appropriately. Hypothyroidism, alcohol consumption, low-molecular-weight heparin, glucocorticoids, psychotropic medications, kidney disease, and lipodystrophy have all been associated with dyslipidemia; however, their effects during pregnancy are poorly characterized. The observed dyslipidemia is independent of diabetes, which is the most common reason for the disturbed lipid metabolism in general.[32] One of the more common reasons for high triglyceride levels during pregnancy is the use of medications. Alcohol, estrogen, oral contraceptives, glucocorticoids, ß-blockers, valproate, sertraline, retinoic acids, cyclosporine, and tacrolimus are a few examples of potential causes. Cocaine use can also cause dyslipidemia. Offending agents should be identified and discontinued, ideally before conception.

Elevated VLDL and chylomicrons levels may occur and are thought to be secondary to a genetic predisposition. Triglyceride levels are typically very high, greater than 2000 mg/dL, increasing the risk of pancreatitis. Clinical features of severe hypertriglyceridemia include eruptive xanthoma, hepatosplenomegaly, abdominal pain, dyspnea, peripheral neuropathy, memory loss, and dementia. These neurologic symptoms need be addressed in pregnant women just as in nonpregnant persons. With severe hypertriglyceridemia, a reduction in fat calories to 15% to 20% daily is usually necessary. Insulin therapy may be used even in the absence of overt diabetes. Fish oil capsules are often used when triglyceride levels are greater than 500 mg/dL. Gemfibrozil or fenofibrate are widely used despite their classification as class C medications. The ultimate goal is to reduce triglyceride levels to less than 400 mg/dL in an effort to reduce the risk of pancreatitis. Other acute therapies reported in case studies include medium-chain triglycerides, niacin, sunflower oil, gene therapy, and plasmapherisis.[33]

All lipid-lowering medications, aside from bile sequestrate and omega-3-fatty acids, should be stopped before conception or immediately when pregnancy occurs unexpected. Lifestyle changes and glycemic control should be instituted where needed. During pregnancy, elevated cholesterol levels can be treated safely with a bile acid sequestrant. Severe hypertriglyceridemia associated with pancreatitis can be treated with omega-3 fatty acids, parenteral nutrition, plasmapheresis, and other lipid-lowering agents in the last trimester of pregnancy, notably gemfibrozil. Monitoring is recommended, at a minimum, every trimester or within 6 weeks of initiating treatment. Close follow-up of the mother with FH or with dysmetabolic issues of pregnancy is strongly recommended.

Women with gestational diabetes and/or preeclampsia are also at increased risk for elevated triglyceride levels, development of chronic hypertension, recurrent gestation diabetes and/or overt diabetes, recurrent preeclampsia, and development of albuminuria later in life. Two registered clinical trials are currently evaluating the effects of lipophilic statins to prevent preeclampsia in pregnancy. The true risk of congenital anomalies caused by statins in pregnancy is not well substantiated in humans. However, because statins are category X, statin use in pregnancy should be conducted only in a research setting until more information is available.[33]

A lipid profile should be obtained before conception and every trimester in women with FH who become pregnant. In these women, N-terminal pro-brain natriuretic peptide has been suggested as a useful marker for possible cardiac ischemia. FH can be treated with lifestyle and bile acid sequestrates, preferably colesevelam. Lastly, mipomersen (class B) and LDL apheresis may be necessary in pregnancy. Evaluation and treatment in a specialized center where facilities are available is recommended.

A thorough understanding of pregnancy and lactation-safe medications is imperative to ensure maternal and fetal safety. Class A and B medications are widely used as needed. Class C medications are often used when the benefit outweighs the risk. The chance for fetal harm is greatest during the first trimester. Category D medications have shown definitive evidence of human fetal risk, although potential benefits may warrant use. For category X medications, however, which have investigational or marketing data showing fetal abnormalities, the risks clearly outweigh the benefit. Class N medications have not been classified. Statins are currently classified as category X, whereas fibrates, ezetimibe, niacin, cholestyramine, and omega-3 are category C. Colesevelam and mipomersen are class B.

## POSTPARTUM CONSIDERATIONS

Postpartum follow-up of women with dyslipidemia during pregnancy includes close observation, specifically for those who experienced preeclampsia and/or diabetes. Compared with women who underwent an uncomplicated pregnancy, women who had preeclampsia were found to have worse cardiometabolic profiles at 1-year postpartum. Given the variety of providers who may participate in a women's antepartum, intrapartum, postpartum, and postpuerperal care, there is often loss of continuity and appropriate follow-up of pregnancy-related conditions. Women often do not lose the weight gained during pregnancy, which frequently goes unrecognized or may not be properly addressed. Overweight and obese women are 6 times more likely to exceed the pregnancy-related weight gain recommendations. These women are predisposed to higher postpartum weight gain and retention after pregnancy, with 13% to 20% of women being 5 kg or more above their preconception weight by 1-year postpartum.[16] The Health, Aging, and Body Composition Study found that the odds ratio for developing CVD was 3.31 for women and infants that were both <2500 gm and preterm compared with women having normal weight infants at term.[34] Weight gain and overweight status during midlife were strong independent predictors of the development of metabolic syndrome, type II diabetes mellitus, and early mortality.[35,36] Additionally, a positive obstetric history for preeclampsia doubles the long-term risk of CVD in the mother.[35] An obstetric history that includes gestational diabetes increases the 10-year risk for developing overt type II diabetes to approximately 40%. The prevalence of a significant and treatable dyslipidemia is approximately one-third in these populations.[36]

Although understanding of maternal dyslipidemia and its impact on the future health and well-being of the mother and her offspring is incomplete, increasing evidence suggests that providers must be more vigilant in assessing and treating CVD risk factors during pregnancy.[36,37] Additional assessments and studies addressing individual and public health consequences of the obesity epidemic are also urgently needed.

## REFERENCES

1. Napoli C, D'Armiento FP, Mancini FP, et al. Fatty streak formation occurs in human fetal aortas and is greatly enhanced by maternal hypercholesterolemia. Intimal accumulation of low density lipoprotein and its oxidation precede monocyte recruitment into early atherosclerotic lesions. J Clin Invest 1997;100(11):2680–90.

2. Woollett LA. Where does fetal and embryonic cholesterol originate and what does it do? Annu Rev Nutr 2008;28:97–114.

3. Woollett LA. Fetal lipid metabolism. Front Biosci 2001;6:D536–45.

4. Woollett LA. Maternal cholesterol in fetal development: transport of cholesterol from the maternal to the fetal circulation. Am J Clin Nutr 2005;82(6): 1155–61.

5. Yoshida S, Wada Y. Transfer of maternal cholesterol to embryo and fetus in pregnant mice. J Lipid Res 2005;46(10):2168–74.

6. Vuorio AF, Miettinen TA, Turtola H, et al. Cholesterol metabolism in normal and heterozygous familial hypercholesterolemic newborns. J Lab Clin Med 2002; 140(1):35–42.

7. Spellacy WN, Ashbacher LV, Harris GK, et al. Total cholesterol content in maternal and umbilical vessels in term pregnancies. Obstet Gynecol 1974; 44(5):661–5.

8. Narverud I, Iversen PO, Aukrust P, et al. Maternal familial hypercholesterolaemia (FH) confers altered haemostatic profile in offspring with and without FH. Thromb Res 2013;131(2):178–82.

9. Palinski W. Maternal-fetal cholesterol transport in the placenta: good, bad, and target for modulation. Circ Res 2009;104(5):569–71.

10. Palinski W, Napoli C. Impaired fetal growth, cardiovascular disease, and the need to move on. Circulation 2008;117(3):341–3.

11. Edison RJ, Berg K, Remaley A, et al. Adverse birth outcome among mothers with low serum cholesterol. Pediatrics 2007;120(4):723–33.

12. Hedderson MM, Darbinian JA, Sridhar SB, et al. Pre-pregnancy cardiometabolic and inflammatory risk factors and subsequent risk of hypertensive disorders of pregnancy. Am J Obstet Gynecol 2012; 207(1):68–9.

13. Salganicoff A, Ranji U, Beamesderfer A, et al. Women and Health Care in the Early Years of the ACA: Key Findings from the 2013 Kaiser Women's Health Survey – Preventive Services – 8590. May

14, 2014. Available at: http://kff.org/report-section/women-and-health-care-in-the-early-years-of-the-aca-key-findings-from-the-2013-kaiser-womens-health-survey-preventive-services/. Accessed March 25, 2015.

14. Ehrenthal DB, Catov JM. Importance of engaging obstetrician/gynecologists in cardiovascular disease prevention. Curr Opin Cardiol 2013;28(5): 547–53.

15. Ventura SJ, Curtin SC, Abma JC, et al. Estimated pregnancy rates and rates of pregnancy outcomes for the United States, 1990-2008. National vital statistics reports, vol. 60 no. 7. Hyattsville, MD: National Center for Health Statistics. 2012.

16. Gunderson EP. Childbearing and obesity in women: weight before, during, and after pregnancy. Obstet Gynecol Clin North Am 2009;36(2):317–32, ix.

17. Napoli C, Glass CK, Witztum JL, et al. Influence of maternal hypercholesterolaemia during pregnancy on progression of early atherosclerotic lesions in childhood: Fate of Early Lesions in Children (FELIC) study. Lancet 1999;354(9186):1234–41.

18. Napoli C, Witztum JL, Calara F, et al. Maternal hypercholesterolemia enhances atherogenesis in normo-cholesterolemic rabbits, which is inhibited by antioxidant or lipid-lowering intervention during pregnancy: an experimental model of atherogenic mechanisms in human fetuses. Circ Res 2000; 87(10):946–52.

19. Palinski W. Effect of maternal cardiovascular conditions and risk factors on offspring cardiovascular disease. Circulation 2014;129(20):2066–77.

20. Goharkhay N, Tamayo EH, Yin H, et al. Maternal hypercholesterolemia leads to activation of endogenous cholesterol synthesis in the offspring. American Journal of Obstetrics and Gynecology 2008; 199(3):273e1–273.e6. http://dx.doi.org/10.1016/j.ajog.2008.06.064.

21. Hanson M, Godfrey KM, Lillycrop KA, et al. Developmental plasticity and developmental origins of non-communicable disease: theoretical considerations and epigenetic mechanisms. Prog Biophys Mol Biol 2011;106(1):272–80.

22. Deruiter M, Alkemade F, Groot A, et al. Maternal transmission of risk for atherosclerosis. Current Opinion in Lipidology 2008;4:333–7.

23. Herrera E. Metabolic adaptations in pregnancy and their implications for the availability of substrates to the fetus. Eur J Clin Nutr 2000; 54(Suppl 1):S47–51.

24. DeRuiter MC, Alkemade FE, Gittenberger-de Groot AC, et al. Maternal transmission of risk for atherosclerosis. Curr Opin Lipidol 2008;19(4):333–7.

25. Reymer PW, Groenemeyer BE, van de Burg R, et al. Apolipoprotein E genotyping on agarose gels. Clin Chem 1995;41(7):1046–7.

26. Reynolds RM, Allan KM, Raja EA, et al. Maternal obesity during pregnancy and premature mortality from cardiovascular event in adult offspring: follow-up of 1 323 275 person years. BMJ 2013; 347:f4539.

27. Hochner H, Friedlander Y, Calderon-Margalit R, et al. Associations of maternal prepregnancy body mass index and gestational weight gain with adult offspring cardiometabolic risk factors: the Jerusalem Perinatal Family Follow-up Study. Circulation 2012; 125(11):1381–9.

28. Potter JM, Nestel PJ. The hyperlipidemia of pregnancy in normal and complicated pregnancies. Am J Obstet Gynecol 1979;133(2):165–70.

29. Wiznitzer A, Mayer A, Novack V, et al. Association of lipid levels during gestation with preeclampsia and gestational diabetes mellitus: a population-based study. Am J Obstet Gynecol 2009;201(5):482–8.

30. Hubel CA, Roberts JM, Taylor RN, et al. Lipid peroxidation in pregnancy: new perspectives on preeclampsia. Am J Obstet Gynecol 1989;161(4):1025–34.

31. Palomba S, Falbo A, Chiossi G, et al. Lipid profile in nonobese pregnant women with polycystic ovary syndrome: a prospective controlled clinical study. Steroids 2014;88:36–43.

32. Toescu V, Nuttall SL, Martin U, et al. Changes in plasma lipids and markers of oxidative stress in normal pregnancy and pregnancies complicated by diabetes. Clin Sci (Lond) 2004;106(1):93–8.

33. Cleary KL, Roney K, Costantine M. Challenges of studying drugs in pregnancy for off-label indications: pravastatin for preeclampsia prevention. Semin Perinatol 2014;38(8):523–7.

34. Catov JM, Newman AB, Roberts JM, et al. Preterm delivery and later maternal cardiovascular disease risk. Epidemiology 2007;18(6):733–9.

35. Brown MC, Best KE, Pearce MS, et al. Cardiovascular disease risk in women with pre-eclampsia: systematic review and meta-analysis. Eur J Epidemiol 2013;28(1):1–19.

36. Nerenberg K, Daskalopoulou SS, Dasgupta K. Gestational diabetes and hypertensive disorders of pregnancy as vascular risk signals: an overview and grading of the evidence. Can J Cardiol 2014; 30(7):765–73.

37. Sattar N, Greer IA. Pregnancy complications and maternal cardiovascular risk: opportunities for intervention and screening? BMJ 2002;325(7356): 157–60.

# Women's Health Considerations for Lipid Management

Robert Wild, MD, MPH, PhD[a],*, Elizabeth A. Weedin, DO[b],
Edward A. Gill, MD, FASE, FAHA, FACC, FACP, FNLA[c]

## KEYWORDS

- Women's health • Lipids • Dyslipidemia • Hypertriglyceridemia

## KEY POINTS

- Understanding opportunities to reduce dyslipidemia before, during, and after pregnancy has major implications for cardiovascular disease risk prevention for the entire population.
- The best time to screen for dyslipidemia is before pregnancy or in the early antenatal period after pregnancy is diagnosed.
- The differential diagnosis of hypertriglyceridemia in pregnancy is the same as in nonpregnant women with the exception that clinical lipidologists need to be aware of the potential obstetric complications associated with hypertriglyceridemia.
- Dyslipidemia discovered during pregnancy should be treated with diet and exercise intervention, as well as glycemic control if indicated.
- A complete lipid profile assessment during each trimester of pregnancy is recommended.

## INTRODUCTION

Although, in general, reducing atherosclerosis and preventing cardiovascular disease (CVD) require the practice and prevention of universal principles common to both genders, the diagnosis and treatment of lipid disorders in women pose unique challenges. Dyslipidemia and sequelae such as atherosclerosis are disease processes that can also affect offspring during a pregnancy and produce long-term comorbidities for both the mother and the child.[1] Acknowledging the principle that lipid awareness is critical throughout the life of the individual is paramount for modern clinical lipidologists. This article discusses some unique women's health issues that are important in lipid management because of the epidemic of obesity in society. Practitioners caring for women of reproductive age are in ideally placed to work toward improving atherosclerosis development for the entire population through examining and controlling lipid levels during gestation.[1]

CVD caused by atherosclerosis of the vessel wall is caused by multiple interrelating factors. Some of the factors relate to lifestyle and are modifiable; others are nonmodifiable. In most women, CVD is recognized an average of 10 years later than in their male counterparts, which leads to an inadvertently decreased emphasis on atherosclerosis prevention in women. Given that most women's health care is practiced by primary care physicians, clinical lipidologists must have a working knowledge of issues important for managing dyslipidemia for women. Recognition of high-risk areas and how

[a] Section of Reproductive Endocrinology and Infertility, Department of Obstetrics and Gynecology, University of Oklahoma Health Sciences Center, 1100 N Lindsay Ave, Oklahoma City, OK 73104, USA; [b] Section of General Obstetrics and Gynecology, Department of Obstetrics and Gynecology, University of Oklahoma Health Sciences Center, 1100 N Lindsay Ave, Oklahoma City, OK 73104, USA; [c] Division of Cardiology, UW Department of Medicine, Harborview Medical Center Echocardiography, University of Washington School of Medicine, Seattle University, 325 Ninth Avenue, Box 359748, Seattle, WA 98104-2499, USA
* Corresponding author.
E-mail address: robert-wild@ouhsc.edu

Cardiol Clin 33 (2015) 217–231
http://dx.doi.org/10.1016/j.ccl.2015.02.003
0733-8651/15/$ – see front matter © 2015 Elsevier Inc. All rights reserved.

lipids are affected by major reproductive issues affecting women's health should be areas of high priority for these physicians.

Understanding opportunities to reduce dyslipidemia before, during, and after pregnancy all have major implication for CVD risk prevention for the entire population. Understanding how contraceptive and hormone choices affect clinical lipid management for women is also essential.

## DETECTION, MANAGEMENT, AND TREATMENT OF DYSLIPIDEMIA IN PREGNANCY
### Lipid Values in Normal and Abnormal Pregnancies

**Fig. 1** shows the average circulating values of total cholesterol, low-density lipoprotein cholesterol (LDL-C), high-density lipoprotein cholesterol (HDL-C), and triglycerides (TG) measured in normal women followed before, during, and after pregnancy in a large cohort of women proceeding through normal pregnancy and delivery. Most of the women are of young reproductive age and as such their values before pregnancy are in the normal range for nonpregnant women. Clinical lipidologists need to understand the pattern throughout pregnancy. Note that in the first trimester, depicted as months since conception, early in gestation there is a noticeable decrease in levels in the first 6 weeks and then a noticeable increase easily discerned by the third month or the end of the first trimester. There begins a steady increase throughout pregnancy in the major lipoprotein lipids. By the third trimester of pregnancy, levels peak to maximize near term.[2] Lipid metabolism favors proper fuel for the fetus

and the natural increase reflects the increasing insulin resistance for the mother as pregnancy progresses through term. Also note that the values noted here do not exceed 250 mg/dL at any time during pregnancy.

Contrast the sequential average fasting lipid and lipoproteins measured in the different population shown in **Fig. 2**.

**Fig. 2** shows the increase in mean lipid levels referred to in **Fig. 1**; however, these measurements also include persons who have complicated pregnancies. Also displayed are the values of triglycerides and total cholesterol seen increasing to term as well; however, average values exceed 300 mg/dL.[3] There is a significant increase in triglyceride content in all circulating lipoprotein fractions in pregnancy.[4]

Assessment of normal values should include specifics of the relevant trimester of pregnancy. When values exceed 250 mg/dL this should alert the clinical lipidologist that an abnormal or complicated pregnancy is underway.

**Fig. 3** shows first trimester maternal triglyceride relationships.

Triglyceride levels exceeding 250 mg/dL during pregnancy are associated with complications of pregnancy-induced hypertension, preeclampsia, gestational diabetes, and large-for-gestational-age babies.[5]

### Optimum Strategies for Detection and Treatment of Dyslipidemia in Pregnancy

Many women have significant undiscovered dyslipidemia before pregnancy. The dyslipidemia is often associated with conditions that make them

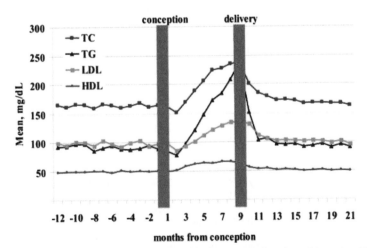

**Fig. 1.** Total cholesterol (TC), triglycerides (TG), high-density lipoprotein (HDL), and low-density lipoprotein (LDL) 1 year before, during, and after pregnancy. (*From* Wiznitzer A, Mayer A, Novack V, et al. Association of lipid levels during gestation with preeclampsia and gestational diabetes mellitus: a population-based study. Am J Obstet Gynecol 2009;201(5):482.e1–8; with permission.)

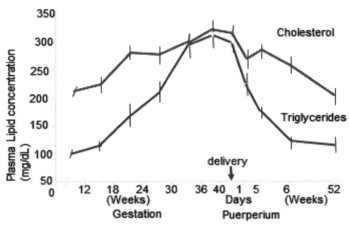

**Fig. 2.** Pregnancy, lipids, and lipoproteins. Fasting lipids were measured serially throughout pregnancy, at delivery, and in the puerperium and at 12 months. Results are ± standard error of the mean and include normal and complicated pregnancies. (*Adapted from* Potter JM, Nestel PJ. The hyperlipidemia of pregnancy in normal and complicated pregnancies. Am J Obstet Gynecol 1979;133(2):165–70; with permission.)

at risk for obstetric and fetal complications should they become pregnant. Uncontrolled diabetes mellitus, polycystic ovarian syndrome (PCOS), and genetic lipid disorders can all be associated with problems for the mother, for the child, and for possible future generations should she conceive. In recent surveys, about one-third of women presenting to obstetrics and Gynecology practices had CVD risk factors that should be diagnosed and reversed if possible. Familial hyperlipidemia (FH) is more common than any of the genetic diseases that are routinely screened for in pregnancy[6] but there are currently no obstetric recommendations in place to screen for FH. Severe hypertriglyceridemia is sometimes encountered because of genetic or acquired conditions. Ultimately, pregnancy can serve as a cardiometabolic stress test for some individuals. Maternal and fetal

The estimated probability for PIH, preeclampsia (PE), and LGA

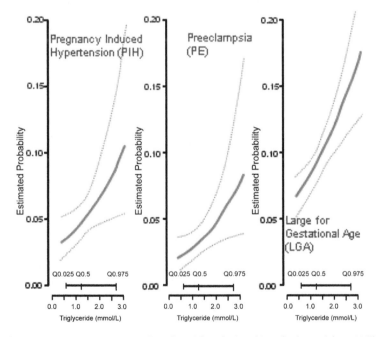

TG levels in the first trimester of pregnancy are a significant, but modest, contributor in the expression of PIH, PE, induced preterm birth, and children to be born Large for Gestational Age. With this observation, inclusion of a lipid profile may be considered early in pregnancy & in the preconception screening.

1 mmol/L of TG = 135 mg/dL
2 mmol/L = 176 mg/dL

Q0.025, Q0.5, and Q0.975 represent the 2.5th, 50.0th, 97.5th percentiles of the studied population.

**Fig. 3.** First trimester maternal triglyceride relationships. (*Adapted from* Vrijkotte TG, Krukziener N, Hutten BA, et al. Maternal lipid profile during early pregnancy and pregnancy complications and outcomes: the ABCD study. J Clin Endocrinol Metab 2012;97(11):3917–25.)

complications can be affected by proper screening and management and taking a detailed metabolic/pregnancy history can provide insight as to the cardiometabolic future risk of mother and child.

The best time to screen for dyslipidemia is before pregnancy or in the early antenatal period after pregnancy is diagnosed. Screening should be performed routinely after the pregnancy is concluded, usually at a minimum by the 6-week routine postpartum visit. Women who experience complications of pregnancy or who gain excessive weight before or during pregnancy are more like to have abnormal cardiometabolic profiles.[7] In patients whose primary provider changes based on development of pregnancy-related complications, continuity and attention to long-term assessment of hyperlipidemia during the puerperal period and beyond is prudent. This potential factor alone can contribute to lack of continuity in proper screening, detection, and management of dyslipidemia in the long term.

### Differential Diagnosis and Evaluation of Hypertriglyceridemia in Pregnancy

The differential diagnosis of hypertriglyceridemia in pregnancy is the same as in a nonpregnant woman with the exception that clinical lipidologists need to be aware of the potential obstetric complications associated with hypertriglyceridemia. Evaluation of hypertriglyceridemia in women preparing for pregnancy or in pregnant women is not different from that in nonpregnant women, with the realization that a 2-fold to 3-fold triglyceride level increase by the third trimester is expected. Furthermore, women with gestational diabetes and preeclampsia often have abnormal triglyceride levels greater than and additive to hypertriglyceridemia associated with obesity before pregnancy. Average values in persons with these disorders exceed 300 mg/dL and levels escalate as pregnancy progresses. What is considered abnormal depends on the trimester in which the triglycerides are measured, with the maximum values usually seen at term. The most common reason for hypertriglyceridemia is poorly controlled or undiscovered diabetes mellitus. Common nondiabetic reasons for increased triglyceride levels are medications that aggravate triglyceride metabolism, particular psychiatric and/or human immunodeficiency virus medications, illicit drugs, and/or alcohol. Hypothyroidism and/or genetic dyslipidemias can also initially be uncovered during pregnancy. Each woman with hypertriglyceridemia needs a careful analysis of family history for hypertriglyceridemia, pancreatitis, diabetes, hypertension, smoking status,

cardiometabolic disease, illicit drugs, or lifestyle issues (including carbohydrate and alcohol intake), as well as use of prescription medicines and supplements. Glycemic, thyroid, hepatic, and renal evaluations are also indicated in this scenario.

### Treatment and Monitoring of Dyslipidemia Associated with Pregnancy

For women with the diagnosis of dyslipidemia before pregnancy, any lipid level–lowering medications aside from bile acid sequestrates and omega-3 fatty acids should be stopped. Recommendations for stopping statins range from 3 months to 1 month before conception. These recommendations are based on expert opinion alone, without definitive evidence. At present, there are 2 ongoing randomized clinical trials to determine whether hydrophilic statins can reduce preeclampsia in pregnancy. Despite this, because of animal data showing that very large doses of lipophilic statins caused birth defects, the US Food and Drug Administration (FDA) has categorized stains as category X. **Box 1** shows the current FDA classification system for medication use in pregnancy. All medication recommendations aside, it is always important to emphasize proper diet and exercise in the given patient scenario.

Even when a medication is labeled as class D, the FDA does not prohibit use but is pointing out that potential benefits may warrant use of the drug in pregnant women despite the risks.

**Table 1** provides the pregnancy classification of widely used lipid level–lowering agents.

Dyslipidemia discovered during pregnancy should be treated with diet and exercise intervention, as well as glycemic control if indicated. Diabetes types I and II during pregnancy can be associated with hypertriglyceridemia. Essential to managing the triglyceride level increases is first to control the diabetes. Common agents used are glyburide and metformin as well as insulin to control blood glucose. Routine glucose screening is an essential component of obstetric care. Hypercholesterolemia can be treated with bile acid sequestrates, notably colesevelam, which is preferred because it is category B.

Severe hypertriglyceridemia (including at levels associated with pancreatitis) can be treated with omega-3 fatty acids, parenteral nutrition, plasmapheresis, or historically with gemfibrozil in the mid to late trimesters (class C medication).[8] It is recommended that lipids be monitored every trimester or within 6 weeks of an intervention to evaluate for compliance, response, and adjustment if needed. Close postpartum follow-up of

---

**Box 1**
**FDA pregnancy drug classifications**

*Category A*

Adequate and well-controlled studies have failed to show a risk to the fetus in the first trimester of pregnancy and there is no evidence of risk in later trimesters.

Examples of drugs or substances: levothyroxine, folic acid, magnesium sulfate, liothyronine.

*Category B*

Animal reproduction studies have failed to show a risk to the fetus and there are no adequate and well-controlled studies in pregnant women.

Examples of drugs: metformin, hydrochlorothiazide, cyclobenzaprine, amoxicillin, pantoprazole.

*Category C*

Animal reproduction studies have shown an adverse effect on the fetus and there are no adequate and well-controlled studies in humans, but potential benefits may warrant use of the drug in pregnant women despite potential risks.

Examples of drugs: tramadol, gabapentin, amlodipine, trazodone, prednisone.

*Category D*

There is positive evidence of human fetal risk based on adverse reaction data from investigational or marketing experience or studies in humans, but potential benefits may warrant use of the drug in pregnant women despite potential risks.

Examples of drugs: lisinopril, alprazolam, losartan, clonazepam, lorazepam.

*Category X*

Studies in animals or humans have shown fetal abnormalities and/or there is positive evidence of human fetal risk based on adverse reaction data from investigational or marketing experience, and the risks involved in use of the drug in pregnant women clearly outweigh potential benefits.

Examples of drugs: atorvastatin, simvastatin, warfarin, methotrexate, finasteride.

*Category N*

FDA has not classified the drug.

Examples of drugs: aspirin, oxycodone, hydroxyzine, acetaminophen, diazepam.

---

**Table 1**
**Lipid level–lowering agents and pregnancy classification**

| Lipid Level–lowering Agent | Pregnancy Class |
| --- | --- |
| Statins | X |
| Fibrates | C |
| Ezetimibe | C |
| Niacin | C |
| Cholestyramine | C |
| Colesevelam | B |
| Mipomersen | B |

mothers and children with FH or dysmetabolic issues of pregnancy is required. States of severe hypertriglyceridemia, hypertension of pregnancy, preeclampsia, gestational diabetes, and/or albuminuria need to be evaluated for residual cardiometabolic risk.

*Familial Hyperlipidemia Monitoring and Treatment*

A complete lipid profile assessment during each trimester of pregnancy is recommended. For women with FH, following brain natriuretic peptide, or B-type natriuretic peptide, as a useful monitor for potential coronary ischemia has been suggested.[9] FH can be treated with lifestyle interventions, bile acid sequestrants (preferably colesevelam, as noted earlier), with monitoring of potential triglyceride level increase in response. If adequate control is not obtained with these regimens, mipomersen (class B medication) and/or low-density lipoprotein (LDL) apheresis may be necessary.[10] Given the complex nature of treatment in such cases, patients with FH are best followed in tertiary care centers with experience in treating these disorders.

### Recommendations for Women with Dyslipidemia Who Are Breastfeeding

Diet and exercise are indicated and tailored to the specific patient scenario. Nutritional consultation is advised. Patients with FH may receive bile acid sequestrates. Lactation may attenuate unfavorable metabolic risk factor changes that occur with pregnancy, with effects apparent after weaning. As a modifiable behavior, lactation may affect women's future risk of cardiovascular and metabolic diseases.[11] For disorders with high triglyceride levels it is advisable to avoid estrogenic oral contraception even with late breastfeeding. However, breastfeeding does not guarantee lactational anovulation and thereby contraception. Approximately 1 in 3 women ovulate during prolonged breast feeding, highlighting the need to advise patients regarding the best contraceptives despite breastfeeding.

### LONG-TERM IMPLICATIONS OF COMPLICATIONS IN PREGNANCY

Recent studies indicate that the endothelial dysfunction incurred during preeclampsia pregnancies may increase the risk of CVD later in life.[12] Contributions of dyslipidemia, obesity, the presence of the metabolic syndrome or insulin-resistance states before pregnancy,[12,13] as well as hypertensive disorders of pregnancy also host important future CVD risk scenarios.

The accumulated weight gain during pregnancies and the inability to effect adequate weight loss during middle age is a well-known risk factor for CVD.[14,15] The increase in lipid components during pregnancy, notably triglycerides and their metabolically dangerous atherogenic particle metabolites, may not be corrected postpartum. Strategies to control blood pressure are well established in the nonpregnant population, and previous preeclampsia and gestational hypertension should be considered as important historical risk factors for stratification of cardiovascular risk and determining the aggressiveness of therapy. Yet to be determined is whether or not blood pressure control in pregnancy has any identifiable long-term benefit.

### Polycystic Ovary Syndrome

PCOS affects 7% to 22% of reproductive-aged women, so an understanding of the diagnosis and therapeutic options for this condition is paramount for lipidologists.[16] Women with PCOS are at increased risk for metabolic syndrome, diabetes mellitus, complications of pregnancy, and endometrial cancer.[13,17] Most individuals with PCOS show insulin resistance, which is intensified by obesity and often the pregnant state, potentially leading to attendant complications. The most common high-risk condition of pregnancy is obesity because it is a foundation for the development of diabetes, preeclampsia, large-for-gestational-age infants, complications of delivery, and neonatal intensive care unit admissions. In addition, women with PCOS are at greater risk for obstetric complications irrespective of whether or not they have developed overt metabolic syndrome.[13]

The most widely used criteria to diagnose PCOS are the Rotterdam criteria, as shown in **Table 2**.

| Table 2 | | | |
|---|---|---|---|
| **Criteria recognized to diagnose PCOS** | | | |
| | **Diagnostic Criteria of PCOS** | | |
| **Criteria** | **NIH 1990 Classic** | **Rotterdam 2003** | **Androgen Excess PCOS** |
| Oligomenorrhea[a] | + | +/− | +/− |
| Clinical or biochemical hyperandrogenism[b] | + | +/− | +/− |
| Polycystic ovaries on ultrasonography[c] | +/− | +/− | +/− |

NIH criteria include both oligomenorrhea and clinical/biochemical hyperandrogenism; Rotterdam criteria include any 2 of the Androgen Excess and Polycystic Ovarian Syndrome Society criteria, presence of clinical/biochemical hyperandrogenism, and 1 other criterion.
[a] Eight or fewer menses per year.
[b] Acne, or hirsutism, or androgenic alopecia.
[c] Ovarian volume greater than 10 mL and/or greater than 12 follicles less than 9 mm in at least 1 ovary.
*Adapted from* Wild RA, Carmina E, Diamanti-Kandarakis E, et al. Assessment of cardiovascular risk and prevention of cardiovascular disease in women with the polycystic ovary syndrome: a consensus statement by the Androgen Excess and Polycystic Ovary Syndrome (AE-PCOS) Society. J Clin Endocrinol Metab 2010;95(5):2038–49.

However, different criteria have evolved in attempts to capture the heterogeneous nature of the condition. The term PCOS originates from the characteristic morphology of the ovary (polycystic ovary), which is derived from the ultrasonographic pathognomonic string-of-pearls sign. This sign results from multiple follicles suspended in similar stages of development. The follicles most often are seen around the periphery as they surround a very endocrinologically active, androgen-secreting inner stroma (**Fig. 4**).

The criteria are based on the presence of at least 2 of the following: androgen excess (clinically in the form of hirsutism, acne, and/or androgenic alopecia, or measured in the blood), ovulatory dysfunction, or the presence of polycystic ovaries (usually assessed by vaginal ultrasonography). The Androgen Excess Society insists that some form of androgen excess is necessary for the diagnosis. The spectrum of the condition can include persons mildly affected to severely affected with androgen excess bordering on severe virilization.

Women with PCOS frequently develop dyslipidemia and/or metabolic syndrome at any age, including at the onset of menses and continuing throughout the adolescent years. Diagnosing PCOS can be difficult at times of physiologic oligomenorrhea commonly observed around menarche as well as menopausal transition. Diagnosing PCOS can be difficult at times of physiologic oligomenorrhea commonly observed around menarche as well as menopausal transition.

## SCREENING FOR ASSOCIATED DYSLIPIDEMIA IN POLYCYSTIC OVARIAN SYNDROME

We recommend that all patients with PCOS, regardless of age, should undergo lipid and diabetes screening given the increased prevalence of dyslipidemia and insulin resistance in this population.[18] We also recommend increased frequency of monitoring for such clinical changes compared with the general population even if initial values are normal because risk of developing these conditions increases with age. Two-year screening intervals have been suggested by some experts. Given that normalizing dyslipidemia and glucose intolerance can reduce atherogenesis, clinical lipidologists need to be familiar with the principles of management for such conditions throughout the reproductive period. We recommend similar, if not tighter, lipid level goals in dyslipidemia as those used in metabolic syndrome. The Androgen Excess Society consensus document recommends the target values shown in **Table 3** in lipid management of women with PCOS.

## TREATMENT OF DYSLIPIDEMIA IN POLYCYSTIC OVARIAN SYNDROME

Diet and exercise are the foundation of intervention. Use of medication to control lipids has special considerations for women with PCOS. Therapy should be focused on reversing all components of the metabolic syndrome through diet, exercise, and medication only if needed.[19] In general, metformin is widely used because of low cost, long-term safety data, and low side effect profile. Unlike the glitazones, metformin is not associated with weight gain or fluid retention and this feature alone leads to wide acceptance. It is often used for its weight loss properties; however, it is not a successful medication for acute weight loss or for reduction of hirsutism. Although diet and exercise have been shown to be superior to metformin in reducing the onset of diabetes,[19] metformin is often used because of ease of improved compliance with the initially once-daily dosing. This dosing profile assists with avoidance of gastrointestinal side effects. In addition, glitazones and metformin are associated with improved ovulation, which may or may not be useful depending on the setting. Ovulation is more likely monofollicular with these agents in women with PCOS, although these medications are not first-line therapy for ovulation induction in women with PCOS who desire pregnancy. Alternatively, because of improved reproductive function

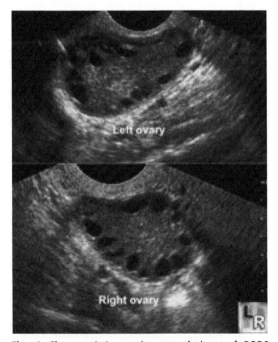

**Fig. 4.** Characteristic ovarian morphology of PCOS revealing the source of the name for the syndrome.

**Table 3**
**PCOS risk categories and lipid target values**

| | Risk | LDL Target Values; mg/dL (mmol/L)[a] | Non-HDL Target Values; mg/dL (mmol/L)[a] |
|---|---|---|---|
| PCOS | At optimal | ≤130 (3.37) | ≤160 (4.14) |
| PCOS (obesity, hypertension, dyslipidemia, cigarette smoking, IGT, subvascular disease | At risk | ≤130 (3.37) | ≤160 (4.14) |
| PCOS with MetS | High risk | ≤100 (2.59) | ≤130 (3.37) |
| PCOS[b] with MetS and T2DM, overt renal disease, or other vascular disease | — | ≤70 (1.81) | ≤100 (2.59) |

Values are based on 12 h fast.
  *Abbreviations:* IGT, impaired glucose tolerance; MetS, metabolic syndrome; T2DM, type 2 diabetes mellitus.
  [a] To convert mg/dL to mmol/L, divide by 39.
  [b] Odds for CVD increase with number of MetS components and with other risk factors, smoking, poor diet, inactivity, obesity, family history of premature CVD (men <55 years old or women <65 years old), and subclinical vascular disease.
  *Adapted from* Wild RA, Carmina E, Diamanti-Kandarakis E, et al. Assessment of cardiovascular risk and prevention of cardiovascular disease in women with the polycystic ovary syndrome: a consensus statement by the Androgen Excess and Polycystic Ovary Syndrome (AE-PCOS) Society. J Clin Endocrinol Metab 2010;95(5);2038–49.

states with these medicines and associated risk of pregnancy in women who require contraception, this fact should always be considered by the primary care provider. As alluded to earlier, glitazones and metformin improve insulin resistance and menstrual irregularity, but they are not first-line agents to enhance fertility.[20]

Of the numerous diet interventions available, Heart Healthy, Mediterranean, and the Dietary Approaches to Stop Hypertension (DASH) diets have shown short-term improved lipid and other biomarker effects for women with PCOS.[21] High-carbohydrate diets tend to aggravate insulin resistance and severely restricting low-carbohydrate diets acutely offer weight loss; however, this is not sustainable with long-term lipid reduction and normalization. Weight loss should be targeted in all overweight women with PCOS through reducing caloric intake in the setting of adequate nutritional intake and healthy food choices, irrespective of diet composition.[22]

Statins are used in women with PCOS to treat their metabolic syndrome as well as to reduce testosterone and androstenedione levels. Statins reduce LDL-C and non–HDL-C levels in women with PCOS. In a high alpha and beta short-term clinical trial, atorvastatin therapy improved chronic inflammation and lipid profile and also reduced the testosterone level in women with PCOS. However, it has also been found to impair insulin sensitivity. Because women with PCOS have an increased risk of developing type 2 diabetes mellitus, the results suggest that statin therapy should be initiated from generally accepted criteria and individual risk assessment of CVD, and not solely in the setting of a PCOS diagnosis.[23] Another challenge with statin use is the pregnancy categorization of X. Although the reliability of the data behind this X recommendation has recently been questioned, the potential teratogenic risk of statin use in women who are pregnant or who are at risk of becoming pregnant must be clearly explained to any person of reproductive age.[24] Reliable forms of contraception and avoidance of statin use in a person who is pregnant are prudent. However, rosuvastatin and pravastatin are water soluble and thus these agents have been suggested to be less likely to cause teratogenic effects. Ongoing multicenter clinical trials are assessing whether such water-soluble statins can reduce preeclampsia when given in the midtrimester of pregnancy. In addition, stains can be useful in treating fatty liver, which is common in women with PCOS who have the metabolic syndrome.[25]

When effectiveness alone is considered, other lipid level–lowering medications have been used successfully in women with PCOS as well. However, given the predominance of women in the reproductive age range when PCOS is diagnosed, teratogenic risks in the scenario of unplanned pregnancy must be acknowledged, which limits the selection of lipid level–lowering agents. This acknowledgment also highlights the importance of contraceptive counseling.

## DYSLIPIDEMIA TREATMENT AND UNIQUE CHALLENGES FOR WOMEN WITH POLYCYSTIC OVARIAN SYNDROME

Therapy for PCOS is complex given the multiorigin cause of the syndrome as well as differing patient concerns. In general, areas to consider are cosmetic (considerations to reduce unwanted hair growth), menstrual regulation (to improve fertility and/or to reduce endometrial cancer risk), as well as metabolic (to control or to prevent diabetes and associated atherogenesis and CVD).

The standard medication used to control menses, to reduce endometrial and ovarian cancer risk, and to reduce hirsutism is the combined oral contraceptive (COC). Acne can accompany the androgen excess, although the true cause is multifactorial, which can also be improved by COC use. In general, the more estrogenic an oral contraceptive compound, the more effective the hirsutism control that will be obtained. In addition, spironolactone is used concomitantly, primarily because of its ability to reduce 5-alpha reductase, the primary enzyme responsible for converting circulating testosterone into the more potent, locally active metabolite, dihydrotestosterone. The topic of contraceptive counseling is also important to review given that 5-alpha reductase inhibitors can cross the placenta and cause ambiguous genitalia in the newborn if used during pregnancy.

Endometrial hyperplasia and ultimately cancer can occur as a result of years of unopposed estrogen. This cycle can begin as early as the teen years in adolescents with PCOS. Given this, the use of oral contraceptives has to be weighed for its contraceptive benefits as well as its cancer prevention abilities even in the adolescent population. The major risk associated with COC use is thrombotic risk and combined oral contraceptives should not be used in women 35 years or older who smoke because of additive stroke and heart attack risk.

In general, the dyslipidemia associated with PCOS reflects the effects of insulin resistance. However, there are other consequences of insulin resistance. The androgen excess seems to occur from effects of insulin on the ovary and/or adrenal glands. Concomitantly, the HDL-C level is often reduced, triglyceride production increases, and circulating atherogenic small LDL particles increase, all of which are further aggravated when women with PCOS become obese. Depending on which COC is chosen for which clinical manifestation of PCOS, triglyceride levels may increase, HDL-C levels may increase, and LDL-C levels may decrease when COCs are given to women with PCOS who have associated dyslipidemia.

Rarely, a genetic lipid disorder is uncovered when screening for dyslipidemia in women with PCOS. Very high triglyceride levels (ie, >500 mg/dL) are rarely caused by PCOS. Using an oral contraceptive can further aggravate hypertriglyceridemia of this magnitude and can precipitate pancreatitis.

Treatment considerations should include sensitivity to all 3 foci of patient concern. Clinical lipidologists need to understand that the choices for lipid control beyond heart-healthy diets and exercise advice depend on all of these considerations.

### Contraception

As outlined earlier, the best time to detect and treat dyslipidemia as it relates to pregnancy is before conception. Understanding the effects of pregnancy on a woman who is or becomes dyslipidemic during pregnancy is relevant for considerations for contraception because family planning in the long run is the best way to optimize pregnancy and maternal outcomes. Avoiding closely timed pregnancies is important to allow return of the body to its baseline metabolic state without prolonged periods of stress-induced hyperlipidemia. Clinical lipidologists need insight into the effects of contraceptive types on lipid metabolism and the effects of lipid management on contraceptive choice, keeping in mind the risk of pregnancy if contraception is not used.

Most surveys show that approximately 50% of pregnancies are unexpected or unwanted.[26] Contraceptive education is important for prevention and the choice of contraceptive method has implications for lipid management. No contraceptive method fits everyone. Each method may have an impact on lipid metabolism and resultant factors relevant to lipid management. The risk of complications associated with pregnancy given the contraceptive choice made include its efficacy in preventing pregnancy (which most often carries greater risk to the mother if the contraceptive is not used or fails) as well as the cardiometabolic impact of the method chosen.

Screening for lipid levels must be kept up to date according to childhood, adolescent, and adult guidelines for population screening (see the National Lipid Association guidelines). Special thought must be used to identify persons with FH, hypertriglyceridemia, or rare genetic forms of hyperlipidemia on routine screening and/or family history. A detailed metabolic/pregnancy history provides insight as to the cardiometabolic future risk of the mother and her children.

## LIPID CHANGES WITH DIFFERENT FORMS OF CONTRACEPTION
### Combined Oral Contraceptives

In order to effect contraception through ovulation inhibition while concomitantly reducing cardiovascular side effects such as myocardial infarction or cardiovascular accident from sex steroids, various formulations of COC have been developed over the years. First-generation COCs were developed exclusively to avoid pregnancy. If used properly, they were effective at pregnancy prevention. Both minor and major side effects were discovered predominantly through population studies. If used perfectly, the first-generation COCs are 99.9% effective in preventing pregnancy, but they are associated with greater risk of thrombotic events. However, when sex steroid content is reduced, efficacy for preventing pregnancy is reduced either through a lower threshold of ovulation inhibition when used perfectly or through the usual use issues with compliance.

Second-generation COCs were primarily designed to reduce heavy or abnormal menstrual bleeding, which is a significant issue for many women. The increased androgen content in second-generation COCs allows improved bleeding control. However, androgenic side effects lead to worse compliance, usually because of side effects such as acne, hair growth, or perceived weight gain. Complaints among women regarding these side effects prompted the creation of third-generations COCs, which are slightly less androgenic.

COCs have multiple tissue effects, including estrogenic, progestational, androgenic, antiestrogenic, and antiandrogenic effects. All forms reduce risk for endometrial and ovarian cancers. The major risk associated with all COCs is thromboembolic disease. Women with various medical comorbidities, older age, and tobacco users are at increased risk for the cardiovascular events. There are 2 types of estrogen (ethinyl-estradiol and mestranol) used in the United States. Various doses of estrogen within COCs are available. Higher doses carry greater risk of thromboembolic events. Few 50-μg estrogen-containing pills are available on the market today for this reason. At present, most COCs contain 35-μg of ethinyl-estradiol or less and there are multiple types of progestins used in the COCs that are marketed today.

The estrogenic effect of COCs increases levels of TGs and HDL-C, and lowers levels of LDL-C. Androgenic progestins (such as norgestrel and levonorgestrel) can increase LDL-C levels and reduce HDL-C levels. The progestational effect is lipid neutral. For example, desogestrel, a third-generation COC that uses low-dose norethindrone, reduces LDL-C levels and increases HDL-C levels. In addition, the more overall estrogenic a COC is, the more it seems to increase triglyceride and high-density lipoprotein (HDL) levels. This effect carries a greater risk of precipitating pancreatitis in scenarios in which baseline triglyceride levels are increased and increase further with estrogenic COC use. However, transdermal or vaginal combination contraceptives (estrogenic plus progestin) do not reduce the risk of a thrombotic event compared with COCs.

There are several medical conditions that require a thorough evaluation of risks, benefits, and alternatives in choosing a contraceptive agent. One example of such a condition is factor V Leiden thrombophilia, an inheritable hypercoagulable state. Detailing each of these conditions is beyond the scope of this article. For each condition of interest the reader is encouraged to access the US Centers for Disease Control and Prevention compendium for medical conditions, which provides recommendations for contraceptive choice for specific comorbidities. **Box 2** shows an example of a recommendation.

## NON–COMBINED ORAL CONTRACEPTIVE METHODS
### Intrauterine Devices

Use of a contraceptive should always include a discussion of risks, benefits, and alternatives, as well as a clear review of proper use. Persons with known hyperlipidemia can be given a progestin-impregnated intrauterine device (IUD) (level 2 recommendation). Less overall bleeding is noted with this method, but breakthrough bleeding is commonly observed. A nonhormonal option is the copper IUD, which can be used for up to 10 years per device. Although this is a

---

**Box 2**
**Classification for clinical recommendations for intrauterine device use are provided in a Likert scale; this scale can be modified for ease of use**

1. A condition for which there is no restriction for use.

2. A condition for which advantages of using the method usually outweigh the theoretic or proven risk.

3. A condition for which the theoretic risk or proven risks usually outweigh the advantages of using the method.

4. A condition posing an unacceptable health risk if the method is used.

lipid-neutral option, most women complain of increased menstrual bleeding with the device.

### Progestin Only

Implantable or injectable progestins are widely used, especially for persons at risk of noncompliance. In general, progestin-only methods are lipid neutral. There is some evidence that injectable Provera is associated with weight gain. Persons at risk for weight gain (eg, persons with PCOS) seem to be at greater risk for this adverse effect. Weight gain is associated with creating or aggravating a current metabolic syndrome with associated risk of diabetes and mixed dyslipidemia. Despite this, implantable and injectable progestin forms of contraception are extremely efficacious for preventing pregnancy. Progestin-only oral contraceptives are available and are often used when estrogenic preparations are contraindicated or when the risk/benefit ratio is a concern with a COC. However, progestin-only formulations are associated with increased breakthrough bleeding and are of decreased contraceptive efficacy.

### Permanent Sterilization

Male and female permanent sterilization procedures are widely used and highly effective forms of contraception. Although nonhormonal and thus lipid neutral, permanent sterilization can unfortunately lead to loss of general-care follow-up as patients are no longer seeking medical care for pregnancy. As primary care providers offering such contraceptive options, it is prudent to recognize the importance of continuing screening for CVD risk factors.

## MENOPAUSE TRANSITION
### Lipid Changes During Menopause

With the onset of waning of ovarian function, lipid changes are noticeable on both a population and an individual basis. The changes tend to occur primarily during the later phases of menopause transition. The magnitude of change toward dyslipidemia is similar to the changes that occur with aging. The relative odds of having an LDL-C level of 130 mg/dL before to after menopause has been reported to be 2.1 (confidence interval [CI], 1.5–2.9).[27]

The changes that occur are presumably related to declining ovarian estradiol production as follicles diminish and secrete less estradiol. Changes in body fat distribution are also observed during this transitional time.[28] In addition, there is a link to an increased prevalence of metabolic syndrome.[29] With expert treatment, it has been shown that carotid atherosclerosis is observed more frequently beginning in the menopause transition, and a significant number of women also possess coronary calcium deposition before this.[30,31]

The absolute risk for CVD increases substantially in midlife for women. Rates associated with a particular adverse effect on lipid metabolism increase at the time of menopause. Those persons with significant risk factors before menopause are additionally affected. It is important for primary care physicians to identify these individuals early to plan for best control of these same risk factors during the menopause transition.[27,32]

**Fig. 5** shows natural changes of the major lipid and apolipoprotein lipid levels using cross-sectional panel design analysis as these women transitioned through the menopause years, studied in the multiethnic Study of Women's Health Across the Nation (SWAN) data set. Note that levels are assessed and measured as annual mean data comparing years before and after the final menstrual period. Menopause is defined in retrospect as 1 year with nonmenses during this transition. Day 0 in the graphs is labeled and standardized as the final menstrual period. Importantly, apolipoprotein (Apo) B levels increase noticeably.

Annual rates of change in carotid intima-media thickness and adventitial diameter have been reported, as noted in **Fig. 6**. The rate of change at the late perimenopausal stage significantly differs from that at the premenopausal stage. The rate of change at the late perimenopausal stage significantly differs from that at the early perimenopausal stage. The rate of change at the postmenopausal stage significantly differs from that at the premenopausal stage (P<.05).

## CURRENT RECOMMENDATIONS FOR HORMONE THERAPY

Menopausal hormone replacement therapy is primarily indicated to control menopause-related quality-of-life issues. Replacement therapy should not be prescribed for cardiovascular purposes (ie, for prevention or treatment of vascular diseases). There is a black box warning by the FDA for women with known coronary artery disease, thromboembolic disorders, or who have had a cerebrovascular accident because these preparations carry thrombotic risk and critical events in persons with these disorders involving thrombotic pathophysiology.

Identifying appropriate candidates for menopausal hormone therapy (HT) is challenging given the complex profile of risks and benefits associated with treatment.[33] Most professional societies agree that HT should not be used for chronic disease prevention.

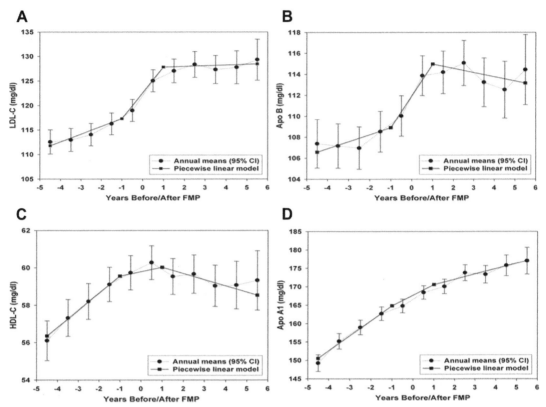

**Fig. 5.** Lipids annual and estimated means patterns of LDL-C (*A*), apolipoprotein (Apo) B (*B*), HDL-C (*C*), and Apo A1 (*D*) across the SWAN study follow-up period. FMP, final menstrual period. (*From* Matthews KA. Are changes in cardiovascular disease risk factors in midlife women due to chronological aging or to the menopausal transition? J Am Coll Cardiol 2009;54(25):2366–73; with permission.)

Recent findings from the Women's Health Initiative and other randomized trials suggest that a woman's age, proximity to menopause, underlying cardiovascular risk factor status, and various biological characteristics may modify health outcomes with HT. An emerging body of evidence suggests that it may be possible to assess individual risk and therefore better predict who is likely to have favorable outcomes versus adverse effects when taking HT. Thus, once a woman is identified as a potential candidate for HT for quality-of-life improvement because of moderate to severe menopausal symptoms or other indications, risk stratification may be an important tool for minimizing patient risk.[33]

This individualized approach holds great promise for improving the safety of HT. Patient-centered outcomes including quality of life and sense of well-being should also be incorporated and will directly affect the risk/benefit ratio as well as compliance. Additional research on hormone dose, formulation, and route of delivery will be important for improving this decision model.

Ultimately, a treatment decision to provide symptom relief should be made with a patient's full understanding of potential risks and benefits, and taking into account her personal preferences. To better integrate patient values, practical considerations, and emerging clinical experience, recent research from observational studies and randomized clinical trials on HT should be considered. Note the results from an analysis of the Women's Health Initiative in which oral estrogen plus progestin and estrogen alone were used in the randomized clinical trial (**Table 4**).

This analysis suggests that persons at higher risk for CVD events (increased dyslipidemia or presence of metabolic syndrome) are more likely to have this risk aggravated by administration of oral hormone replacement therapy. The message is clear: assessing CVD risk before HT is given for menopausal symptoms is prudent to identify persons who may be at increased adverse event risk with oral HT.

There are several biomarkers under study to determine whether they provide incremental risk prediction for CVD in women taking HT. However, thus far none have been shown to provide added risk prediction and currently they are not recommended for clinical use.

A

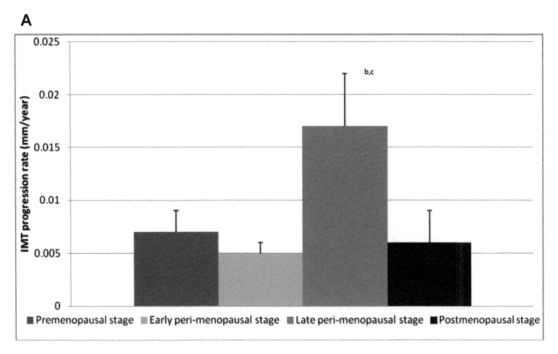

B

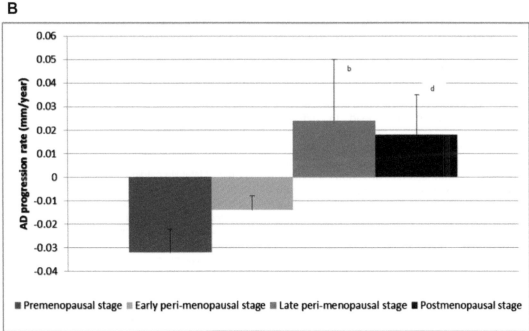

**Fig. 6.** Annual rates of change in (*A*) carotid intima-media thickness (IMT) and (*B*) adventitial diameter (AD). (*From* El Khoudary SR, Wildman RP, Matthews K, et al. Progression rates of carotid intima-media thickness and adventitial diameter during the menopausal transition. Menopause 2013;20(1):8–14; with permission.)

Using the lowest effective dose of HT is recommended, regardless of clinical scenario. In general, doses lower than 0.3 mg of oral conjugated estrogen daily do not control hot flashes for most women. However, this dose is protective against bone loss from estrogen deficiency osteopenia.[34] Delivering the medication transdermally may be associated with fewer adverse events than when given by the oral route.[35] Tissue effects may differ depending on whether there is a first-pass hepatic effect, as is the case with oral estrogen.

With vaginal and transdermal preparations there is less effect on clotting factors, lipid metabolism,

**Table 4**
**CHD risk in the Women's Health Initiative HT trials (estrogen and progestin and estrogen alone) according to baseline levels of biomarkers**

| Biomarker P Value for Interaction | Odds Ratio (95% CI) for HT Treatment Effect | P for Interaction |
|---|---|---|
| **LDL-C (mg/dL)** | | |
| <130 | 0.66 (0.34–1.27) | 0.03 |
| ≥130 | | |
| **LDL-C/HDL-C Ratio** | | |
| <2.5 | 0.66 (0.34–1.27) | 0.002 |
| ≥2.5 | 1.73 (1.18–2.53) | |
| **Hs-CRP(mg/dL)** | | |
| <2.0 | 1.01 (0.63–1.62) | 0.16 |
| ≥2.0 | 1.58 (1.05–2.39) | |
| MetS | 2.26 (1.26–4.07) | 0.03 |
| No MetS | 0.97 (0.58–1.61) | — |

*Abbreviation:* hs-CRP, high-sensitivity C-reactive protein.
*Adapted from* Wild RA, Manson JE. Insights from the Women's Health Initiative: individualizing risk assessment for hormone therapy decisions. Semin Reprod Med 2014;32(6):433–37.

inflammatory biomarkers, and sex hormone–binding globulin synthesis. Differences in dose, route, and formulations, in conjunction with genetic metabolic differences, may lead to different outcomes.

Observational studies, although limited in number, suggest that transdermal delivery may be associated with less risk of venous thromboembolism and stroke than with oral estrogen administration; however, these studies do not prove a cause-effect relationship.[36] Randomized clinical trial evidence is needed to answer this question more definitively.

## REFERENCES

1. Palinski W, D'Armiento FP, Witztum JL, et al. Maternal hypercholesterolemia and treatment during pregnancy influence the long-term progression of atherosclerosis in offspring of rabbits. Circ Res 2001;89(11):991–6.

2. Wiznitzer A, Mayer A, Novack V, et al. Association of lipid levels during gestation with preeclampsia and gestational diabetes mellitus: a population-based study. Am J Obstet Gynecol 2009;201(5):482–8.

3. Potter JM, Macdonald WB. Primary type I hyperlipoproteinaemia–a metabolic and family study. Aust N Z J Med 1979;9(6):688–93.

4. Herrera E. Metabolic adaptations in pregnancy and their implications for the availability of substrates to the fetus. Eur J Clin Nutr 2000; 54(Suppl 1):S47–51.

5. Vrijkotte TG, Krukziener N, Hutten BA, et al. Maternal lipid profile during early pregnancy and pregnancy complications and outcomes: the ABCD study. J Clin Endocrinol Metab 2012;97(11):3917–25.

6. Nordestgaard BG, Chapman MJ, Humphries SE, et al. Familial hypercholesterolaemia is underdiagnosed and undertreated in the general population: guidance for clinicians to prevent coronary heart disease: consensus statement of the European Atherosclerosis Society. Eur Heart J 2013;34(45): 3478–3490a.

7. Smith GN, Walker MC, Liu A, et al. A history of preeclampsia identifies women who have underlying cardiovascular risk factors. Am J Obstet Gynecol 2009;200(1):58.e1–8.

8. Goldberg AS, Hegele RA. Severe hypertriglyceridemia in pregnancy. J Clin Endocrinol Metab 2012; 97(8):2589–96.

9. Tanous D, Siu SC, Mason J, et al. B-type natriuretic peptide in pregnant women with heart disease. J Am Coll Cardiol 2010;56(15):1247–53.

10. Kusters DM, Homsma SJ, Hutten BA, et al. Dilemmas in treatment of women with familial hypercholesterolaemia during pregnancy. Neth J Med 2010;68(1):299–303.

11. Zarrati M, Shidfar F, Moradof M, et al. Relationship between breast feeding and obesity in children with low birth weight. Iran Red Crescent Med J 2013;15(8):676–82.

12. Charlton F, Tooher J, Rye KA, et al. Cardiovascular risk, lipids and pregnancy: preeclampsia and the risk of later life cardiovascular disease. Heart Lung Circ 2014;23(3):203–12.

13. Kjerulff LE, Sanchez-Ramos L, Duffy D. Pregnancy outcomes in women with polycystic ovary syndrome: a metaanalysis. Am J Obstet Gynecol 2011;204(6): 558.e1–6.

14. Gunderson EP. Childbearing and obesity in women: weight before, during, and after pregnancy. Obstet Gynecol Clin North Am 2009;36(2):317–32, ix.

15. Manson JE, Willett WC, Stampfer MJ, et al. Body weight and mortality among women. N Engl J Med 1995;333(11):677–85.

16. Wild RA, Carmina E, Diamanti-Kandarakis E, et al. Assessment of cardiovascular risk and prevention of cardiovascular disease in women with the polycystic ovary syndrome: a consensus statement by the Androgen Excess and Polycystic Ovary Syndrome (AE-PCOS) Society. J Clin Endocrinol Metab 2010; 95(5):2038–49.

17. Barry JA, Azizia MM, Hardiman PJ. Risk of endometrial, ovarian and breast cancer in women with polycystic ovary syndrome: a systematic review and

meta-analysis. Hum Reprod Update 2014;20(5): 748–58.

18. Moran LJ, Misso ML, Wild RA, et al. Impaired glucose tolerance, type 2 diabetes and metabolic syndrome in polycystic ovary syndrome: a systematic review and meta-analysis. Hum Reprod Update 2010;16(4):347–63.

19. Diabetes Prevention Program Research Group, Knowler WC, Fowler SE, et al. 10-year follow-up of diabetes incidence and weight loss in the Diabetes Prevention Program Outcomes Study. Lancet 2009; 374(9702):1677–86.

20. Legro RS, Arslanian SA, Ehrmann DA, et al. Diagnosis and treatment of polycystic ovary syndrome: an Endocrine Society clinical practice guideline. J Clin Endocrinol Metab 2013;98(12):4565–92.

21. Asemi Z, Esmaillzadeh A. DASH diet, insulin resistance, and serum hs-CRP in polycystic ovary syndrome: a randomized controlled clinical trial. Horm Metab Res 2014;47(3):232–8.

22. Moran LJ, Ko H, Misso M, et al. Dietary composition in the treatment of polycystic ovary syndrome: a systematic review to inform evidence-based guidelines. J Acad Nutr Diet 2013;113(4):520–45.

23. Puurunen J, Piltonen T, Puukka K, et al. Statin therapy worsens insulin sensitivity in women with polycystic ovary syndrome (PCOS): a prospective, randomized, double-blind, placebo-controlled study. J Clin Endocrinol Metab 2013;98(12):4798–807.

24. Zarek J, Koren G. The fetal safety of statins: a systematic review and meta-analysis. J Obstet Gynaecol Can 2014;36(6):506–9.

25. Setji TL, Brown AJ. Polycystic ovary syndrome: update on diagnosis and treatment. Am J Med 2014;127(10):912–9.

26. Sanga K, Mola G, Wattimena J, et al. Unintended pregnancy amongst women attending antenatal clinics at the Port Moresby General Hospital. Aust N Z J Obstet Gynaecol 2014;54(4):360–5.

27. Derby CA, Crawford SL, Pasternak RC, et al. Lipid changes during the menopause transition in relation to age and weight: the Study of Women's Health Across the Nation. Am J Epidemiol 2009;169(11): 1352–61.

28. Park JK, Lim YH, Kim KS, et al. Changes in body fat distribution through menopause increase blood pressure independently of total body fat in middle-aged women: the Korean National Health and Nutrition Examination Survey 2007-2010. Hypertens Res 2013;36(5):444–9.

29. Mendes KG, Theodoro H, Rodrigues AD, et al. Prevalence of metabolic syndrome and its components in the menopausal transition: a systematic review. Cad Saude Publica 2012;28(8):1423–37 [in Portuguese].

30. El Khoudary SR, Wildman RP, Matthews K, et al. Progression rates of carotid intima-media thickness and adventitial diameter during the menopausal transition. Menopause 2013;20(1):8–14.

31. Kuller LH, Matthews KA, Sutton-Tyrrell K, et al. Coronary and aortic calcification among women 8 years after menopause and their premenopausal risk factors: the Healthy Women Study. Arterioscler Thromb Vasc Biol 1999;19(9):2189–98.

32. Matthews KA, Gibson CJ, El Khoudary SR, et al. Changes in cardiovascular risk factors by hysterectomy status with and without oophorectomy: Study of Women's Health Across the Nation. J Am Coll Cardiol 2013;62(3):191–200.

33. Wild RA, Manson JE. Insights from the Women's Health Initiative: individualizing risk assessment for hormone therapy decisions. Semin Reprod Med 2014;32(6):433–7.

34. Mizunuma H, Shiraki M, Shintani M, et al. Randomized trial comparing low-dose hormone replacement therapy and HRT plus 1alpha-OH-vitamin D3 (alfacalcidol) for treatment of postmenopausal bone loss. J Bone Miner Metab 2006;24(1):11–5.

35. North American Menopause Society. The 2012 hormone therapy position statement of: The North American Menopause Society. Menopause 2012; 19(3):257–71.

36. Canonico M, Oger E, Plu-Bureau G, et al. Hormone therapy and venous thromboembolism among postmenopausal women: impact of the route of estrogen administration and progestogens: the ESTHER study. Circulation 2007;115(7):840–5.

# Statins and Diabetes

Kevin C. Maki, PhD[a],*, Mary R. Dicklin, PhD[a], Seth J. Baum, MD[b]

## KEYWORDS

- Statins • High intensity statins • Diabetes mellitus • Glucose • Glycemia • Dyslipidemia
- Cardiovascular disease • Coronary heart disease

## KEY POINTS

- Statin use is associated with a modest increase in risk for new-onset type 2 diabetes mellitus compared with placebo or usual care.
- The risk for diabetes seems to be greater for intensive-dosage statin therapy, and to be most evident in those with major risk factors for diabetes.
- The cardiovascular benefits of statin therapy outweigh the potential risk for diabetes development, with several cardiovascular events generally prevented for each excess case of diabetes.
- No changes to clinical practice have been recommended, other than measuring glycated hemoglobin or fasting glucose in patients at elevated diabetes risk before and within 1 year of initiating therapy.
- The American Diabetes Association guidelines should be followed for screening and diagnosis, and lifestyle modification is emphasized for the prevention or delay of diabetes mellitus.

## INTRODUCTION

Statins are first-line drug therapy for the management of dyslipidemia and have been shown to reduce the risks for myocardial infarction, stroke, and cardiovascular death,[1–3] but clinical trial data suggest a modest, yet statistically significant, increase in the incidence of new-onset type 2 diabetes mellitus (T2DM) with statin use.[4–10] Diabetes mellitus is a common condition affecting nearly 10% of the US population[11] and is increasing in prevalence worldwide.[12] In 2012, the US Food and Drug Administration added a statement to the labels of statin medications indicating that increases in glycated hemoglobin (HbA$_{1C}$) and fasting glucose levels have been reported with statin use.[13] In 2014, the National Lipid Association Statin Diabetes Safety Task Force reviewed the published evidence relating statin use to the hazard of diabetes mellitus or worsening glycemia, and provided practical guidance on how to manage this issue in clinical practice.[10] This paper provides a brief overview of the literature regarding statin use and T2DM risk and summarizes the findings and guidance from the National Lipid Association Expert Panel. The terms T2DM and diabetes are used synonymously throughout the article.

## CLINICAL TRIAL EVIDENCE REGARDING STATIN USE AND DIABETES
### West of Scotland Coronary Prevention Study

The West of Scotland Coronary Prevention Study (WOSCOPS) was one of the first clinical trials to draw attention to a possible association, albeit inverse in that trial, between T2DM risk and statin use.[14] An examination of the incidence of new-onset diabetes mellitus among 5974 subjects receiving pravastatin in WOSCOPS indicated that

Disclosures: Dr K.C. Maki discloses that in the past 12 months he has received consulting fees and/or research grants from AbbVie, Amarin, AstraZeneca, and Trygg Pharmaceuticals. Dr M.R. Dicklin has nothing to disclose. Dr S.J. Baum discloses that in the past 12 months he has received consulting/speaking fees from Aegerion, Genzyme, Sanofi, AstraZeneca, and Merck Pharmaceuticals.
[a] Metabolic Sciences, Midwest Center for Metabolic & Cardiovascular Research, 489 Taft Avenue, Suite 202, Glen Ellyn, IL 60137, USA; [b] Division of Medicine, Charles E. Schmidt College of Biomedical Science, Florida Atlantic University, 777 Glades Road, Boca Raton, FL 33431, USA
* Corresponding author.
E-mail address: kmaki@mc-mcr.com

Cardiol Clin 33 (2015) 233–243
http://dx.doi.org/10.1016/j.ccl.2015.02.004
0733-8651/15/$ – see front matter © 2015 Elsevier Inc. All rights reserved.

pravastatin therapy was associated with a lesser risk for development of diabetes mellitus, defined as a blood glucose level of 7.0 mmol/L or greater (126 mg/dL).[14] Subjects assigned to receive pravastatin had a 30% reduction in the risk for developing diabetes, compared with placebo, in multivariate analysis (hazard ratio [HR], 0.70; 95% CI, 0.50–0.99; $P = .042$). Because these analyses were post hoc and not predefined, it was acknowledged that they should be considered hypothesis generating and interpreted with caution.

## Justification for the Use of Statins in Prevention: an Intervention Trial Evaluating Rosuvastatin

The WOSCOPS results sparked interest in pursuing a formal, prospective analysis of the relationship between T2DM risk and statin use. The Justification for the Use of Statins in Prevention: an Intervention Trial Evaluating Rosuvastatin (JUPITER) was a study of 17,802 apparently healthy men and women with low-density lipoprotein cholesterol levels of less than 130 mg/dL and high-sensitivity C-reactive protein levels of 2.0 mg/L or more treated with rosuvastatin 20 mg/d or placebo (n = 8901 in each group) and followed for a median of 1.9 years.[4] The study included protocol-specified comparisons of glucose changes and physician-reported T2DM incidence between treatments. The results of JUPITER indicated that there were no differences between treatment groups in incidence of newly diagnosed glycosuria (rosuvastatin, n = 36; placebo, n = 32) or fasting blood glucose concentrations. A difference between groups in median $HbA_{1C}$ concentration, although small, was detected, with a significantly higher value observed in the rosuvastatin group (5.9% vs 5.8% in the placebo group; $P = .001$). Furthermore, in the rosuvastatin group, there were significantly ($P = .01$) more cases of physician-reported diabetes (not adjudicated by the endpoint committee) among subjects receiving rosuvastatin (270 reports) versus subjects receiving placebo (216 reports; Table 1).

A follow-up analysis from JUPITER included stratification of participants on the basis of whether they had none or at least 1 of the following 4 major risk factors for developing diabetes: the metabolic syndrome, impaired fasting glucose, body mass index of 30 $kg/m^2$ or greater, or $HbA_{1C}$ of greater than 6% (see Table 1).[5] Of the participants, 6095 had no major diabetes mellitus risk factors and 11,508 had at least 1 diabetes risk factor. During follow-up, there were 54 more new cases of T2DM in rosuvastatin-treated subjects with at least 1 diabetes risk factor compared with placebo-treated subjects with at least 1 diabetes risk factor (258 and 204 cases, respectively; $P = .01$). Importantly, all of the excess cases of T2DM with rosuvastatin occurred in patients with at least 1 major diabetes risk factor. There was no difference between treatment groups in the number of new T2DM cases among subjects with no diabetes risk factors (12 cases in each). The HRs (95% CIs) for developing diabetes associated with rosuvastatin use compared with placebo among subjects with none versus at least 1 diabetes risk factor were 0.99 (0.45–2.21) and 1.28 (1.07–1.54), respectively. These results suggest that risk for developing diabetes while on statin therapy may be limited to those with major T2DM risk factors.

Although the risk for developing diabetes was increased modestly, the risk for the primary

**Table 1**
**Risk for developing T2DM with rosuvastatin treatment according to the number of diabetes risk factors in JUPITER**

| Event and Hazard Ratio | Placebo (n = 8901) | Rosuvastatin (n = 8901) | Difference | P-Value |
|---|---|---|---|---|
| New T2DM (All) | 216 (2.4%) | 270 (3.0%) | +54 | .01 |
| New T2DM (0 DM RF) | 12 (0.2%) | 12 (0.2%) | 0 | .99 |
| New T2DM (≥1 DM RF) | 204 (1.7%) | 258 (2.1%) | +54 | .01 |
| HR (95% CI) 0 DM RF | — | 0.99 (0.45, 2.21) | −1% | — |
| HR (95% CI) ≥1 DM RF | — | 1.28 (1.07, 1.54) | +28% | — |

There were 6095 patients with no major diabetes mellitus risk factors and 11,508 with ≥1 risk factor. Diabetes mellitus risk factors included the metabolic syndrome, impaired fasting glucose, body mass index of ≥30 $kg/m^2$, and glycated hemoglobin of >6%.

*Abbreviations:* CI, confidence interval; HR, hazard ratio; JUPITER, Justification for Use of Statins in Prevention: an Intervention Trial Evaluating Rosuvastatin; RF, risk factors; T2DM, type 2 diabetes mellitus.

*Data from* Ridker PM, Pradhan A, MacFadyen JG, et al. Cardiovascular benefits and diabetes risks of statin therapy in primary prevention: an analysis from the JUPITER trial. Lancet 2012;380:565–71.

cardiovascular endpoint (myocardial infarction, stroke, arterial revascularization, hospitalization for unstable angina, or death from cardiovascular causes) in JUPITER was reduced substantially with rosuvastatin overall and in subjects with and without major diabetes risk factors (**Table 2**). In those with at least 1 risk factor, rosuvastatin treatment was associated with a 39% reduction in the primary endpoint (HR, 0.61; 95% CI, 0.47–0.79; $P$ = .0001), and among subjects with no diabetes risk factors, rosuvastatin treatment was associated with a 52% reduction in the primary endpoint (HR, 0.48; 95% CI, 0.33–0.68; $P$ = .0001).[4,5]

## Metaanalyses of Statin Clinical Trials and the Risk:Benefit Ratio

Because of the apparent conflicting findings for new-onset diabetes between the WOSCOPS and JUPITER trials of statin therapy, metaanalyses of clinical trials have been conducted to further examine the association.[7,8,15] Sattar and colleagues[7] identified 13 statin trials with 91,140 participants, of whom 4278 (statin treated [n = 2226] and control treated [n = 2052]) developed diabetes during a mean of 4 years of follow-up (**Fig. 1**). Statin therapy was associated with 9% increased odds for incident diabetes (odds ratio, 1.09; 95% CI 1.02–1.17) with little heterogeneity between trials ($I^2$ = 11%). Although the power was limited to detect differences regarding the association with T2DM among 5 statins—rosuvastatin, atorvastatin, pravastatin, simvastatin, and lovastatin—it is important to recognize that no differences were identified. The number of patients that would need to be treated for 4 years to

produce 1 excess case of T2DM was estimated to be 255 (95% CI, 150–852). The benefit associated with each 1 mmol/L (38.7 mg/dL) decrease in low-density lipoprotein cholesterol over 4 years of statin use, based on an analysis of the Cholesterol Treatment Trialists' group, was reported to be a prevention of 5.4 coronary heart disease events (including myocardial infarction and fatal coronary heart disease).[1] The inclusion of revascularizations and strokes in this analysis roughly doubles the cardiovascular benefit.[2] Thus, when comparing risk and benefit for statin use, as many as 5 to 10 major adverse cardiovascular events might be prevented for each excess case of T2DM associated with use of statin therapy in those with T2DM risk, similar to the average risk among those in the statin trials evaluated.

In another metaanalysis, Preiss and colleagues[8] identified 5 statin trials that compared intensive- with moderate-dosage statin therapy. These included 32,752 participants, of whom 2749 (intensive dosage statin treated [n = 1449] and moderate dosage statin treated [n = 1300]) developed diabetes, and of whom 6684 (intensive dosage statin treated [n = 3134] and moderate dosage statin treated [n = 3550]) experienced a cardiovascular event during a mean follow-up of 4.9 years. The statin therapies defined as intensive dosage in this metaanalysis were atorvastatin 80 mg and simvastatin 80 mg, and the moderate dosage statin therapies were pravastatin 40 mg, simvastatin 10 to 40 mg, and atorvastatin 10 mg. There were 2.0 additional cases of T2DM in the intensive dosage group per 1000 patient-years, and 6.5 fewer cardiovascular events in the intensive dosage group per 1000 patient-years. Odds

**Table 2**
**Risk for the primary cardiovascular endpoint with rosuvastatin treatment according to the number of diabetes risk factors in JUPITER**

| Event and HR | Placebo (n = 8901) | Rosuvastatin (n = 8901) | Difference | P-Value |
|---|---|---|---|---|
| 1° CVD endpoint (All) | 251 (2.8%) | 142 (1.6%) | −109 | .0001 |
| 1° CVD endpoint (0 DM RF) | 91 (1.5%) | 44 (0.7%) | −47 | .0001 |
| 1° CVD endpoint (≥1 DM RF) | 157 (1.3%) | 96 (0.8%) | −61 | .0001 |
| HR (95% CI) 0 DM RF | — | 0.48 (0.33, 0.68) | −52% | |
| HR (95% CI) ≥1 DM RF | — | 0.61 (0.47, 0.79) | −39% | |

There were 6095 patients with no major diabetes mellitus risk factors and 11,508 with ≥1 risk factor. Diabetes mellitus risk factors included metabolic syndrome, impaired fasting glucose, body mass index of ≥30 kg/m², and glycated hemoglobin of >6%.

*Abbreviations:* 1°, primary; CI, confidence interval; CVD, cardiovascular disease; DM, diabetes mellitus; HR, hazard ratio; JUPITER, Justification for Use of Statins in Prevention: an Intervention Trial Evaluating Rosuvastatin; RF, risk factor.

*Data from* Ridker PM, Danielson E, Fonseca FA, et al. JUPITER Study Group. Rosuvastatin to prevent vascular events in men and women with elevated C-reactive protein. N Engl J Med 2008;359:2195–207; and Ridker PM, Pradhan A, Mac-Fadyen JG, et al. Cardiovascular benefits and diabetes risks of statin therapy in primary prevention: an analysis from the JUPITER trial. Lancet 2012;380:565–71.

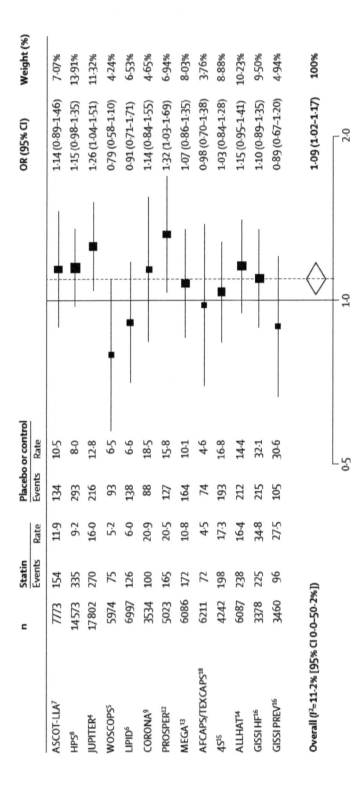

| | n | Statin | | Placebo or control | | OR (95% CI) | Weight (%) |
|---|---|---|---|---|---|---|---|
| | | Events | Rate | Events | Rate | | |
| ASCOT-LLA[7] | 7773 | 154 | 11·9 | 134 | 10·5 | 1·14 (0·89–1·46) | 7·07% |
| HPS[8] | 14573 | 335 | 9·2 | 293 | 8·0 | 1·15 (0·98–1·35) | 13·91% |
| JUPITER[4] | 17802 | 270 | 16·0 | 216 | 12·8 | 1·26 (1·04–1·51) | 11·32% |
| WOSCOPS[5] | 5974 | 75 | 5·2 | 93 | 6·5 | 0·79 (0·58–1·10) | 4·24% |
| LIPID[6] | 6997 | 126 | 6·0 | 138 | 6·6 | 0·91 (0·71–1·71) | 6·53% |
| CORONA[9] | 3534 | 100 | 20·9 | 88 | 18·5 | 1·14 (0·84–1·55) | 4·65% |
| PROSPER[12] | 5023 | 165 | 20·5 | 127 | 15·8 | 1·32 (1·03–1·69) | 6·94% |
| MEGA[13] | 6086 | 172 | 10·8 | 164 | 10·1 | 1·07 (0·86–1·35) | 8·03% |
| AFCAPS/TEXCAPS[18] | 6211 | 72 | 4·5 | 74 | 4·6 | 0·98 (0·70–1·38) | 3·76% |
| 4S[5] | 4242 | 198 | 17·3 | 193 | 16·8 | 1·03 (0·84–1·28) | 8·88% |
| ALLHAT[14] | 6087 | 238 | 16·4 | 212 | 14·4 | 1·15 (0·95–1·41) | 10·23% |
| GISSI HF[16] | 3378 | 225 | 34·8 | 215 | 32·1 | 1·10 (0·89–1·35) | 9·50% |
| GISSI PREV[16] | 3460 | 96 | 27·5 | 105 | 30·6 | 0·89 (0·67–1·20) | 4·94% |
| Overall (I²=11·2% [95% CI 0·0–50·2%]) | | | | | | 1·09 (1·02–1·17) | 100% |

Fig. 1. Statin therapy and incident diabetes in cardiovascular endpoint trials.[7] 4S, Scandinavian Simvastatin Survival Study; AFCAPS/TEXCAPS, Air Force/Texas Coronary Atherosclerosis Prevention Study; ALLHAT, Antihypertensive and Lipid-Lowering Treatment to Prevent Heart Attack Trial; ASCOT-LLA, Anglo-Scandinavian Cardiac Outcomes Trial – Lipid-Lowering Arm; CI, confidence interval; CORONA, Controlled Rosuvastatin Multinational Trial in Heart Failure; GISSI-HF, Gruppo Italiano per lo Studio della Sopravvivenza nell'Insufficienza Cardiaca; JUPITER, Justification for Use of Statins in Prevention: an Intervention Trial Evaluating Rosuvastatin; LIPID, Long-term Intervention with Pravastatin in Ischemic Disease; MEGA, Management of Elevated Cholesterol in the Primary Prevention Group of Adult Japanese; OR, odds ratio; PROSPER, Prospective Study of Pravastatin in the Elderly at Risk; WOSCOPS, West of Scotland Coronary Prevention Study. (*From* Sattar N, Preiss D, Murray HM, et al. Statins and risk of incident diabetes: a collaborative meta-analysis of randomized statin trials. Lancet 2010;375:737; with permission.)

ratios (95% CIs) for new-onset diabetes and cardiovascular events, respectively, for those receiving intensive dosage compared with moderate dosage statin therapy were 1.12 (1.04–1.22) and 0.84 (0.75–0.94; **Fig. 2**). The number of patients who would need to be treated for 1 year with intensive dosage statin therapy versus moderate dosage statin therapy to produce 1 excess case of T2DM was estimated to be 498, and the number of patients that would need to be treated for 1 year with intensive versus moderate dosage statin therapy to prevent 1 cardiovascular event was 155. Accordingly, 3.2 cardiovascular events would be prevented for each excess case of diabetes with intensive versus moderate dosage statin therapy.

The results of these metaanalyses indicate that statin use is associated with a modest, but statistically significant, increase in risk for the development of T2DM of approximately 10% to 12% overall. T2DM risk with statin therapy is somewhat greater for more intensive dosage statin regimens and the increase in risk seems likely to be more pronounced (25%–30%) in those with major T2DM risk factors.[5,8,9] However, available data indicate that several fewer major cardiovascular events should be expected to occur for each excess case of new-onset diabetes associated with statin therapy, or intensification of statin therapy.

The definition of intensity with regard to statin therapies is somewhat complicated. The American College of Cardiology/American Heart Association 2013 cholesterol guidelines[16] defined high-intensity statins as regimens that reduce low-density lipoprotein cholesterol by at least 50%, and included rosuvastatin 20 and 40 mg and atorvastatin 40 and 80 mg (although according to the largest study of atorvastatin, a 40 mg dosage reduced low-density lipoprotein cholesterol by just 48%[17]). Simvastatin 80 mg was placed in the moderate category. This is different from the definition of intensive dosage therapy used in the Preiss metaanalysis.[8]

Three studies have compared 2 dosages of the same statin: Treating to New Targets (80 vs 10 mg atorvastatin),[18] Aggrastat to Zocor (80 vs 20 mg simvastatin),[19] and the Study of the Effectiveness of Additional Reductions in Cholesterol and Homocysteine (80 vs 20 mg simvastatin).[20] However, there are no studies that compare statins at similar degrees of efficacy. Thus, although the available data support the view that higher intensity (efficacy) regimens increase risk for diabetes more than lower intensity (efficacy) regimens, additional research is needed to determine whether there are differences between statins with regard to diabetogenicity at similar degrees of low-density lipoprotein cholesterol reduction.

## Observational Studies of the Relationship Between Statin Use and Diabetes Risk

Data from randomized, clinical trials are very useful for assessing hazards and benefits of therapies, but may have limitations, including relatively short follow-up periods, minimal enrollment of those at greatest risk for ancillary outcomes, and lack of standardized methods for ascertainment of adverse outcomes such as incident T2DM. Therefore, it is also useful to consider results from observational studies. For the association between initiation of statin therapy and new-onset T2DM, the observational data have been consistently supportive of the findings from clinical trials.[21–24] For example, an analysis of electronic medical records from 500 general practices in the UK, including data from 285,864 men and women from 2000 to 2010, indicated that during 1.2 million person-years of follow-up there were 13,455 cases of T2DM, and that statin initiation was associated with increased risk for T2DM (HR [95% CI] of 1.45 [1.39–1.50] before adjusting for potential confounders and 1.14 [1.10–1.19] after adjustment).[21] A systematic review and metaanalysis of 90 observational studies of statin use from 1988 to 2012, which examined the unintended effects of statins, reported an increased risk of diabetes for patients exposed to statins of 31% (odds ratio, 1.31; 95% CI, 0.99–1.73).[24]

Corrao and colleagues[22] investigated the relationship between adherence to statin therapy and risk for developing diabetes in a cohort of 115,708 persons in Italy who started taking statins during 2003 and 2004 and were followed until 2010. Adherence to the statin was assessed by the proportion of days covered with statins (exposure) based on pharmacy refill records. During follow-up, 11,154 subjects were diagnosed with diabetes. Compared with patients with very low adherence (proportion of days covered, <25%), those with low (26%–50%), intermediate (51%–75%), and high (≥75%) adherence to statin therapy had increased risks for developing diabetes (HRs [95% CIs] of 1.12 [1.06–1.18], 1.22 [1.14–1.27], and 1.32 [1.26–1.39], respectively; **Fig. 3**).

The greater risk for diabetes associated with the use of higher intensity statins that has been shown in clinical trials[8] has also been confirmed in observational studies of statin use and diabetes. In an examination of 8 population-based cohort studies and a metaanalysis from 6 Canadian provinces and 2 international databases from the United

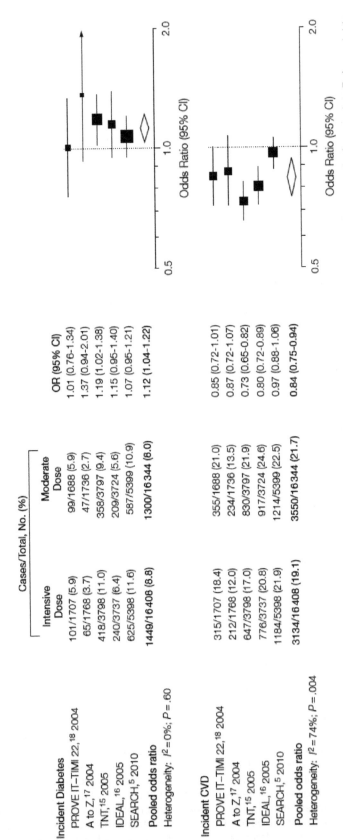

| Cases/Total, No. (%) | | |
| --- | --- | --- |
| | Intensive Dose | Moderate Dose | OR (95% CI) |
| **Incident Diabetes** | | | |
| PROVE IT–TIMI 22,[18] 2004 | 101/1707 (5.9) | 99/1688 (5.9) | 1.01 (0.76-1.34) |
| A to Z,[17] 2004 | 65/1768 (3.7) | 47/1736 (2.7) | 1.37 (0.94-2.01) |
| TNT,[15] 2005 | 418/3798 (11.0) | 358/3797 (9.4) | 1.19 (1.02-1.38) |
| IDEAL,[16] 2005 | 240/3737 (6.4) | 209/3724 (5.6) | 1.15 (0.95-1.40) |
| SEARCH,[5] 2010 | 625/5398 (11.6) | 587/5399 (10.9) | 1.07 (0.95-1.21) |
| Pooled odds ratio | 1449/16408 (8.8) | 1300/16344 (8.0) | 1.12 (1.04-1.22) |
| Heterogeneity: $I^2$ = 0%; $P$ = .60 | | | |
| **Incident CVD** | | | |
| PROVE IT–TIMI 22,[18] 2004 | 315/1707 (18.4) | 355/1688 (21.0) | 0.85 (0.72-1.01) |
| A to Z,[17] 2004 | 212/1768 (12.0) | 234/1736 (13.5) | 0.87 (0.72-1.07) |
| TNT,[15] 2005 | 647/3798 (17.0) | 830/3797 (21.9) | 0.73 (0.65-0.82) |
| IDEAL,[16] 2005 | 776/3737 (20.8) | 917/3724 (24.6) | 0.80 (0.72-0.89) |
| SEARCH,[5] 2010 | 1184/5398 (21.9) | 1214/5399 (22.5) | 0.97 (0.88-1.06) |
| Pooled odds ratio | 3134/16408 (19.1) | 3550/16344 (21.7) | 0.84 (0.75-0.94) |
| Heterogeneity: $I^2$ = 74%; $P$ = .004 | | | |

**Fig. 2.** Metaanalysis of new-onset diabetes and first major cardiovascular events in clinical trials of intensive versus moderate dosage statin therapy. A to Z, Aggrastat to Zocor; CI, confidence interval; CVD, cardiovascular disease; IDEAL, Incremental Decrease in End Points Through Aggressive Lipid Lowering; OR, odds ratio; PROVE IT–TIMI 22, Pravastatin or Atorvastatin Evaluation and Infection Therapy – Thrombolysis in Myocardial Infarction; SEARCH, Study of the Effectiveness of Additional Reductions in Cholesterol and Homocysteine; TNT, Treating to New Targets. (*From* Preiss D, Seshasai SR, Welsh P, et al. Risk of incident diabetes with intensive-dose compared with moderate-dose statin therapy: a meta-analysis. JAMA 2011;305:2560; with permission.)

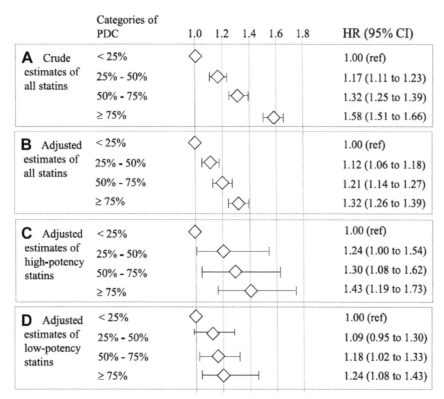

**Fig. 3.** (*A*) Effect of adherence to statin therapy (defined as categories of proportion of days covered) on HRs for the development of diabetes. (*B–D*) Adjusted estimates were made for age (continuous), sex, first-line statin therapy, concomitant use of other drugs, history of cardiovascular disease, categories of Charlson comorbidity index score, number of cholesterolemia tests, and number of outpatient specialist visits. CI, confidence interval; HR, hazard ratio; PDC, proportion of days covered; ref, reference. (*From* Corrao G, Ibrahim B, Nicotra F, et al. Statins and the risk of diabetes: evidence from a large population-based cohort study. Diabetes Care 2014;37:2229; with permission.)

States and the UK, Dormuth and colleagues[23] measured the incremental increase in new-onset diabetes associated with taking higher versus lower intensity statins in 136,966 secondary prevention patients between 1997 and 2011. In the first 2 years of regular statin use, there was a significant increase in the risk of new-onset diabetes with higher intensity statins compared with lower intensity agents (fixed effect rate ratio, 1.15; 95% CI, 1.05–1.26). It was estimated that 342 secondary prevention patients needed to be treated with a higher intensity statin instead of a lower intensity statin for 2 years to produce 1 additional case of diabetes.

## Mechanisms for Causality Between Use of Statins and Increased Diabetes Risk

Major causal factors for T2DM include insulin resistance (peripheral and hepatic) and a defect in the ability of pancreatic β cells to provide sufficient insulin to maintain normal blood glucose levels.[25,26] In combination, these defects result in an imbalance between the rate at which glucose enters the circulation from the liver, intestine, and kidney, and the rate at which glucose is removed from the circulation by the tissues, producing hyperglycemia. To date, there have been relatively few clinical investigations of the effects of statin therapy on determinants of glucose homeostasis.[27–30] Results from studies in animal models and cell cultures suggest a number of cellular mechanisms may be involved, but none of these has been sufficiently demonstrated in humans.[31–33]

In a systematic review and metaanalysis, Baker and colleagues[28] examined the effects of statin treatment on insulin sensitivity in nondiabetic patients, and found no significant class effect of statins in 16 studies. However, subset analyses suggested a modest increase in insulin sensitivity with pravastatin, a modest decrease with simvastatin, and no difference from the comparison conditions for atorvastatin or rosuvastatin. Most of the studies considered in the Baker metaanalysis did not use reference methods for the measurement of insulin sensitivity, and many were also small and likely to be underpowered. A study by Lamendola and colleagues[27] that did use a reference method (modified insulin suppression test) reported no difference in the steady-state plasma glucose concentration for rosuvastatin versus baseline or versus the change with gemfibrozil treatment in 39 insulin-resistant, nondiabetic patients with combined dyslipidemia.

Swerdlow and colleagues[15] recently investigated whether the increase in new-onset T2DM with statin use may be explained by inhibition of 3-hydroxy-3-methylglutaryl coenzyme A reductase (HMGCR). Associations between single nucleotide polymorphisms of the HMGCR gene (rs17238484 and rs12916) that produce lower HMGCR activity and T2DM risk were assessed using data from 223,463 individuals in 43 genetic studies. These HMGCR variants were associated with higher mean (95% CI) plasma glucose concentration (0.23% [95% CI, 0.02–0.44]), and with higher risk of T2DM (odds ratio [95% CI] per rs17238484-G allele of 1.02 [1.00–1.05] and per rs12916-T allele of 1.06 [1.03–1.09]). These findings suggest that the effect of statins on T2DM risk is caused, at least in part, by HMGCR inhibition, and support the hypothesis that the intensity of HMGCR inhibition is important for diabetes risk, but it is unknown whether this effect is independent of the reduction in low-density lipoprotein cholesterol.

At present, the evidence regarding a potential mechanistic link between statin therapy and increased risk for insulin sensitivity or the development of diabetes mellitus are mixed. Additional studies are needed urgently to assess possible influences of statins on hepatic and peripheral insulin sensitivity and pancreatic β cell function, particularly in patients with major T2DM risk factors.

## Impact of Statin Therapy on Glycemic Control in Patients with Diabetes Mellitus

Although there have been many clinical outcomes trials that enrolled subjects with diabetes, relatively few of these have reported the effects of statins on glycemic control.[34–38] In the Heart Protection Study, 40 mg/d simvastatin (n = 10,269) or placebo (n = 10,267) was administered to high-risk patients,[34,35] 5963 of whom had been diagnosed with diabetes. Plasma HbA$_{1C}$ measured at study entry in a random sample of the diabetic subjects (n = 1087) indicated mean (standard error of the mean) values of 6.99% (0.11) for simvastatin and 7.06% (0.10) for placebo; follow-up values 4 to 6 years later were 7.14% (0.06) and 7.17% (0.06),

respectively. There was no difference between groups for the increase in HbA$_{1C}$ (simvastatin 0.15% [0.09] vs placebo 0.12% [0.09]).

In the Collaborative Atorvastatin Diabetes Study, which administered 10 mg/d atorvastatin (n = 1410) or placebo (n = 1428) to patients with T2DM, but without evidence of clinical cardiovascular disease, mean HbA$_{1C}$ increased from 7.9% (1.4) to 8.3% (1.5) and from 7.8% (1.4) to 8.1% (1.5) after 4 years of treatment with atorvastatin and placebo, respectively.[36] This outcome was suggestive of a modestly greater increase in HbA$_{1C}$ with atorvastatin, but the results may have been biased or confounded by dropout or changes in the use of medication(s) for glycemic control. In the Atorvastatin in Factorial with Omega-3 EE90 Risk Reduction in Diabetes trial, which administered atorvastatin 20 mg/d and omega-3-acid ethyl esters 2 g/d, using a 2-by-2 factorial design, to patients with T2DM, but without known cardiovascular disease, mean HbA$_{1C}$ at baseline was 7.0% in both groups, and 4 months later had increased by 0.3% among subjects taking atorvastatin relative to placebo (P<.0001).[37]

In a metaanalysis of 26 randomized, controlled trials of statin therapy in 3232 subjects with T2DM, Zhou and colleagues[38] assessed the influence of statin therapy on glycemic control and reported unremarkable increases in HbA$_{1C}$ (weighted mean difference, 0.04%; 95% CI, -0.08 to 0.16; $I^2$ = 45.7%) and fasting plasma glucose (2.25 mg/dL; 95% CI, -3.50 to 7.99; $I^2$ = 46%). When examined by specific statin, atorvastatin therapy was associated with a modest increase in HbA$_{1C}$ (weighted mean difference, 0.20%; 95% CI, 0.08–0.31), and simvastatin therapy was associated with a modest reduction in HbA$_{1C}$ (weighted mean difference, -0.26%; 95% CI, -0.48 to -0.04). There were no effects observed for cerivastatin, lovastatin, or rosuvastatin (no results for fluvastatin, pravastatin, and pitavastatin were reported).

The JUPITER trial, although it did not include subjects with diabetes, suggested a slightly greater increase from baseline in HbA$_{1C}$ among subjects assigned to rosuvastatin treatment (mean [standard deviation] 0.30% [0.35]) compared with placebo (0.22% [0.40]; P<.001).[4,39] There was no change in fasting serum glucose between the treatment groups (mean [standard deviation] 3 [18.3] mg/dL for rosuvastatin vs 2 [17.3] mg/dL for placebo).

In summary, few data exist regarding the effects of statin therapy on glycemic control in patients with diabetes mellitus. However, the available results suggest that if there is an adverse effect, it is sufficiently small that it is likely to be easily managed by changing the medication regimen for glycemia management. Research is also needed to determine the effects of statin discontinuation on management of glycemic control, that is, if a patient stops taking a statin after statin-associated deterioration in glycemia, would plasma glucose and $HbA_{1C}$ return to their prestatin levels?

## Clinical Guidance

The guidelines for screening and the criteria for the diagnosis of T2DM in the asymptomatic patient as outlined in the *Standards of Medical Care in Diabetes* from the American Diabetes Association,[40,41] and recommended by the National Lipid Association Statin Diabetes Task Force,[10] are listed below.

### Criteria for Screening

- Testing to detect T2DM and prediabetes (fasting glucose, $HbA_{1C}$ or a 75 g oral glucose tolerance test) in asymptomatic, nonpregnant people should be considered in adults of any age who are overweight or obese (body mass index $\geq$25 kg/m$^2$ or $\geq$23 kg/m$^2$ in Asian Americans) and who have 1 or more of the additional risk factors for diabetes listed:
  - Physical inactivity,
  - First-degree relative with T2DM,
  - High-risk race/ethnicity,
  - Hypertension or history of cardiovascular disease,
  - Polycystic ovary syndrome, delivery of a baby weighing greater than 9 pounds, or diagnosed with gestational diabetes,
  - High triglycerides and/or low high-density lipoprotein cholesterol,
  - Impaired fasting glucose, impaired glucose tolerance, or $HbA_{1C}$ of 5.7 or more, and
  - Another condition associated with insulin resistance.
- In those without risk factors, testing should begin at age 45 years.
- If tests are normal, repeat testing at 3-year intervals or less is reasonable. However, testing should be repeated within 1 year of starting a statin.

Screening should occur before initiation of statin therapy in those with at least 1 major diabetes risk factor, although clinicians should not generally delay the initiation of statin therapy to await results from screening tests in a patient for whom statin therapy is indicated. Managing diabetes risk factors to prevent diabetes is of utmost importance whether or not a patient is taking a statin. Medical nutrition therapy directed at weight loss (often 5%–10% of body weight) in those who are overweight or obese and regular physical activity (at least 150 minutes per week of walking or equivalent activities and limiting the amount of time spent being sedentary by breaking up extended amounts of time spent sitting) are central to efforts to prevent diabetes.[40,41] Regularly monitoring weight and preventing weight gain in patients taking a statin are particularly important.

## Potential Use of Nonstatin Add-On Therapy as an Alternative to Statin Intensification in Primary Prevention

The results from the IMProved Reduction of Outcomes: Vytorin Efficacy International Trial (IMPROVE-IT) study supported the cardiovascular benefit of lipid lowering with a Nieman-Pick C1-Like 1 protein inhibitor (ezetimibe) as add-on therapy to a statin in 18,444 patients after acute coronary syndromes.[42,43] The results for ezetimibe as a statin add-on were consistent with effects predicted from studies of statin therapy,[1,44] producing an approximate 10% reduction in major adverse cardiovascular outcomes with a reduction of approximately 0.43 mmol/L (16.7 mg/dL) in low-density lipoprotein cholesterol. Notably, no excess risk for diabetes was observed with ezetimibe plus simvastatin compared with placebo plus simvastatin.[43] These results suggest that the combination of a statin with ezetimibe may be a reasonable alternative to intensification of statin therapy in primary prevention patients with major T2DM risk factors, although it should be emphasized that this strategy has not been tested directly in clinical trials.

## SUMMARY

- Statin use is associated with a modest increase in risk ($\sim$10%–12%) for new-onset T2DM, compared with placebo or usual care.
- Intensive dosage statin therapy seems to increase diabetes risk beyond that of moderate dosage statin therapy.
- Excess risk for diabetes with statin use is most clearly evident in those with major risk factors for diabetes.
- The cardiovascular benefits of statin therapy outweigh the potential risk for diabetes development, with several cardiovascular events prevented for each excess case of diabetes.
- Statin therapy should continue to be recommended when appropriate for the reduction of cardiovascular disease event risk.

- Lifestyle modification should be emphasized to all patients for whom statin therapy is recommended to:
  - Reduce cardiovascular risk, and
  - Attenuate the increase in diabetes risk.
- Patients with risk factors for diabetes should be screened, generally with fasting glucose or HbA$_{1C}$, ideally before starting statin therapy, within 1 year of initiation, and at intervals no longer than 3 years thereafter.

# REFERENCES

1. Cholesterol Treatment Trialists' (CTT) Collaboration, Baigent C, Blackwell L, Emberson J, et al. Efficacy and safety of more intensive lowering of LDL cholesterol: a meta-analysis of data from 170,000 participants in 26 randomised trials. Lancet 2010;376:1670–81.
2. Cholesterol Treatment Trialists' (CTT) Collaborators, Mihaylova B, Emberson J, Blackwell L, et al. The effects of lowering LDL cholesterol with statin therapy in people at low risk of vascular disease: meta-analysis of individual data from 27 randomised trials. Lancet 2012;380:581–90.
3. Taylor R. Banting Memorial Lecture 2012: reversing the twin cycles of type 2 diabetes. Diabet Med 2013;30:267–75.
4. Ridker PM, Danielson E, Fonseca FA, et al, JUPITER Study Group. Rosuvastatin to prevent vascular events in men and women with elevated C-reactive protein. N Engl J Med 2008;359:2195–207.
5. Ridker PM, Pradhan A, MacFadyen JG, et al. Cardiovascular benefits and diabetes risks of statin therapy in primary prevention: an analysis from the JUPITER trial. Lancet 2012;380:565–71.
6. Rajpathak SN, Kumbhani DJ, Crandall J, et al. Statin therapy and risk of developing type 2 diabetes: a meta-analysis. Diabetes Care 2009;32:1924–9.
7. Sattar N, Preiss D, Murray HM, et al. Statins and risk of incident diabetes: a collaborative meta-analysis of randomized statin trials. Lancet 2010;375:735–42.
8. Preiss D, Seshasai SR, Welsh P, et al. Risk of incident diabetes with intensive-dose compared with moderate-dose statin therapy: a meta-analysis. JAMA 2011;305:2556–64.
9. Waters DD, Ho JE, DeMicco DA, et al. Predictors of new-onset diabetes in patients treated with atorvastatin: results from 3 large randomized clinical trials. J Am Coll Cardiol 2011;57:1535–45.
10. Maki KC, Ridker PM, Brown WV, et al. An assessment by the statin diabetes safety task force: 2014 update. J Clin Lipidol 2014;8:S17–29.
11. National Center for Chronic Disease Prevention and Health Promotion. Division of Diabetes Translation. National Diabetes Statistics Report. 2014. Available at: http://www.cdc.gov/diabetes/pubs/statsreport14/ national-diabetes-report-web.pdf. Accessed February 24, 2015.
12. International Diabetes Federation. IDF Diabetes Atlas. 6th edition. 2014. Available at: http://www.idf.org/sites/default/files/Atlas-poster-2014_EN.pdf. Accessed February 24, 2015.
13. Food and Drug Administration. FDA drug safety communication: important safety label changes to cholesterol lowering statin drugs. Available at: http://www.fda.gov/Drugs/DrugSafety/ucm293101.htm. Accessed November 6, 2013.
14. Freeman DJ, Norrie J, Sattar N, et al. Pravastatin and the development of diabetes mellitus: evidence for a protective treatment effect in the West of Scotland Coronary Prevention Study. Circulation 2001;103:357–62.
15. Swerdlow DJ, Preiss D, Kuchenbaecker KB, et al. HMG-coenzyme A reductase inhibition, type 2 diabetes, and bodyweight: evidence from genetic analysis and randomised trials. Lancet 2015;385:351–61.
16. Stone NJ, Robinson JG, Lichtenstein AH, et al. 2013 ACC/AHA guideline on the treatment of blood cholesterol to reduce atherosclerotic cardiovascular risk in adults: a report of the American College of Cardiology/American Heart Association Task Force on Practice Guidelines. J Am Coll Cardiol 2014;63(25 Pt B):2889–934.
17. Jones PH, Davidson MH, Stein EA, et al. Comparison of the efficacy and safety of rosuvastatin versus atorvastatin, simvastatin, and pravastatin across doses (STELLAR Trial). Am J Cardiol 2003;92:152–60.
18. LaRosa JC, Grundy SM, Waters DD, et al. Intensive lipid lowering with atorvastatin in patients with stable coronary disease. N Engl J Med 2005;352:1425–35.
19. de Lemos JA, Blazing MA, Wiviott SD, et al. Early intensive vs a delayed conservative simvastatin strategy in patients with acute coronary syndromes: phase Z of the A to Z trial. JAMA 2004;292:1307–16.
20. Study of the Effectiveness of Additional Reductions in Cholesterol and Homocysteine (SEARCH) Collaborative Group, Armitage J, Bowman L, et al. Intensive lowering of LDL cholesterol with 80 mg versus 20 mg simvastatin daily in 12,064 survivors of myocardial infarction: a double-blind randomised trial. Lancet 2010;376:1658–69.
21. Danaei G, Garcia Rodriquez LA, Fernandez Cantero O, et al. Statins and risk of diabetes: an analysis of electronic medical records to evaluate possible bias due to differential survival. Diabetes Care 2013;36:1236–40.
22. Corrao G, Ibrahim B, Nicotra F, et al. Statins and the risk of diabetes: evidence from a large population-based cohort study. Diabetes Care 2014;37:2225–32.
23. Dormuth CR, Filion KB, Paterson JM, et al. Canadian network for observational drug effect studies investigators. Higher potency statins and the risk of new

diabetes: multicenter, observational study of administrative databases. BMJ 2014;348:g3244.

24. Macedo AF, Taylor FC, Casas JP, et al. Unintended effects of statins from observational studies in the general population: systematic review and meta-analysis. BMC Med 2014;12:51.

25. Gerich JE. Measurements of renal glucose release. Diabetes 2001;50:905.

26. DeFronzo RA. Banting Lecture. From the triumvirate to the ominous octet: a new paradigm for the treatment of type 2 diabetes mellitus. Diabetes 2009; 58:773–95.

27. Lamendola C, Abbasi F, Chu JW, et al. Comparative effects of rosuvastatin and gemfibrozil on glucose, insulin, and lipid metabolism in insulin-resistant, nondiabetic patients with combined dyslipidemia. Am J Cardiol 2005;95:189–93.

28. Baker WL, Talati R, White CM, et al. Differing effect of statins on insulin sensitivity in non-diabetics: a systematic review and meta-analysis. Diabetes Res Clin Pract 2010;87:98–107.

29. Abbas A, Milles J, Ramachandran S. Rosuvastatin and atorvastatin: comparative effects on glucose metabolism in non-diabetic patients with dyslipidemia. Clin Med Insights Endocrinol Diabetes 2012;5: 13–30.

30. Sato H, Carvalho G, Sato T, et al. Statin intake is associated with decreased insulin sensitivity during cardiac surgery. Diabetes Care 2012;35:2095–9.

31. Sampson UK, Linto MF, Fazio S. Are statins diabetogenic? Curr Opin Cardiol 2011;26:342–7.

32. Banach M, Malodobra-Mazur M, Gluba A, et al. Statin therapy and new-onset diabetes: molecular mechanisms and clinical relevance. Curr Pharm Des 2013;19:4904–12.

33. Goldstein MR, Mascitelli L. Do statins cause diabetes? Curr Diab Rep 2013;13:381–90.

34. Heart Protection Study Collaborative Group. MRC/BHF Heart Protection Study of cholesterol lowering with simvastatin in 20,536 high-risk individuals: a randomised placebo-controlled trial. Lancet 2002; 360:7–22.

35. Collins R, Armitage J, Parish S, et al, Heart Protection Study Collaborative Group. MRC/BHF Heart Protection Study of cholesterol lowering with simvastatin in 5963 people with diabetes: a randomized placebo-controlled trial. Lancet 2003;361:2005–16.

36. Colhoun HM, Betteridge DJ, Durrington PN, et al, CARDS Investigators. Primary prevention of cardiovascular disease with atorvastatin in type 2 diabetes in the Collaborative Atorvastatin Diabetes Study (CARDS): multicenter randomized placebo-controlled trial. Lancet 2004;364:685–96.

37. Holman RR, Paul S, Farmer A, et al, Atorvastatin in Factorial with Omega 3 EE90 Risk Reduction in Diabetes Study Group. Atorvastatin in Factorial with Omega-3 EE90 Risk Reduction in Diabetes (AFORRD): a randomised controlled trial. Diabetologia 2009;52:50–9.

38. Zhou Y, Yuan Y, Cai RR, et al. Statin therapy on glycaemic control in type 2 diabetes: a meta-analysis. Expert Opin Pharmacother 2013;14:1575–84.

39. Astra Zeneca. Clinical briefing document – Endocrine and Metabolic Drugs Advisory Committee meeting for rosuvastatin (Crestor). Available at: http://www.fda.gov/downloads/AdvisoryCommittees/CommitteesMeetingMaterials/Drugs/Endocrinologicand MetabolicDrugsAdvisoryCommittee/UCM193833.pdf. Accessed November 5, 2013.

40. American Diabetes Association. Standards of medical care in diabetes – 2014. Diabetes Care 2014; 37(Suppl 1):S14–80.

41. American Diabetes Association. Standards of medical care in diabetes – 2015. Diabetes Care 2015; 38(Suppl 1):S1–90.

42. Katsiki N, Theocharidou E, Karagiannis A, et al. Ezetimibe therapy for dyslipidemia: an update. Curr Pharm Des 2013;19:3107–14.

43. Cannon CP on behalf of the IMPROVE IT Investigators. IMPROVE-IT Trial: A comparison of ezetimibe/simvastatin versus simvastatin monotherapy on cardiovascular outcomes after acute coronary syndromes. Late-breaking clinical trial abstracts and clinical science special reports abstracts from the American Heart Association's Scientific Sessions 2014. Circulation. 2014;130:2105–2126.

44. Cholesterol Treatment Trialists' (CTT) Collaborators, Baigent C, Keech A, Kearney PM, et al. Efficacy and safety of cholesterol-lowering treatment: prospective meta-analysis of data from 90,056 participants in 14 randomised trials of statins. Lancet 2005;366:1267–78.

# Statins and Cognitive Side Effects
## What Cardiologists Need to Know

Carlos Rojas-Fernandez, BSc (Pharm), PharmD[a,b,c,*],
Zain Hudani, BPharm, MSc Candidate[d],
Vera Bittner, MD, MSPH, FNLA[e]

## KEYWORDS

- Statins • Cognition • Memory • Adverse drug effects • Iatrogenesis • Drug safety

## KEY POINTS

- Adverse cognitive effects such as amnesia, concentration difficulties, confusion, and other complaints have been reported and attributed to statins in the lay press, the scientific literature, and by the US Food and Drug Administration (FDA) by way of spontaneous reports.
- Spontaneous reports from the FDA's Adverse Event Reporting System do not allow appropriate causality assessment.
- The weight of the evidence to date does not support the position that statins have a propensity to meaningfully or commonly contribute to adverse cognitive effects.
- Clinicians should not dismiss patient-reported cognitive effects. A thorough assessment should be conducted to rule out other potential causes.
- Baseline assessment of cognition before initiating a statin drug is not recommended at this time.

## INTRODUCTION

Since the approval of the first statin, lovastatin, on September 1, 1987 by the United States Food Drug Administration (FDA),[1] statins have revolutionized the primary and secondary prevention of atherosclerotic cardiovascular disease. A series of meta-analyses by the Cholesterol Treatment Trialists (CTT) summarizes the clinical trials evidence and documents significant reductions in nonfatal myocardial infarction and coronary death;

fatal and nonfatal stroke; coronary revascularizations; coronary mortality; and, importantly, in total mortality with statin therapy.[2] Statin benefits in these trials were proportional to the degree of reduction in low-density lipoprotein cholesterol levels in post-hoc analyses, were seen in patients across the spectrum of cardiovascular risk, and were largely independent of the baseline lipid profile.[2–4] Absolute risk reductions were greater in high-risk versus low-risk subjects.[2] In high-risk subjects with coronary disease, high-intensity

Disclosures: Dr C. Rojas-Fernandez receives research grant support from AstraZeneca, Pfizer, Bristol-Myers Squibb, Medisystems Pharmacy, and Remedy's Rx Pharmacies; Dr V. Bittner receives research support from Amgen, Astra Zeneca, Bayer Healthcare, Janssen Pharmaceuticals, Pfizer, and Sanofi Aventis, and is a consultant for Amgen and Eli Lilly.
<sup>a</sup> Schlegel-UW Research Institute for Ageing & School of Pharmacy, University of Waterloo, Waterloo, Ontario, Canada; <sup>b</sup> School of Public Health and Health Systems, Faculty of Applied Health Sciences, University of Waterloo, Waterloo, Ontario, Canada; <sup>c</sup> Michael G. DeGroote School of Medicine, Department of Family Medicine, McMaster University, Hamilton, Ontario, Canada; <sup>d</sup> University of Waterloo School of Pharmacy, 10 Victoria St S, Kitchener, Ontario N2G 1C5, Canada; <sup>e</sup> Division of Cardiovascular Disease, University of Alabama at Birmingham, LHRB 310, 701 19th Street South, Birmingham, AL 35294, USA
* Corresponding author. Schlegel Research Chair in Geriatric Pharmacotherapy, University of Waterloo School of Pharmacy, 10 Victoria St S, Room 7004, Kitchener, ON N2G 1C5.
E-mail address: carlos.rojas-fernandez@uwaterloo.ca

Cardiol Clin 33 (2015) 245–256
http://dx.doi.org/10.1016/j.ccl.2015.02.008
0733-8651/15/$ – see front matter © 2015 Elsevier Inc. All rights reserved.

statin therapy provides incremental benefits compared with moderate-intensity statin therapy.[5]

Despite these well-documented benefits, statins in general and high-intensity statins in particular remain underused. The most recent report based on the National Health and Nutrition Survey reveals that in 2011 to 2012, 29% of individuals with diagnosed cardiovascular disease and 37% of those with diabetes did not report using any lipid level–lowering medications.[6] This underuse is in part driven by concerns among clinicians and patients about statin safety. In the CTT meta-analyses, there was no increase in cancer incidence. Subsequent analyses of the clinical trials database showed an increase in the incidence of diabetes mellitus with statin use.[7] Statin myopathy is also well described, although the true incidence is a matter of controversy.[8,9] Both statin-induced diabetes and statin myopathy seem to be related to the intensity of statin therapy.[8,9]

Statin benefits and risks were carefully considered in the 2013 American College of Cardiology/American Heart Association Cholesterol Treatment Guidelines, which concluded that benefits outweigh risks for the 4 statin benefit groups and individuals with a risk of future cardiovascular events of more than 7.5% over the next 10 years, but the guidelines also emphasize the importance of individual benefit/risk discussions during the clinician-patient encounter.[10]

More recently, data from 2 randomized trials, 1 challenge-dechallenge study, and multiple case reports have suggested a potential association between statins and cognitive impairment.[11,12] In 2012, the FDA extended the warning section of statin labels to include a statement that statin use may contribute to "...notable, but ill defined memory loss or impairment that was reversible upon discontinuation of statin therapy."[13] The FDA stated that the data on which this statement was predicated did not suggest these cognitive changes to be common, or that they lead to clinically significant cognitive decline or impairment. Because statin drugs are widely used, these potential side effects need to be carefully considered and put in the context of available scientific evidence as well as the established benefits of statins.

## COGNITIVE IMPAIRMENT DEFINED AND IMPLICATIONS FOR IATROGENESIS

Cognition can be generally described under 4 domains: executive function, memory, language, and visuospatial ability. The risk-benefit profile of statins in relation to cognitive impairment is best considered with knowledge of the spectrum of cognitive disorders. Cognitive impairment can be defined as impairment in any of the aforementioned domains. Mild cognitive impairment (MCI) is a state between normal cognition and dementia, the latter being defined as cognitive impairment involving 2 domains and being sufficiently severe to interfere with daily activities and leading to a progressive loss of independence.[14] Clinically, patients with MCI have difficulties performing objective cognitive tasks, but the difficulties are not severe enough to impair instrumental activities of daily living. The distinction between MCI and dementia is often hazy because the demands of activities of daily living vary considerably depending on age, education, occupation, family situation, and other factors.

When considering potential cognitive effects of statins, clinicians should remember that MCI and dementia are common in individuals more than 65 years of age and can have a variety of causes, including neurodegenerative conditions such as Alzheimer disease, frontotemporal dementia, Parkinson disease, and dementia with Lewy bodies. Cognitive impairment may also be attributable to other conditions, including depression, infections, metabolic disturbances, inflammatory or vascular diseases, and anoxic injury, or may be secondary to various medications, or may occur in conjunction with general anesthesia or cardiopulmonary bypass. In addition, MCI/dementia may be the result of primary and secondary causes combined.[15] Although mixed dementias with primary and secondary causes are frequent, there is no gold standard for diagnosing these disorders.[16] In addition, variability exists in the clinical course of dementing illnesses. Some dementias progress slowly, some more rapidly, whereas others progress in spurts or at intermediate rates. The variable course of illness progression makes it difficult to interpret case reports of putative statin-induced cognitive adverse effects, because the duration and extent of follow-up vary across reports. In contrast, iatrogenic cognitive impairment from drugs that are well known to contribute to, or cause, cognitive impairment (**Table 1**) can be observed soon after the causative drug is started and are easily attributable to these medications from their clinical pharmacology.[17]

Considering the proportion of the population receiving statins, uncommon adverse effects have the potential to affect a large number of people. For example, it was estimated that, in 2002, 7.8% of the Canadian population was taking a statin.[18] If the incidence of statin-associated cognitive impairment were 0.1%, it would currently affect about 2500 people in Canada. In the United States, approximately 41% of adults 45 years of

**Table 1**
**Drugs associated with adverse cognitive effects**

| Mechanism | Common Examples[a] |
|---|---|
| GABAergic benzodiazepine receptor agonists | Alprazolam, diazepam, lorazepam, clonazepam, zolpidem, zaleplon, eszopiclone |
| Opioids | Codeine, morphine, hydromorphone, oxycodone, hydrocodone |
| Anticholinergic | Bladder relaxant drugs: oxybutynin, tolterodine, darifenacin<br>Some antidepressants: amitriptyline, imipramine, paroxetine<br>Some drugs for Parkinson disease: benztropine, trihexyphenidyl |
| First-generation histamine $H_1$ antagonists | Chlorpheniramine, hydroxyzine, diphenhydramine, dimenhydrinate, promethazine |
| Mixed mechanisms | Some antipsychotics: olanzapine, quetiapine, thioridazine, chlorpromazine |

*Abbreviation:* GABA, gamma aminobutyric acid.
[a] This is not an exhaustive list; for detailed review see Ref.[17]
*Adapted from* Rojas-Fernandez CH, Goldstein L, Levey A, et al. An assessment by the Statin Cognitive Safety Task Force: 2014 Update. J Clin Lipidol 2014;8:S10; with permission.

age or older reported using a statin in 2005 and 2008, which represents approximately 126 million people (based on the 2010 census).[19] In turn, if 0.1% of these statin users developed some form of cognitive adverse effect, it would affect 126,600 people. Furthermore, in a recent informal poll in the United States, cognitive decline ranked second only to cancer among leading health concerns in adults aged 45 to 65 years.[20] Thus, cognitive impairment secondary to pharmacotherapy is an important medical issue because it may contribute to decreased quality of life and functional deficits, and because it can be rectified.

In 2012, the first published review of statin-associated cognitive impairment concluded that the benefits of statins outweigh any potential (and rare) cognitive adverse effects, based on the evidence to date.[12] Given the central role of statins in cardiovascular pharmacotherapy it is critical that clinicians have access to valid and reliable information regarding the cognitive safety of these drugs.

## OBJECTIVE

Since publication of the 2012 review by Rojas-Fernandez and Cameron,[12] there have been 2 systematic reviews, 1 Cochrane Review of statins for the treatment of dementia, 1 review article of cognitive effects of statins, 1 review of neuropsychiatric side effects of statins, and 1 expert consensus panel report published assessing statins and putative adverse cognitive effects.[21–25] The placebo-controlled trials available to date that were analyzed in the systematic review and the expert consensus report are summarized in **Table 2**, and a summary of observational studies

is given in **Table 3**. The reviews published since 2012 are summarized in **Table 4**.

Individually and collectively, these reports consistently conclude that, overall, there is a lack of consistent quality evidence of an effect of statins on cognition (adverse or beneficial). In addition, there are important considerations within these reports. The 2013 Cochrane Review specifically selected randomized, double-blind, placebo-controlled trials of lipophilic statins in patients with possible or probable Alzheimer disease as per National Institute of Neurological and Communicative Disorders and Stroke/Alzheimer's Disease and Related Disorders Association or National Institute of Neurological Disorders and Stroke/Association Internationale pour la Recherché et l'Enseignement en Neurosciences criteria.[23] A total of 748 participants with mild to moderate Alzheimer disease were included in this analysis, which concluded that there was no evidence that statins had detrimental effects on cognition. These findings are important, because they show that use of statins in a high-risk population does not result in cognitive worsening. The systematic review by Richardson and colleagues[21] also provides intriguing insights. As part of their systematic review, they conducted an independent analysis of the FDA postmarketing surveillance database and reported that over the marketed lifetime of statins, losartan, and clopidogrel, rates (per 1 million prescriptions) of cognitive adverse events were 1.9, 1.6, and 1.9, respectively (see Table 2 in Richardson and colleagues[21]). It is noteworthy that losartan and clopidogrel have not been hitherto associated with cognitive impairment, and studies have not suggested an association of these drugs with adverse cognitive effects.

**Table 2**
**Summary of placebo-controlled clinical trials of statins and cognition**

| Study | Statins | Population, Sample Size | Duration | Randomized Study | Effects on Cognition |
|---|---|---|---|---|---|
| Harrison et al[49] | Sim 40 Prav 40 | Healthy N = 25 | 4 wk | Y | None |
| Kostis et al[50] | Lov 40 Prav 40 | N = 22 | 6 wk | Y | None |
| Cutler et al[51] | Sim 20 Prav 40 | N = 24/arm (crossover) | 4 wk | Y | None |
| Gengo et al[52] | Lov 40 Prav 40 | N = 24/arm (crossover) | 4 wk | Y | DSST better for statins vs placebo |
| Santanello et al[53] | Lov 20 Lov 40 | N = 431 | 6 mo | Y | None |
| Muldoon et al[54] | Lov 20 | N = 209 | 6 mo | Y | None |
| Gibellato et al[55] | Lov 40 Prav 40 | N = 80 | 4 wk | DK | None |
| Muldoon et al[56] | Sim 10 Sim 40 | N = 308 | 6 mo | Y | Placebo improved on Elithorn mazes and recurrent words, whereas Sim did not; no difference on grooved pegboard, digit vigilance, or mirror tracing; Four-Word Memory Test showed detrimental effects with sim |
| Golomb et al[57] | Prav Sim | N = 1016 | 6 mo | Y | None |
| Parale et al[58] | Ator 10 | N = 55 | 6 mo | N | Positive |
| Summers et al[59] | Ator 10 | N = 57 | 12 wk | Y | None |
| Berk-Planken et al[60] | Ator 10 Ator 80 | N = 30 | 30 wk | N | Positive |
| Shepherd et al[61] | Prav | N = 5804 70–82 y | 3.2 y | Y | None |
| Collins et al[62] | Sim 40 | N = 20,536 | 5.3 y | Y | None |

*Abbreviations:* Ator, atorvastatin; DK, do not know; DSST, digit symbol substitution testing; Lov, lovastatin; N, no; Prav, pravastatin; Sim, simvastatin; Y, yes.
*From* Rojas-Fernandez CH, Goldstein L, Levey A, et al. An assessment by the Statin Cognitive Safety Task Force: 2014 Update. J Clin Lipidol 2014;8:S9; with permission.

The Statin Cognitive Safety Task Force report published in 2014 represents a comprehensive assessment of the cognitive safety of statins, which used all available evidence from 1966 to December 2013 to address the issue of potential adverse cognitive effects attributable to statins.[8] The expert panel, which was composed of 2 neurologists, a preventive cardiologist, a basic vascular scientist with expertise in statin metabolism, and a clinical pharmacologist with expertise in geriatrics and neuropsychopharmacology, concluded that, as a class, statins are not associated with adverse cognitive effects. Other key questions were also addressed and specific recommendations were provided for clinicians, patients, and for future research (**Tables 5** and **6**).

## POSSIBLE MECHANISMS

Plausible neurobiological explanations for the reported cognitive effects of statins are presently elusive. Most cholesterol in the central nervous system (CNS) is produced by de novo synthesis, and thus one theory posits that reduced cholesterol synthesis in oligodendrocytes below a critical level, leading to inhibition of myelination in the CNS, may cause neurocognitive deficits.[8] This hypothesis has been supported by preclinical studies showing inhibition of remyelination by statins in mice after chemically induced demyelination.[26,27] However, there is cause for skepticism regarding this proposed mechanism, because animal models are difficult to generalize to humans (with or without dementia) for multiple reasons. For example, in the aforementioned studies, neuronal damage was chemically induced, and therefore the reported effects of statins on remyelination represent a scenario that is dissimilar from patients taking statins.[26,27] In addition, cognitive symptoms have been reported to occur from 1 to 60 days (although data for time to onset were only available for 30 cases) after patients began taking statins.[28,29] The rate of cholesterol turnover in the brain is very low, with an estimated half-life of about 8 months.[30] The time frame of reported adverse effects as well as the slow turnover of brain cholesterol therefore bring into question putative near-term adverse effects of statins via alterations in CNS cholesterol.[30] Preclinical data also exist that show differential effects of different statins (ie, simvastatin vs pravastatin) on expression of Alzheimer disease–related genes in astrocytes and neuronal cells.[31] These data suggest that it is possible that cholesterol delivery to neurons is decreased, leading to impaired maintenance and function of synapses, and that this effect is more pronounced with simvastatin, which is lipophilic and readily crosses the blood-brain barrier (BBB), versus pravastatin, a hydrophilic statin. Additional mechanisms have also been recently suggested, including effects of statins on Rho GTPase, mitochondrial function, increased tau phosphorylation, and enhancement of arachidonic acid release.[24] These preclinical findings are difficult to put into context, because the underlying theory for statin effects is predicated on long-term statin use, and, as previously mentioned, the reported side effects have generally appeared early in therapy; in addition, use of lipophilic statins in patients with dementia has thus far failed to produce documented adverse cognitive effects. In addition, preclinical data exist that show beneficial effects of statins on brain health, making it clear that further study is necessary to better understand what effect, if any, these drugs have on cognition and/or CNS physiology.[31]

## LIMITS AND STRENGTHS OF CURRENT DATA AND CONSIDERATIONS FOR VASCULAR RISK FACTOR CONTROL

Despite the limits of currently available data, which are outlined in the 2014 Statin Cognitive Task Force report, note that the expert panel used stringent methods in their review of currently available data and used contemporary methods to grade the scientific evidence and their clinical recommendations. The consistency of independent findings of all recent reviews further shows that, to date, the evidence does not suggest an adverse effect of statin drugs on cognitive function. Furthermore, these adverse effects seem to be rare, and likely represent some yet-to-be defined vulnerability in susceptible individuals.

Regarding vascular risk factor control, recent observational studies have provided intriguing insights regarding the potential for vascular risk factor control to slow cognitive decline.[32,33] For example, Li and colleagues[33] followed 837 patients with MCI at baseline for 5 years, and observed that patients who had all their vascular risk factors treated had a lower risk for dementia than those who had some vascular risk factors treated; when individual risk factors were analyzed, treatment of hyperlipidemia was associated with a decreased hazard for Alzheimer disease, with an adjusted hazard ratio (HR) 0.88 (95% confidence interval, 0.83, 0.93). Similarly, Deschaintre and colleagues[32] followed 301 patients with Alzheimer disease but without cerebrovascular disease for an average of 2.3 years, and those who had all their vascular risk factors treated declined less than those with no treated vascular risk factors, an effect that was largely driven by treatment of hypercholesterolemia. These findings should be considered preliminary given the observational study design, but they lend some support to the contention that treatment of hyperlipidemia in patients at risk for cognitive impairment is a reasonable action; a view that is shared by the 2011 statement from the American Heart Association/ American Stroke Association.[34]

## SUGGESTIONS FOR CLINICIANS

Statins have important benefits in patients with, or at high risk of, cardiovascular and/or cerebrovascular events that far outweigh the putative risks of cognitive dysfunction as an adverse effect (also see **Tables 3** and **4**). It is possible that cognitive side effects of statins may occur in rare individuals, but the evidence supporting a causal effect is weak at best, or nonexistent at worst. The true incidence of these adverse effects cannot be determined with currently available data. Nevertheless, because of the potentially serious nature of cognitive dysfunction, the widespread use of statins, and the high prevalence of cognitive impairment caused by any number of causes (particularly with aging and with concomitant cardiovascular and cerebrovascular diseases), patient reports regarding cognition should be taken seriously and appropriately evaluated. Specifically, if a patient taking a statin presents with cognitive complaints that they attribute to statin use, then the clinician should systematically evaluate this complaint. This evaluation should include

**Table 3**
Summary of observational studies

| Reference | Design | Drug | Patients | Cognitive Assessment | Results |
|---|---|---|---|---|---|
| Jick (2000)[63] | Nested case control | Atorvastatin, cerivastatin, fluvastatin, pravastatin, simvastatin | N = 1364; age 50–89 y; patients with dementia and controls | Diagnosis of dementia | Statin users had lower risk of developing dementia vs nonusers (adjusted relative risk, 0.29; 95% CI, 0.13–0.63; P = .002) |
| Hajjar (2002)[64] | Case control and retrospective | Not specified | N = 655; age 52–98 y (mean 78.7 y); 74% women; dyslipidemia or patients with dementia and controls | MMSE, Clock Drawing Test, Geriatric Depression Scale | Patients on statins were less likely to have dementia (OR composite dementia: 0.23; 95% CI, 0.1–0.56; P = .001. OR Alzheimer disease: 0.37; 95% CI, 0.19–0.74; P = .005. OR vascular dementia: 0.25; 95% CI, 0.08–0.85; P = .027); patients on statins also had improved MMSE score vs decline in controls (OR for no change or improvement: 2.81; 95% CI, 1.02–8.43; P = .045) and scored higher on the Clock Drawing Test (difference of 1.5 ± 0.1; P = .036) |
| Rockwood (2002)[65] | Cohort and case control | Not specified | N = 1315; age ≥65 y; patients with dementia and controls | MMSE | Adjusted analysis found that the protective effect of statin (or other lipid level–lowering agent) was observed for dementia in those <80 y old (OR, 0.24; 95% CI, 0.07–0.80), but not for those >80 y old (OR, 0.43; 95% CI, 0.11–1.58) |
| Yaffe (2002)[66] | Cohort subanalysis | Simvastatin, atorvastatin, pravastatin, lovastatin, fluvastatin | N = 1037; age <80 y; postmenopausal women, CAD | Modified MMSE | Statin users had higher mean modified MMSE scores vs nonusers (93.7 ± 6.1 vs 92.7 ± 7.1; P = .02) and a trend toward lower likelihood of cognitive impairment (OR, 0.67; 95% CI, 0.42–1.05) |

| Study | Study type | Statin | N / Population | Cognitive test | Results |
|---|---|---|---|---|---|
| Starr (2004)[67] | Retrospective cohort | Not specified | N = 478; no dementia; tested at ages 11 and 80 y | Moray House Test of Intelligence | A relative improvement in IQ was observed among statin users at ages 11 and 80 y vs nonusers; statins had a beneficial effect on lifelong cognitive change (F = 5.78; P = .017; partial $\eta^2$ = 0.013) |
| Agostini (2007)[68] | Observational cohort | Atorvastatin, lovastatin, pravastatin, simvastatin | N = 756; age ≥65 y | Trail Making B | Statin nonusers performed worse on the Trail Making B outcome (11.0-s difference; P = .05) |
| Redelmeier (2008)[69] | Cohort analysis | Atorvastatin, simvastatin, pravastatin, lovastatin, fluvastatin, rosuvastatin, cerivastatin | N = 284,158; age ≥65 y; admitted for elective surgery | International Classification of Disease codes 293.0–293.9 (delirium) | Patients on statins before elective surgery had ~30% higher risk of postoperative delirium (95% CI, 15%–47%; 14 per 1000) vs those not taking statins (11 per 1000; P<.001) |
| Glasser (2010)[70] | Cohort | Atorvastatin, simvastatin, lovastatin | N = 24,595; age ≥45 y | Six-item Screener | Cognitive impairment in 8.6% of statin users vs 7.7% of nonusers (P = .014); after adjustment for confounders, impairment no longer found (OR, 0.98; 95% CI, 0.87–1.10); no association between statin type and cognition (OR, 1.03; 95% CI, 0.86–1.24) |
| Benito-León (2010)[71] | Cross-sectional cohort | Pravastatin, simvastatin, lovastatin, fluvastatin, atorvastatin | N = 5278; age ≥65 y | 37 item MMSE, Trail Making Test A, Verbal Fluency, Six Objects Test, Story Recall Task, Word Accentuation Test | After adjustment for confounders, no significant difference between statin users and nonusers on neuropsychological test scores |

*Abbreviations:* CAD, coronary artery disease; CI, confidence interval; IQ, intelligence quotient; MMSE, Mini-Mental State Examination; OR, odds ratio.

*From* Rojas-Fernandez CH, Cameron JC. Is statin associated cognitive impairment clinically relevant? A narrative review and clinical recommendations. Ann Pharmacother 2012;46(4):549–57.

**Table 4**
**Reviews published since 2012**

| | Reference | Publication Type | Number of Reports Included[a] | Main Findings |
|---|---|---|---|---|
| 1 | Swiger et al,[22] 2013 | Systematic review and meta-analysis | 27 | Short-term data indicated no adverse effect of statins on cognition and long-term data indicated 29% reduction in incident dementia in patients on statins (HR, 0.71; 95% CI, 0.61–0.82) |
| 2 | Richardson et al,[21] 2013 | Systematic review and meta-analysis | 27 | 1. Meta-analyses of RRs from cohort studies:<br>• Association between statin users and dementia: adjusted RR, 0.87 (95% CI, 0.82–0.92)<br>• Association between statin users and Alzheimer disease: adjusted RR, 0.79 (95% CI, 0.63–0.99)<br>• Association between statin users and MCI: adjusted RR, 0.66 (95% CI, 0.51–0.86)<br>2. Meta-analyses of RRs from case-control studies:<br>• Association between statin users and dementia: adjusted RR, 0.25 (95% CI, 0.14–0.46)<br>• Association between statin users and Alzheimer disease: adjusted RR, 0.56 (95% CI, 0.41–0.78)<br>• Association between statin users and MCI: adjusted RR, 0.37 (95% CI, 0.16–0.84)<br>3. Meta-analyses of RRs from cross-sectional studies:<br>• Association between statin users and dementia: adjusted RR, 0.54 (95% CI, 0.22–1.33)<br>• Association between stain users and Alzheimer disease: adjusted RR, 0.45 (95% CI, 0.35–0.58) |
| 3 | Rojas-Fernandez et al,[8] 2014 | Semisystematic review/expert panel consensus | 23 | Statins as a class are not associated with adverse effects on cognition |
| 4 | Kelley & Glasser,[24] 2014 | Review | 35 | Review of literature does not reliably show a robust association between incident cognitive impairment and statin use; study findings are mixed. Some studies report an increased risk and others report no association or a protective effect |
| 5 | Tuccori et al,[25] 2014 | Descriptive | 30 | Most studies reviewed found no adverse or protective effects of statins on cognition |

*Abbreviations:* HR, hazard ratio; RR, risk ratio.
[a] Includes randomized controlled studies, case reports, case series, case-control studies, and cohort studies.

searching for other potential causes or contributors to cognitive impairment, and considering using the Montreal Cognitive Assessment Test or another cognitive screening instrument to document the affected cognitive domains and magnitude of impairment. The patient should also be asked to describe the specific cognitive problems noted, and the severity and frequency. If the clinician reasonably suspects that, independent of other causes, the statin is suspected of contributing to cognitive symptoms, it would be reasonable for the drug to be discontinued for 1 to 2 months and then to consider a rechallenge. The patient should be reassessed every 1 to 2 months with the same cognitive screening tool that was used to document the affected cognitive domains until the patient no longer reports cognitive symptoms before considering a rechallenge with another statin or a lower dose of the same statin. A repeat assessment would clearly be

**Table 5**
**Clinical questions addressed by the 2014 Statin Cognitive Safety Task Force**

| Questions | Answer | Strength of Recommendation | Quality of Evidence |
|---|---|---|---|
| 1. Should a baseline cognitive assessment be performed before beginning a statin? | No | E (expert opinion) | Low |
| 2. Are statins as a class associated with adverse effects on cognition? | No | A (strong recommendation) | Low to moderate |
| 3. What should the provider do if a patient reports cognitive symptoms after beginning a statin? | Cognitive testing should be conducted and the risk of stopping statin should be assessed | E (expert opinion) | Low |

*Adapted from* Rojas-Fernandez CH, Goldstein L, Levey A, et al. An assessment by the Statin Cognitive Safety Task Force: 2014 Update. J Clin Lipidol 2014;8:S5–15.

useful in documenting improvement and/or a normal result. Patients who have had a recent stroke represent an important exception to statin discontinuation, because statin withdrawal in this setting increases the risk of recurrence and poorer outcomes.[35–37]

Whether rechallenge with a statin is appropriate should be determined and discussed with the patient based on their individual characteristics, expected benefits from resuming statin therapy, and patient preferences. Which statin to subsequently use is a salient question facing the clinician. Controversy exists regarding whether or not hydrophilic drugs like pravastatin can enter the brain, and the CNS pharmacokinetics of statins are not well delineated.[38] Some lipophilic statins, such as lovastatin and simvastatin, cross the BBB via passive diffusion, whereas others, such as pravastatin, depend on low-affinity transport systems. Mixed data for CNS penetration of atorvastatin and cerivastatin have been reported. Peripheral lactonization represents an additional mechanism that may facilitate atorvastatin and simvastatin penetrating into the CNS.[39,40] Animal data suggest that CNS levels of statins correspond, at least in part, with their lipophilicity in the rank order of simvastatin>lovastatin>pravastatin.[41–44] Data also support the suggestion that rosuvastatin, like pravastatin, has low potential to penetrate the BBB.[45] Furthermore although mechanisms for the apparently rapid elimination of statins from the brain remain elusive, it is possible that different statins are eliminated via different transporters, such as P-glycoprotein (statins are ligands for P-glycoprotein).[38]

The aforementioned preclinical study by Dong and colleagues[31] might lend additional support for the preferential use of hydrophilic statins such as pravastatin or rosuvastatin.

**Table 6**
**Recommendations from the cognitive expert panel**

| Recommendations to Clinicians | Recommendations to Patients |
|---|---|
| Benefits of statins in patients at risk of cardiovascular events far outweigh the risk of cognitive dysfunction | Information from case reports is inconclusive, not reliable, and has not been proved in a cause-and-effect manner |
| Cognitive side effects of statins are rare and evidence to support causality is weak or nonexistent | Many other causes of memory complaints exist, including normal aging, the effect of certain medications, and effects of other conditions such as anxiety, depression, and sleep apnea |
| Complaints associated with memory in patients whose cognitive symptoms persist even after statin discontinuation should be taken seriously and evaluated with appropriate neuropsychological testing | Patients should discuss any cognitive symptoms with health care professionals before discontinuing statin therapy |

*Adapted from* Rojas-Fernandez CH, Goldstein L, Levey A, et al. An assessment by the Statin Cognitive Safety Task Force: 2014 Update. J Clin Lipidol 2014;8:S5–15.

In addition, the potential role of a dysfunctional BBB should also be considered. The aforementioned considerations may be altered by factors that are commonly present in older people. For example, the permeability of the BBB increases with normal aging, hypertension, diabetes, and hyperlipidemia[46,47] These observations are further complicated by the effects of stroke, including lacunar infarcts (which are often silent), which account for 25% of ischemic stroke.[47] The aforementioned insults have been associated with a compromised BBB, which allows greater penetrance of drugs into the brain, which would be expected to lead to greater risk for CNS adverse drug effects.

If a statin is reinitiated, clinicians should use the lowest dose to achieve the treatment goal, and may consider using a statin that may theoretically be less likely to contribute to CNS effects (ie, a statin such as pravastatin or rosuvastatin).[12,48] However, at present there is insufficient evidence to unequivocally recommend substitution of hydrophilic rather than lipophilic statins.[8,43] In patients whose symptoms persist despite statin discontinuation, a prompt search for alternate causes should be undertaken, and consideration should be given to referral to a specialist such as a geriatrician or neurologist.

Patients should be reassured that, although cognitive symptoms have been reported by some statin users, information from such case reports cannot be considered to be reliable, is not conclusive, and has not been proven in a cause-and-effect manner. Patients should understand that there are many other causes of cognitive symptoms, including normal aging; the effect of many commonly used medications (eg, sedative-hypnotics, over-the-counter antihistamines, or pain medications); and the effects of many comorbidities, such as anxiety, depression, or sleep apnea. Patients should first discuss any cognitive concerns with their health care providers before considering discontinuing their statin.

## SUMMARY

Since 2012, the issue of statin-induced cognitive impairment has received much attention in the literature and in the lay press, and has probably fueled much dialogue between patients and clinicians regarding the risk/benefit profile of statins. Anecdotally, misinformation exists among health care professionals regarding this issue, which may be affecting appropriate use of statins in patients who need these medications. Furthermore, premature closure (ie, attribution of cognitive dysfunction to a statin to the exclusion of other

diagnoses) can result in patient harm. The current evidence does not support a causal association between the use of statin medications and incident cognitive symptoms; cognitive considerations should not play a role in decision making for most patients for whom statins are indicated.

## REFERENCES

1. Tobert JA. Lovastatin and beyond: the history of the HMG-CoA reductase inhibitors. Nat Rev Drug Discov 2003;2(7):517–26.
2. Baigent C, Keech A, Kearney PM, et al. Efficacy and safety of cholesterol-lowering treatment: prospective meta-analysis of data from 90,056 participants in 14 randomised trials of statins. Lancet 2005;366(9493): 1267–78.
3. Cholesterol Treatment Trialists' (CTT) Collaborators, Mihaylova B, Emberson J, et al. The effects of lowering LDL cholesterol with statin therapy in people at low risk of vascular disease: meta-analysis of individual data from 27 randomised trials. Lancet 2012;380(9841):581–90.
4. Cholesterol Treatment Trialists' (CTT) Collaborators, Kearney PM, Blackwell L, et al. Efficacy of cholesterol-lowering therapy in 18,686 people with diabetes in 14 randomised trials of statins: a meta-analysis. Lancet 2008;371(9607):117–25.
5. Cholesterol Treatment Trialists' (CTT) Collaboration, Baigent C, Blackwell L, et al. Efficacy and safety of more intensive lowering of LDL cholesterol: a meta-analysis of data from 170,000 participants in 26 randomised trials. Lancet 2010;376(9753):1670–81.
6. Gu Q, Paulose-Ram R, Burt VL, et al. Prescription cholesterol-lowering medication use in adults aged 40 and over: United states, 2003-2012. NCHS Data Brief 2014;(177):1–8.
7. Sattar N, Preiss D, Murray HM, et al. Statins and risk of incident diabetes: a collaborative meta-analysis of randomised statin trials. Lancet 2010;375(9716): 735–42.
8. Rojas-Fernandez CH, Goldstein LB, Levey AI, et al, The National Lipid Association's Safety Task, Force. An assessment by the statin cognitive safety task force: 2014 update. J Clin Lipidol 2014;8(3 Suppl):S5–16.
9. Rosenson RS, Baker SK, Jacobson TA, et al, The National Lipid Association's Muscle Safety Expert, Panel. An assessment by the statin muscle safety task force: 2014 update. J Clin Lipidol 2014; 8(3 Suppl):S58–71.
10. Stone NJ, Robinson JG, Lichtenstein AH, et al. 2013 ACC/AHA guideline on the treatment of blood cholesterol to reduce atherosclerotic cardiovascular risk in adults: a report of the American College of Cardiology/American Heart Association Task Force on Practice Guidelines. J Am Coll Cardiol 2014; 63(25 Pt B):2889–934.

11. Padala KP, Padala PR, McNeilly DP, et al. The effect of HMG-CoA reductase inhibitors on cognition in patients with Alzheimer's dementia: a prospective withdrawal and rechallenge pilot study. Am J Geriatr Pharmacother 2012;10(5):296–302.

12. Rojas-Fernandez CH, Cameron JC. Is statin-associated cognitive impairment clinically relevant? A narrative review and clinical recommendations. Ann Pharmacother 2012;46(4):549–57.

13. US Food and Drug Administration. FDA drug safety communication: important safety label changes to cholesterol-lowering statin drugs. Available at: http://www.fda.gov/drugs/drugsafety/ucm293101.htm. Accessed November 6, 2013.

14. Petersen RC. Clinical practice. Mild cognitive impairment. N Engl J Med 2011;364(23):2227–34.

15. Feldman H, Levy AR, Hsiung GY, et al. A Canadian Cohort Study of Cognitive Impairment and Related Dementias (ACCORD): study methods and baseline results. Neuroepidemiology 2003;22(5): 265–74.

16. Hachinski V, Iadecola C, Petersen RC, et al. National institute of neurological disorders and stroke–Canadian Stroke Network vascular cognitive impairment harmonization standards. Stroke 2006;37(9): 2220–41.

17. Tannenbaum C, Paquette A, Hilmer S, et al. A systematic review of amnestic and non-amnestic mild cognitive impairment induced by anticholinergic, antihistamine, GABAergic and opioid drugs. Drugs Aging 2012;29(8):639–58.

18. Neutel CI, Morrison H, Campbell NR, et al. Statin use in Canadians: trends, determinants and persistence. Can J Public Health 2007;98(5):412–6.

19. Centers for Disease Control and Prevention. National center for health statistics. health, united states, 2010: With special feature on death and dying. Available at: http://www.cdc.gov/nchs/data/hus/hus10.pdf. Accessed February 5, 2014.

20. Anderson S. Upbeat boomers say they're not old yet. USA today. July 14, 2011. Available at: http://usatoday30.usatoday.com/news/health/healthcare/health/healthcare/prevention/story/2011/07/For-boomers-old-isnt-what-it-used-to-be/49375968/1. Accessed October 2, 2013.

21. Richardson K, Schoen M, French B, et al. Statins and cognitive function: a systematic review. Ann Intern Med 2013;159(10):688–97.

22. Swiger KJ, Manalac RJ, Blumenthal RS, et al. Statins and cognition: a systematic review and meta-analysis of short- and long-term cognitive effects. Mayo Clin Proc 2013;88(11):1213–21.

23. McGuinness B, O'Hare J, Craig D, et al. Cochrane Review on 'statins for the treatment of dementia'. Int J Geriatr Psychiatry 2013;28(2):119–26.

24. Kelley BJ, Glasser S. Cognitive effects of statin medications. CNS Drugs 2014;28(5):411–9.

25. Tuccori M, Montagnani S, Mantarro S, et al. Neuropsychiatric adverse events associated with statins: Epidemiology, pathophysiology, prevention and management. CNS Drugs 2014;28(3):249–72.

26. Miron VE, Zehntner SP, Kuhlmann T, et al. Statin therapy inhibits remyelination in the central nervous system. Am J Pathol 2009;174(5):1880–90.

27. Klopfleisch S, Merkler D, Schmitz M, et al. Negative impact of statins on oligodendrocytes and myelin formation in vitro and in vivo. J Neurosci 2008; 28(50):13609–14.

28. Evans MA, Golomb BA. Statin-associated adverse cognitive effects: survey results from 171 patients. Pharmacotherapy 2009;29(7):800–11.

29. Wagstaff LR, Mitton MW, Arvik BM, et al. Statin-associated memory loss: analysis of 60 case reports and review of the literature. Pharmacotherapy 2003; 23(7):871–80.

30. Saher G, Simons M. Cholesterol and myelin biogenesis. Subcell Biochem 2010;51:489–508.

31. Dong W, Vuletic S, Albers JJ. Differential effects of simvastatin and pravastatin on expression of Alzheimer's disease-related genes in human astrocytes and neuronal cells. J Lipid Res 2009;50(10): 2095–102.

32. Deschaintre Y, Richard F, Leys D, et al. Treatment of vascular risk factors is associated with slower decline in Alzheimer disease. Neurology 2009; 73(9):674–80.

33. Li J, Wang YJ, Zhang M, et al. Vascular risk factors promote conversion from mild cognitive impairment to Alzheimer disease. Neurology 2011;76(17): 1485–91.

34. Gorelick PB. Statin use and intracerebral hemorrhage: evidence for safety in recurrent stroke prevention? Arch Neurol 2012;69(1):13–6.

35. Flint AC, Kamel H, Navi BB, et al. Statin use during ischemic stroke hospitalization is strongly associated with improved poststroke survival. Stroke 2012;43(1):147–54.

36. Flint AC, Kamel H, Navi BB, et al. Inpatient statin use predicts improved ischemic stroke discharge disposition. Neurology 2012;78(21):1678–83.

37. Blanco M, Nombela F, Castellanos M, et al. Statin treatment withdrawal in ischemic stroke: a controlled randomized study. Neurology 2007;69(9):904–10.

38. Wood WG, Eckert GP, Igbavboa U, et al. Statins and neuroprotection: a prescription to move the field forward. Ann N Y Acad Sci 2010;1199:69–76.

39. Shepardson NE, Shankar GM, Selkoe DJ. Cholesterol level and statin use in Alzheimer disease: II. Review of human trials and recommendations. Arch Neurol 2011;68(11):1385–92.

40. Jacobsen W, Kuhn B, Soldner A, et al. Lactonization is the critical first step in the disposition of the 3-hydroxy-3-methylglutaryl-CoA reductase inhibitor atorvastatin. Drug Metab Dispos 2000;28(11):1369–78.

41. Johnson-Anuna LN, Eckert GP, Keller JH, et al. Chronic administration of statins alters multiple gene expression patterns in mouse cerebral cortex. J Pharmacol Exp Ther 2005;312(2):786–93.

42. Thelen KM, Rentsch KM, Gutteck U, et al. Brain cholesterol synthesis in mice is affected by high dose of simvastatin but not of pravastatin. J Pharmacol Exp Ther 2006;316(3):1146–52.

43. Tsuji A, Saheki A, Tamai I, et al. Transport mechanism of 3-hydroxy-3-methylglutaryl coenzyme A reductase inhibitors at the blood-brain barrier. J Pharmacol Exp Ther 1993;267(3):1085–90.

44. Saheki A, Terasaki T, Tamai I, et al. In vivo and in vitro blood-brain barrier transport of 3-hydroxy-3-methylglutaryl coenzyme A (HMG-CoA) reductase inhibitors. Pharm Res 1994;11(2):305–11.

45. Nezasa K, Higaki K, Matsumura T, et al. Liver-specific distribution of rosuvastatin in rats: comparison with pravastatin and simvastatin. Drug Metab Dispos 2002;30(11):1158–63.

46. Farrall AJ, Wardlaw JM. Blood-brain barrier: ageing and microvascular disease–systematic review and meta-analysis. Neurobiol Aging 2009;30(3):337–52.

47. Zeevi N, Pachter J, McCullough LD, et al. The blood-brain barrier: geriatric relevance of a critical brain-body interface. J Am Geriatr Soc 2010;58(9):1749–57.

48. Schachter M. Chemical, pharmacokinetic and pharmacodynamic properties of statins: an update. Fundam Clin Pharmacol 2005;19(1):117–25.

49. Harrison RW, Ashton CH. Do cholestrol-lowering agents affect brain activity? A comparison of simvastatin, pravastatin, and placebo in healthy volunteers. Br J Clin Pharmacol 1994;37:231–6.

50. Kostis JB, Rosen RC, Wilson AC. Central nervous system effects of HMG CoA reductase inhibitors: lovastatin and pravastatin on sleep and cognitive performance in patients with hypercholesterolemia. J Clin Pharmacol 1994;34:989–96.

51. Cutler N, Sramek J, Veroff A, et al. Effects of treatment with simvastatin and pravastatin on cognitive function in patients with hypercholesterolaemia. Br J Clin Pharmacol 1995;39:333–6.

52. Gengo F, Cwudzinski D, Kinkel P, et al. Effects of treatment with lovastatin and pravastatin on daytime cognitive performance. Clin Cardiol 1995;18:209–14.

53. Santanello NC, Barber BL, Applegate WB, et al. Effect of pharmacologic lipid lowering on health-related quality of life in older persons: results from the Cholesterol Reduction in Seniors Program (CRISP) Pilot Study. J Am Geriatr Soc 1997;45:8–14.

54. Muldoon MF, Barger SD, Ryan CM, et al. Effects of lovastatin on cognitive function and psychological well-being. Am J Med 2000;108:538–46.

55. Gibellato MG, Moore JL, Selby K, et al. Effects of lovastatin and pravastatin on cognitive function in military aircrew. Aviat Space Environ Med 2001;72:805–12.

56. Muldoon MF, Ryan CM, Sereika SM, et al. Randomized trial of the effects of simvastatin on cognitive functioning in hypercholesterolemic adults. Am J Med 2004;117:823–9.

57. Golomb BA, Dimsdale JE, White HL, et al. Do Low Dose Statins Affect Cognition? Results of the UCSD Statin Study. Circulation 2006;114:II–289.

58. Parale GP, Baheti NN, Kulkarni PM, et al. Effects of atorvastatin on higher functions. Eur J Clin Pharmacol 2006;62:259–65.

59. Summers MJ, Oliver KR, Coombes JS, et al. Effect of atorvastatin on cognitive function in patients from the Lipid Lowering and Onset of Renal Disease (LORD) trial. Pharmacotherapy 2007;27:183–90.

60. Berk-Planken I, de Konig I, Stolk R, et al. Atorvastatin, diabetic dyslipidemia, and cognitive functioning. Diabetes Care 2002;25:1250–1.

61. Shepherd J, Blauw GJ, Murphy MB, et al. Pravastatin in elderly individuals at risk of vascular disease (PROSPER): a randomised controlled trial. Lancet 2002;360:1623–30.

62. Collins R, Armitage J, Parish S, et al. Effects of cholesterol-lowering with simvastatin on stroke and other major vascular events in 20536 people with cerebrovascular disease or other high-risk conditions. Lancet 2004;363:757–67.

63. Jick H, Zornberg GL, Jick SS, et al. Statins and the risk of dementia. Lancet 2000;356:1627–31.

64. Hajjar I, Schumpert J, Hirth V, et al. The impact of the use of statins on the prevalence of dementia and the progression of cognitive impairment. J Gerontol A Biol Sci Med Sci 2002;57:M414–8.

65. Rockwood K, Kirkland S, Hogan DB, et al. Use of lipid-lowering agents, indication bias, and the risk of dementia in community-dwelling elderly people. Arch Neurol 2002;59:223–7.

66. Yaffe K, Barrett-Connor E, Lin F, Grady D. Serum lipoprotein levels, statin use, and cognitive function in older women. Arch Neurol 2002;59:378–84.

67. Starr JM, McGurn B, Whiteman M, et al. Life long changes in cognitive ability are associated with prescribed medications in old age. Int J Geriatr Psychiatry 2004;19:327–32.

68. Agostini JV, Tinetti MR, Han L, et al. Effects of statin use on muscle strength, cognition, and depressive symptoms in older adults. J Am Geriatr Soc 2007;55:420–5.

69. Redelmeier DA, Thiruchelvam D, Daneman N. Delirium after elective surgery among elderly patients taking statins. CMAJ 2008;179:645–52.

70. Glasser SP, Wadley V, Judd S, et al. The association of statin use and statin type and cognitive performance: analysis of the reasons for geographic and racial differences in stroke (REGARDS) study. Clin Cardiol 2010;33:280–8.

71. Benito-León J, Louis ED, Vega S, et al. Statins and cognitive functioning in the elderly: a population-based study. J Alzheimers Dis 2010;21:95–102.

# Statins and the Liver

Cynthia Herrick, MD[a],*, Samira Bahrainy, MD[b],
Edward A. Gill, MD, FASE, FAHA, FACC, FACP, FNLA[c]

## KEYWORDS

- Dyslipidemia • Chronic liver disease • Statins • Hepatic transaminases

## KEY POINTS

- Transaminase elevations are a class effect of statins and do not represent liver toxicity in the absence of bilirubin elevation or synthetic dysfunction.
- Routine monitoring of liver enzymes on statin therapy is no longer recommended because severe toxicity is rare and idiosyncratic.
- Statins reduce cardiovascular disease risk in patients with mild liver disease, do not seem to worsen liver disease, and may improve the underlying liver problem.
- Statins, with appropriate consideration for drug interactions, are considered safe after liver transplantation.

## INTRODUCTION

Statins are the foundation of lipid-lowering therapy, resulting in a significant reduction in major vascular events and all-cause mortality in men and women. According to the most recent meta-analysis using patient-level data on 174,149 patients from 27 randomized, controlled trials, each 1 mmol/L (39 mg/dL) reduction in low-density lipoprotein cholesterol (LDL-C) reduced major vascular events approximately 20% (women: rate ratio [RR], 0.84 [99% CI, 0.78–0.91]; men: RR, 0.78 [99% CI, 0.75–0.81]) and all-cause mortality around 10% (women: RR, 0.91 [99% CI, 0.84–0.99]; men: RR, 0.90 [99% CI, 0.86–0.95]).[1]

Concern with using statins in patients with liver disease stems from their mechanism (inhibiting a key step in cholesterol synthesis in the liver), metabolism (frequently involving the cytochrome p450 system in the liver), and class effect in increasing transaminases. However, there is now sufficient information available supporting the use of statins in at least mild liver disease,

with no differences in peak or steady state statin levels in patients with Child Class A cirrhosis.[2,3] With the obesity epidemic, there are a rising number of patients with nonalcoholic fatty liver disease (NAFLD) and nonalcoholic steatohepatitis (NASH) that may have concurrent liver enzyme and lipid abnormalities who could benefit from the cardiovascular risk–lowering properties of statins.

There are currently 7 US Food and Drug Administration (FDA)–approved statin medications. Their principle metabolic pathways are delineated in **Table 1**. For patients in whom drug interactions are a particular concern, pravastatin, rosuvastatin, and pitavastatin are preferred therapies given that they have no metabolism through CYP3A4. Further, it has been noted in multiple trials that statins have a class effect on transaminases that does not seem to be associated with liver damage. **Box 1** elucidates these class effects further. One key point is that, according to Hy's law, synthetic dysfunction and bilirubin elevation signal true drug toxicity rather than transaminase elevation alone.

[a] Division of Endocrinology, Metabolism and Lipid Research, Department of Medicine, Washington University School of Medicine, Campus Box 8127, 660 South Euclid, St Louis, MO 63110, USA; [b] VA Medical Center, Puget Sound, 1660 South Columbian Way, Seattle, WA 98104, USA; [c] Harborview Medical Center, University of Washington School of Medicine, 325 Ninth Avenue, Box 359748, Seattle, WA 98104, USA
* Corresponding author.
*E-mail address:* cherrick@dom.wustl.edu

Cardiol Clin 33 (2015) 257–265
http://dx.doi.org/10.1016/j.ccl.2015.02.005
0733-8651/15/$ – see front matter © 2015 Elsevier Inc. All rights reserved

**Table 1**
**Metabolism of FDA-approved statin medications**

| Not by CYP 450 system | CYP2C9 | CYP3A4 |
|---|---|---|
| Pravastatin[a] | Fluvastatin | Lovastatin |
| | Rosuvastatin[a] (minimal) | Simvastatin |
| | | Atorvastatin |
| | Pitavastatin[a] (minimal) | |

[a] Fewer drug interactions.
*Adapted from* Neuvonen PJ, Niemi M, Backman JT. Drug interactions with lipid-lowering drugs: mechanisms and clinical relevance. Clin Pharmacol Ther 2006;80:565–81.

## Patient Evaluation Overview

Reviews of adverse event databases indicate that rates of fulminant liver failure (2 per 1 million with lovastatin) and liver transplants (3 in 51,741) attributable to statin use occur rarely with currently marketed statins.[7] **Box 2** highlights the lack of benefit of routine monitoring of liver function tests during statin therapy, endorsed by both the US FDA and National Lipid Association (NLA), with the exception of a single liver function panel before initiation of therapy.

The NLA Statin Liver Safety Task Force recommends a tiered approach to considering statin use in patients with abnormal liver enzymes at baseline or if assessed for other reasons at some point during treatment. This approach is guided by the degree of transaminase elevation and the presence or absence of bilirubin elevation if the alanine aminotransferase/aspartate aminotransferase (ALT/AST) levels are less than or equal to 3 times the upper limit of normal (ULN; **Box 3**).

**Box 1**
**Class effects of statins on liver enzymes**

- Transaminases increase, ALT > AST, during first 3 months
  - Often return to baseline without adjustment of statin dose
  - May not increase again with rechallenge with the same statin
- Persistent elevation >3× ULN occurs in <1% of the general population and 2%–3% of patients on 80 mg/d or combination therapy with ezetemibe
- Transaminase elevations alone are not associated with histopathologic change
- Hy's law: Drug toxicity is unlikely if bilirubin is ≤2× ULN

*Abbreviations:* ALT, alanine aminotransferase; AST, aspartate aminotransferase; ULN, upper limit of normal.

*Adapted from* Refs.[3–6]

**Box 2**
**Lack of benefit of routine monitoring**

- Irreversible liver damage is rare
- Routing monitoring will miss idiosyncratic reactions
- Routine LFTs no longer recommended by FDA or NLA statin safety task force
- No unexpected safety concerns raised since this recommendation was made

*Abbreviations:* FDA, US Food and Drug Administration; LFT, liver function test; NLA, National Lipid Association.

*Adapted from* Refs.[3,4,8]

**Box 3**
**Evaluation of elevated transaminases**

ALT/AST > ULN but ≤3× ULN

- Total bilirubin normal, CK normal → likely NAFLD, OK to start or not hold statin
- Old indirect bilirubin elevation, CK normal → Gilbert's + likely NAFLD, OK to start or not hold statin
- New indirect or direct bilirubin elevation → stop or hold statin while evaluating[a]

ALT/AST > 3× ULN

- Stop or hold statin while evaluating[a]

[a] Further Evaluation includes: stopping other drugs with potential liver toxicity; evaluating synthetic function: albumin, PT, and CBC; and lifestyle modification if obese. Consider laboratory evaluation for viral hepatitis, autoimmune hepatitis, primary biliary cirrhosis, hemochromatosis, α-1 antitrypsin deficiency, Wilson's disease as appropriate. Consider evaluation for anatomic abnormalities with abdominal ultrasonography. Other imaging or liver biopsy if no resolution and evaluation unrevealing.

*Abbreviations:* ALT, alanine aminotransferase; AST, aspartate aminotransferase; CBC, complete blood count; CK, creatinine kinase; NAFLD, nonalcoholic fatty liver disease; PT, prothrombin time; ULN, upper limit of normal.

*Adapted from* Bays H, Cohen DE, Chalasani N, et al. An assessment by the statin liver safety task force: 2014 update. J Clin Lipidol 2014;8:S47–57.

## Pharmacologic Treatment Options and Complications

One limitation in the ability to recommend statins in patients with liver disease has historically been a lack of evidence on the use of statins in this population in randomized, controlled trials. **Table 2** summarizes the available evidence from the largest available prospective trials evaluating the use of pravastatin, atorvastatin, and pitavastatin in patients with abnormal liver enzymes and underlying liver disease at baseline. As demonstrated, studies vary in terms of drug dose and combination used, presence or absence of a control group, duration of follow-up, and severity of underlying liver disease. Despite these differences, all studies demonstrated no significant worsening in liver abnormalities among patients in the statin therapy groups and many demonstrated improvement in liver biochemical and imaging endpoints after the use of a statin.

**Table 2**
**Evidence of statin safety in liver disease**

| Statin | Liver Disease: Baseline Transaminases | Liver Endpoints | Comment |
|---|---|---|---|
| **Pravastatin** | | | 1 prospective placebocontrolled RCT |
| 80 mg vs placebo[9] | HCV, NAFLD/NASH, or other Baseline ALT/AST $\leq$ 5× ULN | No difference in ALT doubling Mean ALT reduction from baseline with pravastatin | 36 wk (N = 326) |
| **Atorvastatin** | | | 5 prospective studies |
| 10–20 mg vs 1–4 mg pitavastatin[13] | Non-EtOH, nonviral ALT $\geq$ 1.25 ULN, $\leq$ 2.5 ULN | ~5% w/ALT > 100 at 12 wk Reduced GGT at 12 wk Reduced CT fat accumulation | 12 wk (N = 189) |
| 20 mg vs 200 mg fenofibrate or combo[14] | NAFLD + MetS ALT/AST > ULN, $\leq$ 3× ULN | 40% reduction in ALT 67% reduction in biochemical + US NAFLD | 54 wk (N = 186) |
| 20 mg + vitamins C/E vs placebo[10] | NAFLD or no liver disease ALT/AST $\leq$ 1.5× ULN | Lower CT evidence of NASH 4.4% vs 70.4% (OR, 0.29; 95% CI, 0.15–0.57) | ~3.6 y (N = 455) Post hoc analysis |
| 10–80 mg vs no control[11] | Any liver disease, most NAFLD ALT/AST > ULN, $\leq$ 3× ULN | ALT, 35% reduction AST, 47% reduction | ~3 y (N = 437) Post hoc analysis |
| 80 mg vs 20–40 mg simvastatin[12] | 1081 ALT $\geq$ ULN but <3× ULN, 7782 ALT < ULN | Significant reduction in ALT from baseline in both groups Greater reductions in major CV event with atorvastatin in patients with ALT $\geq$ ULN | Mean ~4.8 y (N = 8863) Post hoc analysis |
| **Pitavastatin** | | | 1 prospective active drug-controlled RCT |
| 1–4 mg vs 10–20 mg atorvastatin[13] | Non-EtOH, nonviral ALT $\geq$ 1.25 ULN, $\leq$ 2.5 ULN | ~5% w/ALT >100 at 12 wk Reduced GGT and ALT at 12 wk Reduced CT fat accumulation | 12 wk (N = 189) |

*Abbreviations:* ALT, alanine aminotransferase; AST, aspartate aminotransferase; CV, cardiovascular; EtOH, alcohol induced liver disease; GGT, gamma glutamyltransferase; HCV, hepatitis C virus; MetS, metabolic syndrome; NAFLD, nonalcoholic fatty liver disease; NASH, nonalcoholic steatohepatitis; RCT, randomized, controlled trial; ULN, upper limit of normal; US, ultrasonography.

The study of pravastatin 80 mg versus placebo remains the best evidence on the use of statins in patients with liver disease as this was a multicenter, prospective, placebo-controlled, randomized, trial including patients with baseline ALT/AST up to 5 times the ULN, and the drug was only stopped if ALT/AST reached 10 times the ULN or there was evidence of synthetic dysfunction, patients were followed for 9 months and patients with many different types of liver disease were included.[9] The post-hoc analysis of the St. Francis Heart study, which included patients with fatty liver disease on Atorvastatin, as well as the post-hoc analyses of the Greek Atorvastatin and Coronary Heart Disease Evaluation (GREACE) and Incremental Decrease in End Points Through Aggressive Lipid Lowering (IDEAL) studies provide longer term follow-up information, supporting safety of statins in the population with liver disease over more than three years.[10–12] Atorvastatin and pitavastatin seem to have similar effects on liver parameters, although pitavastatin decreased significantly ALT at 12 weeks whereas atorvastatin did not.[13]

Beyond evidence from prospective trials specifically focusing on patients with liver disease, a meta-analysis of randomized, controlled trials examining low- to moderate-dose statin for primary and secondary prevention of cardiovascular disease, including 13 trials and 49,390 patients, demonstrated that statin therapy, except for fluvastatin, was not associated with an increased odds of having liver function test (LFT) abnormalities (odds ratio [OR], 1.26; 95% CI, 0.99–1.62; $P = .07$).[15] High-dose statin trials not included in this analysis do note higher rates of LFT abnormalities in the statin treated groups, although that may not actually equate with hepatotoxicity because these patients did not have concurrent synthetic dysfunction.

In a retrospective study comparing cohorts with and without liver enzyme elevations either on or off of statin therapy, investigators found that, among those with elevated liver enzymes at baseline, there were no differences between those on and off statin medication in mild to moderate ($\leq10\times$ ULN) or severe ($>10\times$ ULN) liver enzyme elevations at 6 months follow-up.[16] In a similarly designed study looking specifically at lovastatin, a significantly higher percentage of patients with elevated liver enzymes not on lovastatin experienced severe elevations in liver enzymes, than those who were prescribed lovastatin, over the 12-month follow-up period.[17] In both of these studies, although those with increased liver enzymes at baseline had more mild to moderate increases in liver enzymes during follow-up on a statin than those without elevated baseline liver enzymes, they did not have significantly higher rates of severe elevations.

## Evaluation of Outcome and Recommendations in Specific Liver Diseases

**Table 3** summarizes findings with regard to statin use in specific liver diseases as well as the special

**Table 3**
**Effects of statins in specific liver diseases**

| Liver Disease | Statin Effects |
|---|---|
| Hepatitis C | Less severe liver enzyme elevations[18]<br>Greater decline in transaminases[19]<br>Improved HCV virologic response[20] |
| NAFLD/NASH | Pilot studies in atorvastatin, pravastatin, rosuvastatin<br>   Reduced transaminases[21–26]<br>   Improved steatosis/necroinflammation[22–24,26]<br>Other studies have shown no difference in transaminases or steatosis with<br>   statins[27,28] |
| Primary biliary cirrhosis | Simvastatin and atorvastatin had no significant liver adverse effects[29–31]<br>Statins with ezetemibe over 3-y of follow-up had no significant ALT<br>   changes[32] |
| Autoimmune hepatitis | No problems per safety task force as long as there is no synthetic dysfunction[3]<br>Reports of statin-induced autoimmune hepatitis are likely idiosyncratic |
| Liver transplantation | Immunosuppressive therapy can worsen lipid abnormalities[33,34]<br>CYP3A4 interactions are of concern with immunosuppressives, hence,<br>   pravastatin, pitavastatin, rosuvastatin or fluvastatin may be better<br>   choices[35,36] |

*Abbreviations:* ALT, alanine aminotransferase; HCV, hepatitis C virus; NAFLD, nonalcoholic fatty liver disease; NASH, nonalcoholic steatohepatitis.

case of statin use after liver transplantation. Further details for each are provided elsewhere in this article.

## Hepatitis C

Hepatitis C affects almost 2% of the US population, leading to liver disease–related morbidity and mortality. A retrospective cohort of 830 patients found that hepatitis C virus (HCV)-positive patients on statins are less likely to have severe liver biochemical abnormalities (AST or ALT > 10× ULN or bilirubin > 3) than those not on a statin, but more likely to have mild to moderate LFT abnormalities.[18] Another retrospective cohort study of 20 HCV-positive statin users compared with 64 matched, HCV-positive, nonstatin users demonstrated greater transaminase declines among the statin users over 6 to 12 months.[19]

HCV depends on host lipid metabolism in a number of ways. First, HCV particles use the LDL-C receptor to enter the hepatocyte. Viral particle replication then depends on geranylgeranylation, which requires a product of the cholesterol synthesis pathway. 3-hydroxy-3-methylglutaryl coenzyme A reductase inhibitors may have some antiviral efficacy by disrupting this process.[37] Finally, HCV secretion is linked to secretion of apolipoprotein B. A recent cohort study demonstrated that HCV infection is associated with lower LDL-C levels after adjustment for race, sex and BMI and that successful treatment for HCV is associated with rising LDL-C levels.[38]

These associations between HCV and lipid metabolism suggest a role for statins in HCV therapy. A meta-analysis of 5 studies including 454 patients over 48 weeks demonstrated improvement in sustained virologic response among patients receiving statins with IFN and ribavirin compared with IFN and ribavirin alone (OR, 2.02; 95% CI, 1.38–2.94) without increasing adverse event rates.[20] Randomized, controlled trials have been conducted using fluvastatin, rosuvastatin, and pitavastatin with the most consistent effect on sustained virologic response seen in studies with fluvastatin.[39,40] Further, a retrospective analysis of 3070 patients receiving pegylated interferon and ribavirin found that high pretreatment LDL-C and statin use significantly predicted sustained virologic response in a multivariable regression model.[41]

## Nonalcoholic Fatty Liver Disease and Nonalcoholic Steatohepatitis

The prevalence of NAFLD and NASH has increased dramatically with the increase in obesity. Approximately 9% to 37% of people worldwide have

NAFLD and 3% to 5% have NASH, with rates in obese patients undergoing bariatric surgery estimated to be more than 60% and 25% to 30%, respectively.[42] Individuals with these conditions are likely to have cardiovascular risk factors requiring lipid-lowering therapy and the liver disease itself may benefit from statin therapy.

In addition to larger studies on statin safety, which included patients with NAFLD, there are a number of pilot studies in the literature that specifically address the use of statins in NAFLD or NASH. Over a 6- to 24-month period, atorvastatin was associated with transaminase reduction in pilot studies including fewer than 50 patients.[21–24] Liver biopsies done before and after therapy showed significant improvement in steatosis and necroinflammatory grade, although there was no change in fibrosis grade.[22–24] Small studies in patients on pravastatin and rosuvastatin have shown similar reductions in transaminases and pravastatin-treated patients also had reductions in steatosis and inflammation on posttreatment biopsy.[25,26] Among 137 patients with NAFLD in another study, 68 had follow-up biopsy results (51 without statin and 17 receiving a statin). Statin-treated patients in this cohort demonstrated a decline in steatosis over time.[43]

In contrast to the above studies, a 16 patient pilot study randomizing patients with NASH to simvastatin or placebo found no significant differences in cholesterol levels, biopsy results or transaminases, but was underpowered for such findings, and showed no adverse events in the treatment group.[27] Moreover, a cross-sectional analysis of 2287 patients from the Dallas Heart Study, matching patients on a statin with those who used no lipid-lowering agent by ethnicity, gender, age, waist circumference and IR HOMA demonstrated no significant difference in hepatic steatosis (as measured by H-NMR spectroscopy) or ALT levels between groups.[28] While the studies may be limited by small sample size, cross-sectional design, sample bias, or lack of placebo control, they suggest potential benefit and lack of harm from statin therapy in patients with NAFLD and NASH.

## Primary Biliary Cirrhosis and Cholestatic Liver Disease

Primary biliary cirrhosis (PBC) is a rare autoimmune cholestatic liver disease, predominantly affecting women, that alters cholesterol metabolism. Cholestasis reduces bile acid secretion, leading to decreased bile acid synthesis and reduced hepatic cholesterol synthesis. There is a concurrent reduction in functional LDL receptors as hepatocytes fail and intestinal cholesterol absorption declines. LDL cholesterol increases as disease progresses, but the predominant lipoprotein in cholestatic liver disease is LP-x, which is actually thought to inhibit LDL oxidation, possibly reducing the risk of atherosclerosis. High-density lipoprotein levels are variable in PBC and triglycerides tend to be high. A systematic review from 2007 cited 3 prospective studies of cardiac disease in PBC, each following between 300 and 600 patients for up to 14 years, and found no difference in cardiovascular risk among patients with PBC and those without.[44]

There are few studies of lipid-lowering medications in PBC. Statins could be useful in slowing PBC disease progression through antiinflammatory properties, but there is no clear evidence that this occurs. Those studies that have been conducted include very small numbers of patients, usually lack a control group, may be retrospective, or have short follow-up if prospective. A randomized, controlled trial of simvastatin versus placebo in 21 patients with PBC found significant reduction in LDL-C without adverse effect on liver function in the simvastatin group, although statins had no clear effects on inflammation or endothelial function.[29] Nineteen patients with PBC on 10 mg of atorvastatin (no control group) followed for 1 year demonstrated a 35% reduction in LDL-C, improved endothelial function, and no significant change in liver parameters.[30] A retrospective study of 15 PBC patients on atorvastatin compared with age- and gender-matched controls found a significant reduction in LDL-C, although there was no change in inflammatory parameters or liver enzymes.[31] PBC patients on statins or ezetemibe from a single center followed for a mean duration for 41 months had significant cholesterol reduction and without significant adverse effects or ALT changes.[32] Finally, an early description of 6 PBC patients on simvastatin reflected reduction in LDL-C as well as improvement in alkaline phosphatase, gamma glutamyltransferase, and immunoglobulin M.[45] This limited literature suggests that statins are safe and effective for lipid lowering in PBC, although PBC alone does not seem to increase cardiovascular risk.

## Liver Transplantation

Liver transplantation poses many challenges to lipid-lowering therapy. Immunosuppressive medications can predispose to dyslipidemia and other conditions associated with cardiovascular risk, such as insulin resistance and diabetes. Important drug interactions exist between lipid-lowering agents and immunosuppressive agents. Finally, the risk of therapy to the transplanted organ is also important to weigh.

A single-center, retrospective cohort study of 598 liver or liver–kidney transplant recipients showed hyperlipidemia prevalence increased from 12% pretransplant to 22% at 7 years posttransplant, although this study was limited by use of diagnostic codes and loss to follow-up.[33] Another review of cardiovascular risk factors after transplant found hyperlipidemia incidence rates varying from 29% to 50%.[34] The biggest risk factors for the development of hyperlipidemia were use of sirolimus and glucocorticoids. Sirolimus increases adipose tissue lipase activity, decreases lipoprotein lipase, and increases triglycerides and very low-density lipoprotein cholesterol levels. Glucocorticoids increase acetyl coenzyme A carboxylase, free fatty acid synthetase, and 3-hydroxy-3-methylglutaryl coenzyme A reductase activity. They also stimulate appetite and increase risk for obesity predisposing to dyslipidemia. Cyclosporine leads to hyperlipidemia by reducing conversion of cholesterol to bile salts and decreasing lipoprotein lipase. Tacrolimus seems to be the immunosuppressive agent least associated with hyperlipidemia. A prospective study of 13 patients converted from cyclosporine to tacrolimus found a consistent and significant reduction in total cholesterol at 6 months and significant reduction in triglycerides at 1 month.[46] In a randomized, controlled trial of 110 liver transplant patients, rapid tapering of steroids to tacrolimus monotherapy reduced rates of hypercholesterolemia at 6 months (10% vs 41%; $P = .002$) but not at 5 years (24% vs 16%; $P = .412$).[47]

Drug interactions among lipid-lowering drugs and immunosuppressive agents are concerning. Many immunosuppressives used in liver transplantation (cyclosporine, sirolimus, tacrolimus) are metabolized through CYP3A4 and statins metabolized through the same enzyme (lovastatin, simvastatin, atorvastatin) may alter levels of immunosuppressive medications or be cleared less rapidly, predisposing to increased risks for hepatotoxicity or myopathy. Nonetheless, statins are still considered the cornerstone of therapy for hyperlipidemia in liver transplant patients along with lifestyle modifications. A retrospective review of patients on lipid-lowering agents after transplantation (including statins and fibrates) found that 90% of patients reached target lipid levels and none had a significant increase in LFTs. Of the fewer than 10% who had myalgia or myopathy (none with myositis or rhabdomyolysis), all of these patients were also on cyclosporine, a CYP3A4 inhibitor.[35] An early, prospective cohort study of 98 patients with 2 risk factors for coronary disease given pravastatin 20 mg daily after transplantation found a decrease in total cholesterol in patients on cyclosporine with 2% of patients experiencing mild elevation in creatine phosphokinase and no increase in hepatotoxicity.[36] A randomized, cross-over trial of 16 patients, more than 2 years posttransplantation on cyclosporine or tacrolimus, who received pravastatin 10 mg and cerivastatin 0.1 mg for 6 weeks, each found that both drugs significantly reduced LDL-C from baseline and neither drug adversely affected LFT or creatinine kinase levels or required a change in immunosuppressive dose.[48] The compilation of these trials provides evidence that statins are safe in the setting of liver transplantation, even those that inhibit CYP3A4. Given the totality of CYP3A4 inhibitors amongst the immunosuppressive agents, it does seem prudent to avoid CYP3A4 inhibiting statins unless more aggressive lipid lowering is indicated.

## SUMMARY/DISCUSSION

Statins are critically important for primary and secondary cardiovascular risk reduction and may be used safely in patients with mild liver disease. Routine monitoring of liver enzymes is not recommended given that (1) severe hepatotoxicity is rare and idiosyncratic and (2) mild transaminase elevations are a known class effect of statins, typically resolve without statin interruption, do not recur with rechallenge, and do not seem to be associated with hepatotoxicity in the absence of bilirubin elevation and other signs of synthetic dysfunction. If baseline transaminases are elevated but less than or equal to 3 times the ULN, it is generally safe to continue statin therapy as long as there is not a new or direct bilirubin elevation. In this case, or if baseline transaminases are more than 3 times the ULN, further evaluation for underlying liver disease should proceed according to the NLA liver safety task force algorithm. Transaminase abnormalities should not be assumed automatically to be statin related. The quality of studies of statins in liver disease varies, but pravastatin, atorvastatin, and pitavastatin have been studied in prospective trials, demonstrating lipid-lowering benefit and no liver harm. A meta-analysis and retrospective trials echo these findings. The use of statins specifically in HCV, NAFLD/NASH, PBC, autoimmune hepatitis, and liver transplantation seems to be safe, and in the case of HCV and NAFLD/NASH may also benefit the underlying liver disease. Future research must focus on obtaining long-term follow-up data on the use of statins in patients with liver disease as well as comparing statin therapies in large,

prospective, placebo-controlled, randomized trials in this population.

## REFERENCES

1. Cholesterol Treatment Trialists (CTT) Collaboration. Efficacy and safety of LDL-lowering therapy among men and women: meta-analysis of individual data from 174,000 participants in 27 randomised trials. Lancet 2015. http://dx.doi.org/10.1016/S0140-6736(14)61368-4 [pii:S0140–6736(14)61368-4].
2. Simonson SG, Martin PD, Mitchell P, et al. Pharmacokinetics and pharmacodynamics of rosuvastatin in subjects with hepatic impairment. Eur J Clin Pharmacol 2003;58:669–75.
3. Bays H, Cohen DE, Chalasani N, et al. An assessment by the statin liver safety task force: 2014 update. J Clin Lipidol 2014;8:S47–57.
4. Cohen DE, Anania FA, Chalasani N. An assessment of statin safety by hepatologists. Am J Cardiol 2006; 97:77C–81C.
5. Tzefos M, Olin JL. 3-hydroxyl-3-methylglutaryl coenzyme A reductase inhibitor use in chronic liver disease: a therapeutic controversy. J Clin Lipidol 2011;5:450–9.
6. Riley P, Bakir MA, O'Donohue J, et al. Prescribing statins to patients with nonalcoholic fatty liver disease: real cardiovascular benefits outweigh theoretical hepatotoxic risk. Cardiovasc Ther 2009;27:216–20.
7. Chalasani N. Statins and hepatotoxicity: focus on patients with fatty liver. Hepatology 2005;41:690–5.
8. FDA Drug Safety Communication. Important safety label changes to cholesterol-lowering statin drugs. Available at: http://www.fda.gov/drugs/drugsafety/ucm293101.htm. Accessed May 31, 2013.
9. Lewis JH, Mortensen ME, Zweig S, et al. Efficacy and safety of high-dose pravastatin in hypercholesterolemic patients with well-compensated chronic liver disease: results of a prospective, randomized, double-blind, placebo-controlled, multicenter trial. Hepatology 2007;46:1453–63.
10. Foster T, Budoff MJ, Saab S, et al. Atorvastatin and antioxidants for the treatment of nonalcoholic fatty liver disease: the St. Francis Heart Study randomized clinical trial. Am J Gastroenterol 2011;106: 71–7.
11. Athyros VG, Tziomalos K, Gossios TD, et al. Safety and efficacy of long-term statin treatment for cardiovascular events in patients with coronary heart disease and abnormal liver tests in the Greek Atorvastatin and Coronary Heart Disease Evaluation (GREACE) study: a post-hoc analysis. Lancet 2010; 376:1916–22.
12. Tikkanen MJ, Fayyad R, Paergeman O, et al, for the IDEAL Investigators. Effect of intensive lipid lowering with atorvastatin on cardiovascular outcomes in coronary heart disease patients with mild-to-moderate

baseline elevations in alanine aminotransferase levels. Int J Cardiol 2013;168:3846–52.

13. Han KH, Rha SW, Kang HJ, et al. Evaluation of short-term safety and efficacy of HMG-CoA reductase inhibitors in hypercholesterolemic patients with elevated serum alanine transaminase concentrations: PITCH study (PITavastatin versus atorvastatin to evaluate the effect on patients with hypercholesterolemia and mild to moderate hepatic damage). J Clin Lipidol 2012;6:340–51.

14. Athyros VG, Mikhailidis DP, Didangelos TP, et al. Effect of multifactorial treatment on non-alcoholic fatty liver disease in metabolic syndrome: a randomised study. Curr Med Res Opin 2006;22:873–83.

15. deDenus S, Spindelr SA, Miller K, et al. Statins and Liver Toxicity: a meta-analysis. Pharmacotherapy 2004;24:584–91.

16. Chalasani N, Aljadhey H, Kesterson J, et al. Patients with elevated liver enzymes are not at higher risk for statin hepatotoxicity. Gastroenterology 2004;126:1287–92.

17. Vuppalanchi R, Teal E, Chalasani N. Patients with elevated baseline liver enzymes do not have higher frequency of hepatotoxicity from lovastatin than those with normal baseline liver enzymes. Am J Med Sci 2005;329:62–5.

18. Khorashadi S, Hasson NK, Cheung RC. Incidence of statin hepatotoxicity in patients with hepatitis C. Clin Gastroenterol Hepatol 2006;4:902–7.

19. Henderson LM, Patel S, Giordano TP, et al. Statin therapy and serum transaminases among a cohort of HCV-infected veterans. Dig Dis Sci 2010;55:190–5.

20. Zhu Q, Li N, Han Q, et al. Statin therapy improves response to interferon alfa and ribavirin in chronic hepatitis C: a systematic review and meta-analysis. Antiviral Res 2013;98:373–9.

21. Gomez-Dominguez E, Gisbert JP, Moreno-Monteagudo JA, et al. A pilot study of atorvastatin treatment in dyslipidemic, non-alcoholic fatty liver patients. Aliment Pharmacol Ther 2006;23:1643–7.

22. Hatzitolios A, Savopoulos C, Lazarski G, et al. Efficacy of omega-3 fatty acids, atorvastatin and orlistat in non-alcoholic fatty liver disease with dyslipidemia. Indian J Gastroenterol 2004;23:131–4.

23. Kimura Y, Hyogo H, Yamagishi SI, et al. Atorvastatin decreases serum levels of advanced glycation end-products (AGEs) in nonalcoholic steatohepatitis (NASH) patients with dyslipidemia: clinical usefulness of AGEs as a biomarker for the attenuation of NASH. J Gastroenterol 2010;45:750–7.

24. Hyogo H, Tazuma S, Arihiro K, et al. Efficacy of atorvastatin for the treatment of nonalcoholic steatohepatitis with dyslipidemia. Metabolism 2008;57:1711–8.

25. Antonopoulos S, Mikros S, Mylonopoulou M, et al. Rosuvastatin as a novel treatment of non-alcoholic fatty liver disease in hyperlipidemia patients. Atherosclerosis 2006;184:233–4.

26. Rallidis LS, Drakoulis CK. Pravastatin in patients with nonalcoholic steatohepatitis: results of a pilot study. Atherosclerosis 2004;174:193–6.

27. Nelson A, Torres D, Morgan AE, et al. A pilot study using simvastatin in the treatment of nonalcoholic steatohepatitis: a randomized placebo-controlled trial. J Clin Gastroenterol 2009;43:990–4.

28. Browning JD. Statins and hepatic steatosis: perspectives from the Dallas Heart Study. Hepatology 2006;44:466–71.

29. Cash WJ, O'Neill S, O'donnell ME, et al. Randomized controlled trial assessing the effect of simvastatin in primary biliary cirrhosis. Liver Int 2013;33:1–9.

30. Stojakovic T, Claudel T, Putz-Bankuti C, et al. Low dose atorvastatin improves dyslipidemia and vascular function in patients with primary biliary cirrhosis after one year of treatment. Atherosclerosis 2010;209:178–83.

31. Stanca CM, Bach N, Allina J, et al. Atorvastatin does not improve liver biochemistries or Mayo Risk Score in Primary Biliary Cirrhosis. Dig Dis Sci 2008;53:1988–93.

32. Rajab MA, Kaplan MM. Statins in Primary Biliary Cirrhosis: are they safe? Dig Dis Sci 2010;55:2086–8.

33. Parekh J, Corley DA, Feng S. Diabetes, hypertension, and hyperlipidemia: prevalence over time and impact on long-term survival after liver transplantation. Am J Transplant 2012;12:2182–7.

34. Desai S, Hong JC, Saab S. Cardiovascular risk factors following orthotopic liver transplantation: predisposing factors, incidence and management. Liver Int 2010;30:948–57.

35. Martin J, Cavanaugh T, Trumbull L, et al. Incidence of adverse events with HMG-CoA reductase inhibitors in liver transplant patients. Clin Transplant 2008;22:113–9.

36. Ingawa D, Dawson S, Holt C, et al. Hyperlipidemia after liver transplantation: natural history and treatment with the hydroxy-methylglutaryl-coenzyme A reductase inhibitor pravastatin. Transplantation 1996;62:934–42.

37. Ye J, Wang C, Sumpter R, et al. Disruption of hepatitis C virus RNA replication through inhibition of host protein geranylgeranylation. Proc Natl Acad Sci U S A 2003;100:15865–70.

38. Corey KE, Kane E, Munroe C, et al. Hepatitis C virus infection and its clearance alter circulating lipids: implications for long-term follow-up. Hepatology 2009;50:1030–7.

39. Kondo C, Atsukawa M, Tsubota A, et al. An open-label randomized controlled study of pegylated interferon/ribavirin combination therapy for chronic hepatitis C with versus without fluvastatin. J Viral Hepat 2012;19:615–22.

40. Shimada M, Yoshida S, Masuzaki R, et al. Pitavastatin enhances antiviral efficacy of standard pegylated

interferon plus ribavirin in patients with chronic hepatitis C: a prospective randomized pilot study. J Hepatol 2012;56:298–302.

41. Harrison SA, Rossaro L, Hu KQ, et al. Serum cholesterol and statin use predict virological response to pegintereron and ribavirin therapy. Hepatology 2010;52:864–74.

42. Rafiq N, Bai C, Fang Y, et al. Long-term follow-up of patients with nonalcoholic fatty liver. Clin Gastroenterol Hepatol 2009;7:234–8.

43. Ekstedt M, Franzen LE, Mathiesen UL, et al. Statins in non-alcoholic fatty liver disease and chronically elevated liver enzymes: a histopathological follow-up study. J Hepatol 2007;47:135–41.

44. Sorokin A, Brown JL, Thompson PD. Primary biliary cirrhosis, hyperlipidemia, and atherosclerotic risk: a systematic review. Atherosclerosis 2007;194:293–9.

45. Ritzel U, Leonhardt U, Nather M, et al. Simvastatin in primary biliary cirrhosis: effects on serum lipids and distinct disease markers. J Hepatol 2002;36: 454–9.

46. Roy A, Kneteman N, Lilly L, et al. Tacrolimus as intervention in the treatment of hyperlipidemia after liver transplant. Transplantation 2006;82: 494–500.

47. Weiler N, Thrun I, Hoppe-Lotichius M, et al. Early steroid free immunosuppression with FK506 after liver transplantation: long-term results of a prospectively randomized double-blinded trial. Transplantation 2010;90:1562–6.

48. Zachoval R, Gerbes AL, Schwandt P, et al. Short-term effects of statin therapy in patients with hyperlipoproteinemia after liver transplantation: results of a randomized cross-over trial. J Hepatol 2001;35: 86–91.

# Genetic Testing in Hyperlipidemia

Ozlem Bilen, MD[a,1], Yashashwi Pokharel, MD, MSCR[b,c,1], Christie M. Ballantyne, MD[c,d,e],*

## KEYWORDS

- Dyslipidemia • Hereditary lipid disorder • Familial hypercholesterolemia • Genetic testing

## KEY POINTS

- Cascade screening of family members with lipid profile should be widely implemented for identification of familial hypercholesterolemia (FH) cases.
- Using cholesterol levels and other clinical information for FH diagnosis and screening can be specific but less sensitive.
- Some existing FH diagnostic criteria already incorporate genetic information for FH diagnosis. Identification of specific mutation or mutations in the affected individual with a focused screening of the mutation in family members can be quick and less expensive.
- Employment and insurance implications of genetic screening are important.
- Randomized clinical trials and cost-effectiveness analyses comparing the incremental benefit of genetic testing with clinical criteria are needed.

## INTRODUCTION

Levels of certain plasma lipids and lipoproteins, such as low-density lipoprotein (LDL) cholesterol (LDL-C) and lipoprotein(a) (Lp[a]), are key risk factors for cardiovascular disease (CVD).[1,2] Although plasma lipids are determined largely by environmental and genetic factors, for some individuals levels are primarily determined by genotype. The Fredrickson classification of lipid disorders was based on common phenotypes (ie, abnormal lipid and lipoprotein subclasses) (**Table 1**).[3] Some of these phenotypes are frequently due to monogenic defects that directly affect lipoproteins and their function, and others are associated with polygenic abnormalities with multiple genetic variations.[3]

Familial hypercholesterolemia (FH), which most commonly has a Fredrickson IIa phenotype, is the most common hereditary lipid disorder, resulting in elevated blood cholesterol levels

Disclosures: O. Bilen: Nothing to disclose. Y. Pokharel: Supported by American Heart Association SWA Summer 2014 Postdoctoral Fellowship Award. C.M. Ballantyne: Grant/Research support (All paid to institution, not individual): Abbott Diagnostic, Amarin, Amgen, Eli Lilly, Esperion, GlaxoSmithKline, Merck, Novartis, Pfizer, Regeneron, Roche Diagnostic, Sanofi-Synthelabo, National Institutes of Health, American Heart Association. Consultant: Abbott Diagnostics, Amarin, Amgen, Astra Zeneca, Cerenis, Esperion, Genentech, Genzyme, Kowa, Merck, Novartis, Pfizer, Regeneron, Sanofi-Synthelabo. Advisory panel: Merck, Pfizer.

[a] Department of Medicine, Baylor College of Medicine, 3131 Fannin Street, Houston, TX 77030, USA; [b] Section of Cardiovascular Research, Department of Medicine, Baylor College of Medicine, 6565 Fannin Street, Suite B157, Houston, TX 77030, USA; [c] Center for Cardiovascular Disease Prevention, Methodist DeBakey Heart and Vascular Center, 6565 Fannin Street, M.S. A-601, Houston, TX 77030, USA; [d] Section of Cardiovascular Research, Department of Medicine, Baylor College of Medicine, 6565 Fannin Street, M.S. A-601, Suite 656, Houston, TX 77030, USA; [e] Section of Cardiology, Department of Medicine, Baylor College of Medicine, 6565 Fannin Street, M.S. A-601, Suite 656, Houston, TX 77030, USA
[1] Both authors contributed equally.
* Corresponding author. 6565 Fannin Street, M.S. A-601, Suite 656, Houston, TX 77030.
*E-mail address:* cmb@bcm.edu

**Table 1**
**Genetics underlying Fredrickson phenotypes**

| ICD 10 Codes | Fredrickson Phenotype | ↑ Lipid(s) | ↑ Lipoprotein(s) | Genetic Mutations |
|---|---|---|---|---|
| E78.3 Hyperchylomicronemia | I | TG | CM | Monogenic; autosomal recessive: *LPL, APOC2*; other forms: *APOA5, LMF1, ?GPIHBP1* |
| E78.0 Pure hypercholesterolemia | IIa | Chol | LDL | ~90% polygenic, ~10% monogenic; heterozygous: *LDLR, APOB, PCSK9*; homozygous: *LDLR, LDLRAP1* |
| E78.2 Mixed hyperlipidemia | IIb | Chol, TG | VLDL, LDL | Polygenic; some cases due to *USF1, APOB, LPL*; ~35% have *APOA5* S19W or −1131T>C |
| E78.2 Mixed hyperlipidemia | III | Chol, TG | IDL | Polygenic; *APOE* or homozygosity for E2 allele of *APOE* necessary but not sufficient; ~40% have *APOA5* S19W or −1131T>C |
| E78.1 Pure hyperglyceridemia | IV | TG | VLDL | Polygenic; ~35% have *APOA5* S19W or −1131T>C |
| E78.3 Hyperchylomicronemia | V | Chol, TG | VLDL, CM | Polygenic; ~10%: *LPL, APOC2, APOA5*; ~55% have *APOA5* S19W or −1131T>C; small effects from *APOE, TRIB1, CHREBP, GALNT2, GCKR, ANGPTL3* |

*Abbreviations:* 1131T>C, a T-to-C conversion at position −1131; *ANGPTL3*, angiopoietin-like 3; *APOA5*, apolipoprotein A-V; *APOB*, apolipoprotein B; *APOC2*, apolipoprotein C-II; *APOE*, apolipoprotein E; Chol, cholesterol; *CHREBP*, carbohydrate response element binding protein (also known as *MLX/PL*); CM, chylomicron; *GALNT2*, UDP-N-acetyl-α-D-galactosamine:polypeptide *N*-acetylgalactosaminyltransferase 2; *GCKR*, glucokinase regulator; HLP, hyperlipoproteinemia; IDL, intermediate-density lipoprotein; *LDLRAP1*, LDL receptor adaptor protein 1 (also known as *ARH*); *LPL*, lipoprotein lipase; *PCSK9*, proprotein convertase subtilisin/kexin type 9; S19W, serine to tryptophan conversion at amino acid 19; TG, triglyceride; *TRIB1*, tribbles homologue 1 (*Drosophila*); *USF1*, upstream transcription factor 1; VLDL, very low density lipoprotein.

and premature atherosclerotic disease. FH has an autosomal-dominant inheritance with rare autosomal-recessive forms also described.[4] The most common cause of FH is mutation in the LDL receptor (LDL-R), with greater than 1600 different genetic mutations associated with FH.[5] Other causes include defects in apolipoprotein B (apoB), gain-of-function mutations in proprotein convertase subtilisin/kexin 9 (PCSK9), and other rare genetic abnormalities resulting in the FH phenotype.[6–8] FH can be heterozygous (HeFH), affecting only one allele; homozygous (HoFH), affecting 2 identical alleles; or compound heterozygous, affecting 2 different alleles. HeFH is among the most common metabolic disorders, affecting 1 in 300 to 1 in 500 individuals.[9] In founder populations such as French Canadians, Dutch, and Lebanese, HeFH is even more prevalent (1 in 50 to 1 in 100 individuals).[10–12] FH has a gene-dose effect such that in patients with HoFH, LDL-C level often exceeds 500 mg/dL. Patients with HeFH typically have LDL-C levels greater than 160 mg/dL as children and greater than 190 mg/dL as adults.[13] In addition to lifestyle changes, high-intensity statins are the pharmacotherapy of first choice, and if adequate response is not obtained, other lipid-lowering medications and LDL apheresis are available. In general, response to cholesterol-lowering medications that lead to increased LDL-R activity is determined by the degree of LDL-R function.[14]

In patients with HeFH, the risk of premature coronary heart disease increases by about 20-fold compared with individuals without FH.[15] Very often, a myocardial infarction is the first presenting sign in FH patients.[16] Approximately 20% of myocardial infarctions before the age of 45 years and 5% before the age of 60 years can be attributed to FH.[14] It is estimated that the risk of having CVD before age 50 is about 50% in men and 30% in women with FH. Despite the risk burden, most individuals with FH remain undiagnosed and either untreated or inadequately treated.[9,17] Furthermore, it has been shown that after FH patients attain optimal LDL-C levels by using lifestyle and pharmacologic therapies (such as high-intensity statins), the risk for ischemic events is reduced to that in non-FH populations.[18,19] Therefore, an improved screening and diagnostic tool for FH would be of immense public health value.

Lp(a) is another atherogenic lipoprotein, and higher levels increase the risk for ischemic cardiovascular events independent of other risk factors, including LDL-C.[20] Elevated Lp(a) is also one of the most commonly inherited dyslipidemias and is primarily genetically determined, but unfortunately, no approved therapies that lower Lp(a) also lower ischemic vascular events.[21] Currently, there is no clear role of genetic testing in routine practice in the management of individuals with elevated levels of Lp(a).

In this article genetic testing in the management of lipid disorders is reviewed, with a focus on FH.

## GENETIC TESTING IN FAMILIAL HYPERCHOLESTEROLEMIA
### Current Clinical Criteria for Diagnosis of Familial Hypercholesterolemia

It is currently estimated that only about 15% to 20% of patients with FH are actually diagnosed.[9] There are no internationally accepted criteria for FH diagnosis. However, the 3 commonly used criteria are the Dutch, Simon Broome, and US MedPed criteria (**Table 2**). Unlike the US criteria, which use total cholesterol levels and family history of FH, the Simon Broome and the Dutch criteria integrate personal and family lipid profiles, history of premature CVD (onset in men before age 55 years and in women before age 65 years), physical examination findings such as tendon xanthomas for the index person and family members, and genetic information.[22–24] The Simon Broome and the Dutch criteria classify definitive, probable, and possible FH. According to the Simon Broome criteria, to make a definitive FH diagnosis, either a positive genetic test or elevated cholesterol levels accompanied by tendon xanthomas in self or family are needed, whereas according to the Dutch criteria (which uses a scoring system), either a positive genetic test or a constellation of the aforementioned nongenetic criteria qualify for a definitive FH diagnosis (see **Table 2**).

The first steps in the assessment of a hereditary dyslipidemia in a clinic are to take a thorough history, including family history that covers at least 3 generations' history of CVD (including premature onset) and risk factors, family members' lipid profile (if available), performing a focused physical examination, and ordering a lipid profile. The presence of tendon xanthomas should be sought by careful inspection and palpation of the tendons commonly affected, such as the Achilles, finger extensor, and patellar tendons. Corneal arcus, if present in a patient under the age of 45 years, can indicate FH. Similarly, xanthelasma or tuberous xanthomas in a young patient should raise a concern for FH, although these are not FH specific.

### Genetic Testing to Improve Diagnostic Accuracy

It is obvious that identification of the mutated gene or genes provides a definite diagnosis of FH, which

**Table 2**
**Clinical criteria in diagnosis of familial hypercholesterolemia**

| Simon Broome Familial Hypercholesterolemia Register Diagnostic Criteria for Familial Hypercholesterolemia: Criteria (Description) | |
| --- | --- |
| • TC >290 mg/dL in adults or >260 mg/dL in children aged <16 y, or LDL-C >190 mg/dL in adults or >155 mg/dL in children (A)<br>• Tendinous xanthomata in the patient or a first-degree relative (B)<br>• Positive DNA test (C)<br>• Family history of premature CVD (D)<br>• Family history of: TC >290 mg/dL in a first-degree or second-degree relative or >260 mg/dL in child or sibling aged <16 y (E) | Definitive FH: A and B or C<br>Probable FH: A and D or A and E |

| Dutch Lipid Clinic Network Diagnostic Criteria for Familial Hypercholesterolemia: Criteria (Points) | |
| --- | --- |
| • First-degree relative with known premature (men <55 y; women <60 y) coronary and vascular disease, or first-degree relative with known LDL-C above the 95th percentile (1)<br>• First-degree relative with tendinous xanthomata and/or arcus cornealis, or children aged <18 y with LDL-C above the 95th percentile (2)<br>• Patient with premature CAD (2)<br>• Patient with premature CVD or PVD (1)<br>• Tendinous xanthoma (6)<br>• Arcus cornealis before age 45 y (4)<br>• LDL-C ≥329 (8), 251–329 (5), 193–251 (3), 155–193 (1)<br>• Functional mutation in LDLR gene (8) | Definite FH: ≥8 points<br>Probable FH: 6–8 points<br>Possible FH: 3–5 points |

| US MedPed Program Diagnostic Criteria for Probable Heterozygous Familial Hypercholesterolemia | | | | |
| --- | --- | --- | --- | --- |
| | **Total Cholesterol (mg/dL)** | | | |
| Age (y) | First-Degree Relative with FH | Second-Degree Relative with FH | Third-Degree Relative with FH | General Population |
| <20 | 220 | 230 | 240 | 270 |
| 20–29 | 240 | 250 | 260 | 290 |
| 30–39 | 270 | 280 | 290 | 340 |
| ≥40 | 290 | 300 | 310 | 360 |

is not always the case with a clinical diagnosis of FH. Clinical criteria are, in general, more specific than sensitive because they usually identify individuals with an extreme phenotype, such as those with very high LDL-C levels.[24] Although the clinical criteria are low cost and easy to assess, they lack sensitivity for several reasons. Some FH patients may not have severely elevated LDL-C levels and can be easily missed by using these clinical criteria.[25] The cholesterol levels used in these clinical criteria are off-treatment levels; however, most FH patients seen in a clinic are usually on cholesterol-lowering medications and therefore it is frequently difficult to obtain untreated total cholesterol and LDL-C levels in routine practice. Similarly, physical examination findings may not be as helpful in the modern era. Not only are findings such as corneal arcus and xanthelasma not specific to FH but common in the general aging population,[26] but more importantly, FH-specific findings such as tendon xanthoma, which results from lifelong cholesterol accumulation on tendons, are frequently not present when statins are used in FH patients since very early in life. Furthermore, family history may not be reliable in regard to premature CVD with improved medical therapy. Furthermore, women with FH usually manifest disease later than men. Therefore, it is possible that a male proband may present with premature onset of coronary heart disease, while his mother may have high levels of LDL-C but no history of an ischemic cardiac event. Genetic testing in the mother will be very helpful in this situation so that a proactive prevention strategy can be used to lower LDL-C for both the mother and her offspring, who may inherit the mutated genes. In all these situations, given its high sensitivity and specificity,[27,28] genetic testing can be of value in diagnosing FH.[24] Clearly, in both the Simon Broome and the Dutch criteria, a positive genetic test alone is sufficient to make the diagnosis of FH, whereas many individuals who would clinically have an autosomal-dominant pattern of high LDL-C and heart disease no longer meet these criteria.

## Genetic Testing in Screening for Familial Hypercholesterolemia

Cascade screening involves stepwise diagnosis of all first-degree relatives of FH patients and it then extends to second-degree and third-degree relatives. Data from the United Kingdom suggest that cascade screening was associated with FH diagnosis at a younger age and led to higher rates of statin therapy in FH patients.[29] As mentioned previously, the institution of statin therapy in FH patients has been associated with a reduction in incident coronary heart disease.[18,30]

Cascade screening can be performed using clinical criteria, which rely mostly on cholesterol levels, or by using genetic testing. A mutation can be identified in up to 80% of the screened population depending on the clinical criteria used for FH diagnosis and sensitivity of the genetic test used. Once a mutation is found in the index case, genetic testing in first-degree relatives is quick, less expensive, and very sensitive and specific.[31] Although the cost of genetic testing may be of concern, cascade genetic testing has been shown to be the most effective strategy in screening for FH.[32,33]

The first successful model of a national genetic cascade screening program came from the Netherlands; since it started in 1994, more than 9000 FH patients have been identified.[32] Initially, without genetic testing, only 39% of these individuals were on cholesterol-lowering medications, and after 2 years of genetic screening, 85% were on medications. Other countries that followed similar strategies include Norway, Spain, Australia, New Zealand, and Wales. In general, mutation detection ranged from 36% to 59%, and the rates differed based on the original likelihood for having an FH diagnosis and on the methods used for genetic screening.[34–36] The National Institute for Health and Clinical Excellence in the United Kingdom recommends genetic cascade screening of close biological relatives of people with a clinical diagnosis of FH to identify additional FH patients effectively.[37,38] It should be noted that FH screening using a genetic approach has not been compared directly with using clinical FH criteria in a randomized controlled trial, and therefore, data are lacking on the potential benefit of a genetic approach compared with clinical criteria for FH diagnosis and screening. Furthermore, because FH remains underdiagnosed and cascade screening has been shown to be effective, it is very important to adopt wide implementation of cascade screening of family members (using cholesterol levels and clinical criteria) first.

In the United States as elsewhere, FH is underdiagnosed, indicating a need for better screening.[9] The American College of Cardiology/American Heart Association guidelines to treat cholesterol identified individuals with off-treatment LDL-C of 190 mg/dL or greater (individuals with FH usually have LDL-C >190 mg/dL) as a group that would benefit from statin therapy regardless of the underlying cause.[39] The National Lipid Association Expert Panel published clinical guidelines to address screening, diagnosis, and management of FH and recommended cascade screening with clinical criteria and using genetic testing in cases of diagnostic uncertainty.[40] The Familial Hypercholesterolemia Foundation recently established a multicenter registry in the United States, Cascade Screening for Awareness and Detection of Familial Hypercholesterolemia (CASCADE-FH), to improve awareness and eventually screening and outcomes in FH patients.[41] As cascade screening progresses in the United States, using genetic testing can be complementary to diagnosis and in certain situations may provide additional valuable information that may influence treatment decisions and outcomes.[40]

## Genetic Testing in the Treatment of Familial Hypercholesterolemia

The presence of specific genetic mutations can be informative in FH treatment, especially given that currently there are numerous classes of approved and investigational therapies submitted for regulatory approval that work via different mechanisms.[40] Genetic sequencing may also identify new and unknown mutations, which may lead to novel therapeutic targets. Mutations in the PCSK9 gene were first identified in 2 French families who had phenotypic FH, and ultimately, led to the discovery that gain-of-function mutations in PCSK9 can cause FH.[7] Conversely, loss-of-function mutations were associated with lower LDL-C levels and lower risk of CVD.[42] These genetic data led to the development of a number of monoclonal antibodies against PCSK9 as a therapeutic target, which are currently under investigation in phase 3 trials, with 2 already submitted for regulatory approval.[43] In addition, response to lipid lowering, with some patients showing excellent response and others very resistant to treatment with statins,[44] may be predicted by genetic information in patients who are clinically thought to have HoFH, as shown in the Trial Evaluating PCSK9 Antibody in Subjects with LDL Receptor Abnormalities, in which the efficacy of evolocumab, a monoclonal antibody against PCSK9, for reducing LDL-C levels in clinically defined HoFH patients was dependent on LDL-R mutations without complete loss of function, suggesting that genetic data can provide incremental information to assess response to treatment.[45] Other studies have shown association of certain alleles with response to statins and CVD outcomes.[46–50]

Another use of genetic information is in pharmacogenomics. In addition to the usefulness in assessing response to certain medications as described previously, certain genetic variants may be associated with increased likelihood of having an adverse effect from a certain medication, such as SLCO1B1 with high-dose simvastatin,[51] although testing for such mutations has not been firmly established in lipid disorders.[13]

## OTHER POTENTIAL USES OF GENETIC TESTING

Numerous biomarkers have been tested for CVD risk prediction,[52,53] and a growing area of interest is the identification of common genetic variants associated with the development of CVD.[54,55] Pilot studies have shown that single-nucleotide polymorphism data can assist in prediction of CVD risk.[55,56] Common variants at 9p21 exhibit the strongest and most reproducible associations with CVD in genome-wide association studies.[54,55,57] In the Atherosclerosis Risk in Communities study, the 9p21 allele was added to a base model with traditional risk factors to assess the incremental value of 9p21 variants to predict CVD and to assess potential reclassification of individuals among risk categories. The hazards ratio for incident CVD was 1.2 per allele ($P<.0003$), and 12.1% and 12.6% of the low-intermediate and high-intermediate groups were appropriately reclassified, respectively.[58] However, the addition of 9p21 variants to a conventional risk factor model in the Women's Health Study did not change the C statistic or improve calibration, and the net reclassification improvement was modest (2.7%, $P<.02$).[59] Therefore, these data suggest that the 9p21 variation is associated with modestly increased risk for CVD; however, the net reclassification improvement was less than that provided by imaging tests or assessment of biomarkers.

## GENETIC TESTING IN HYPERTRIGLYCERIDEMIA

Another important plasma lipid is triglyceride. Mild-to-moderate hypertriglyceridemia, as commonly encountered in clinical practice, is typically lifestyle related, but can also be polygenic and result from the cumulative burden of common and rare variants in several genes.[60] Familial chylomicronemia syndrome is a monogenic autosomal-recessive disorder caused by 2 mutant alleles of the genes encoding lipoprotein lipase, apoC-II, apoA-V, lipase maturation factor 1, glycosylphosphatidylinositol-anchored high-density lipoprotein binding protein 1, or glycerol-3-phosphate dehydrogenase 1.[60] Because of clustering of susceptibility alleles and lifestyle-related factors in families, biochemical screening and counseling for family members are essential, but routine genetic testing is not warranted.[60]

## DISADVANTAGES OF GENETIC TESTING

The yield of genetic testing varies by referral criteria used and the population studied. Up to 10% to 30% of individuals may lack a mutation, especially in populations without founder effects and with significant ancestral heterogeneity such as the US population.[61] Most of these individuals are thought to have polygenic disease. Mutation detection rates are also lower in individuals classified as having possible or probable FH than in those with definite FH. Although the specificity for genetic testing is very high, false-positive cases may be seen with nonpathogenic sequences.

Cost of genetic testing can be a potential problem, although the price of genetic testing for patients with severe hypercholesterolemia has substantially decreased over time (**Table 3**). The psychological or emotional impact of "labeling" on patients and family members should also be considered. Legal ramifications regarding insurance or employment can be important and are covered in the United States by the Genetic Information Nondiscrimination Act (GINA), which prohibits the use of genetic information in health insurance and employment.[62] However, it should be noted that GINA does not apply to employers with less than 15 employees. The protection in employment does not extend to the US military, nor does it apply to health insurance through the Tricare Military Health System, the Indian Health Service, the Veterans Health Administration, or the Federal Employees Health Benefits Program. Finally, the law does not cover long-term care insurance, life insurance, and disability insurance.[63]

**Table 3**
**Laboratories offering genetic testing in the United States and costs of the tests**

| Gene | % of FH | No. of Mutations/Cost | US Laboratories |
|------|---------|----------------------|-----------------|
| LDLR | 60%–80% | • >1000 mutations<br>○ Whole gene analysis<br>■ ~$1400<br>○ Deletion/duplication test<br>■ ~$2030 | • 7 in USA: (20 International)<br>○ Ambry Genetics (CA)<br>○ Correlagen Diagnostics (MA)<br>○ Athena Diagnostics (MA)<br>○ Mayo Clinic (MN)<br>○ Baylor College of Medicine (TX)<br>○ Progenika (MA)<br>○ Prevention Genetics (WI) |
| ApoB | 1%–10% | • 1 common mutation<br>○ Targeted mutation analysis<br>■ ~$400 | • 2 in USA: (6 International)<br>○ Ambry Genetics (CA)<br>○ ARUP Laboratories (UT) |
| PCSK9 | <5% | • 1 common mutation<br>○ Targeted mutation analysis<br>■ ~$1400 | • 1 in USA: (2 International)<br>○ Ambry Genetics (CA) |

NOTE: Subsequent testing in family members is inexpensive once causal variant is already identified (~$250–$400). The costs for genetic tests may or may not be covered by health insurance.

Interpretation of genetic test results may appear confusing to physicians and can require specialized expertise unless presented in simplified form. In addition, "incidentally found mutations" without known phenotypic associations can be confusing to both patients and health care providers.

## CURRENT TESTS AVAILABLE

Currently available tests and testing centers can be identified from the Gene Tests Web site (see **Table 3**).[64] **Table 3** summarizes currently available US laboratories that offer specific genetic tests.

## SUMMARY

FH is a common disorder in which early diagnosis and treatment can prevent the development of CVD in most individuals. Unfortunately, this common disorder is underdiagnosed and undertreated. Using clinical screening and diagnostic tools, such as CASCADE-FH, screening can be very effective and should be widely adopted. As advances in human genome sequencing are being made, there is increasing evidence that genetic information can be helpful in screening, diagnosis, and treatment of FH. However, randomized trials and cost-effectiveness studies to assess the incremental benefit of genetic testing over clinical criteria for screening and diagnosis of FH are needed to provide definitive answers for wider implementation of genetic testing in clinical practice.

## ACKNOWLEDGMENTS

We thank Kerrie Jara for her editorial assistance.

## REFERENCES

1. Lusis AJ. Atherosclerosis. Nature 2000;407:233–41.
2. Rader DJ, Daugherty A. Translating molecular discoveries into new therapies for atherosclerosis. Nature 2008;451:904–13.
3. Hegele RA. Plasma lipoproteins: genetic influences and clinical implications. Nat Rev Genet 2009;10:109–21.
4. Tada H, Kawashiri MA, Nohara A, et al. Autosomal recessive hypercholesterolemia: a mild phenotype of familial hypercholesterolemia: insight from the kinetic study using stable isotope and animal studies. J Atheroscler Thromb 2014. [Epub ahead of print].
5. Brown MS, Goldstein JL. A receptor-mediated pathway for cholesterol homeostasis. Science 1986;232:34–47.
6. Innerarity TL, Weisgraber KH, Arnold KS, et al. Familial defective apolipoprotein B-100: low density lipoproteins with abnormal receptor binding. Proc Natl Acad Sci U S A 1987;84:6919–23.
7. Abifadel M, Varret M, Rabes JP, et al. Mutations in PCSK9 cause autosomal dominant hypercholesterolemia. Nat Genet 2003;34:154–6.
8. Garcia CK, Wilund K, Arca M, et al. Autosomal recessive hypercholesterolemia caused by mutations in a putative LDL receptor adaptor protein. Science 2001;292:1394–8.
9. Nordestgaard BG, Chapman MJ, Humphries SE, et al. Familial hypercholesterolaemia is underdiagnosed

and undertreated in the general population: guidance for clinicians to prevent coronary heart disease: consensus statement of the European Atherosclerosis Society. Eur Heart J 2013;34:3478–3490a.

10. Moorjani S, Roy M, Gagne C, et al. Homozygous familial hypercholesterolemia among French Canadians in Quebec Province. Arteriosclerosis 1989;9: 211–6.

11. Seftel HC, Baker SG, Jenkins T, et al. Prevalence of familial hypercholesterolemia in Johannesburg Jews. Am J Med Genet 1989;34:545–7.

12. Fahed AC, Nemer GM. Familial hypercholesterolemia: the lipids or the genes? Nutr Metab (Lond) 2011;8:23.

13. Bays HE, Jones PH, Brown WV, et al. National Lipid Association annual summary of clinical lipidology 2015. J Clin Lipidol 2014;8:S1–36.

14. Hopkins PN, Toth PP, Ballantyne CM, et al. Familial hypercholesterolemias: prevalence, genetics, diagnosis and screening recommendations from the National Lipid Association Expert Panel on Familial Hypercholesterolemia. J Clin Lipidol 2011;5:S9–17.

15. Watts GF, Lewis B, Sullivan DR. Familial hypercholesterolemia: a missed opportunity in preventive medicine. Nat Clin Pract Cardiovasc Med 2007;4: 404–5.

16. Wu NQ, Guo YL, Xu RX, et al. Acute myocardial infarction in an 8-year old male child with homozygous familiar hypercholesterolemia: laboratory findings and response to lipid-lowering drugs. Clin Lab 2013;59:901–7.

17. Neil HA, Hammond T, Huxley R, et al. Extent of underdiagnosis of familial hypercholesterolaemia in routine practice: prospective registry study. BMJ 2000;321:148.

18. Versmissen J, Oosterveer DM, Yazdanpanah M, et al. Efficacy of statins in familial hypercholesterolaemia: a long term cohort study. BMJ 2008;337: a2423.

19. Rees A. Familial hypercholesterolaemia: underdiagnosed and undertreated. Eur Heart J 2008;29:2583–4.

20. Emerging Risk Factors. Lipoprotein(a) concentration and the risk of coronary heart disease, stroke, and nonvascular mortality. JAMA 2009;302:412–23.

21. Koschinsky ML, Boffa MB. Lipoprotein(a): an important cardiovascular risk factor and a clinical conundrum. Endocrinol Metab Clin North Am 2014;43:949–62.

22. Civeira F, International Panel on Management of Familial Hypercholesterolemia. Guidelines for the diagnosis and management of heterozygous familial hypercholesterolemia. Atherosclerosis 2004;173: 55–68.

23. Scientific Steering Committee on behalf of the Simon Broome Register Group. Risk of fatal coronary heart disease in familial hypercholesterolaemia. BMJ 1991;303:893–6.

24. Williams RR, Hunt SC, Schumacher MC, et al. Diagnosing heterozygous familial hypercholesterolemia using new practical criteria validated by molecular genetics. Am J Cardiol 1993;72:171–6.

25. Graadt van Roggen JF, van der Westhuyzen DR, Coetzee GA, et al. FH Afrikaner-3 LDL receptor mutation results in defective LDL receptors and causes a mild form of familial hypercholesterolemia. Arterioscler Thromb Vasc Biol 1995;15:765–72.

26. Kotulak JC, Brungardt T. Age-related changes in the cornea. J Am Optom Assoc 1980;51:761–5.

27. National Institute for Health and Care Excellence. Identification and Management of Familial Hypercholesterolaemia (NICE clinical guideline 71). London; 2008. Available at: http://www.guidance.nice.org.uk/cg71. Accessed February 23, 2015.

28. Humphries SE, Norbury G, Leigh S, et al. What is the clinical utility of DNA testing in patients with familial hypercholesterolaemia? Curr Opin Lipidol 2008;19: 362–8.

29. Ballantyne CM, Pazzucconi F, Pintó X, et al. Efficacy and tolerability of fluvastatin extended-release delivery system: a pooled analysis. Clin Ther 2001; 23:177–92.

30. Neil A, Cooper J, Betteridge J, et al. Reductions in all-cause, cancer, and coronary mortality in statin-treated patients with heterozygous familial hypercholesterolaemia: a prospective registry study. Eur Heart J 2008;29:2625–33.

31. The Task Force for the management of dyslipidaemias of the European Society of Cardiology (ESC) and the European Atherosclerosis Society (EAS). ESC/EAS Guidelines for the management of dyslipidaemias. Eur Heart J 2011;32:1769–818.

32. Leren TP. Cascade genetic screening for familial hypercholesterolemia. Clin Genet 2004;66:483–7.

33. Marks D, Wonderling D, Thorogood M, et al. Screening for hypercholesterolaemia versus case finding for familial hypercholesterolaemia: a systematic review and cost-effectiveness analysis. Health Technol Assess 2000;4:1–123.

34. Austin MA, Breslow JL, Hennekens CH, et al. Low-density lipoprotein subclass patterns and risk of myocardial infarction. JAMA 1988;260:1917–21.

35. Muir LA, George PM, Laurie AD, et al. Preventing cardiovascular disease: a review of the effectiveness of identifying the people with familial hypercholesterolaemia in New Zealand. N Z Med J 2010;123: 97–102.

36. Aviram M, Lund-Katz S, Phillips MC, et al. The influence of the triglyceride content of low density lipoprotein on the interaction of apolipoprotein B-100 with cells. J Biol Chem 1988;263: 16842–8.

37. Ned RM, Sijbrands EJ. Cascade screening for familial hypercholesterolemia (FH). PLoS Curr 2011; 3:RRN1238.

38. Austin MA. Plasma triglyceride as a risk factor for coronary heart disease: the epidemiologic evidence and beyond. Am J Epidemiol 1989;129:249–59.

39. Stone NJ, Robinson JG, Lichtenstein AH, et al. 2013 ACC/AHA guideline on the treatment of blood cholesterol to reduce atherosclerotic cardiovascular risk in adults: a report of the American College of Cardiology/American Heart Association Task Force on Practice Guidelines. J Am Coll Cardiol 2014;63: 2889–934.

40. Goldberg AC, Hopkins PN, Toth PP, et al. Familial hypercholesterolemia: screening, diagnosis and management of pediatric and adult patients: clinical guidance from the National Lipid Association Expert Panel on Familial Hypercholesterolemia. J Clin Lipidol 2011;5:133–40.

41. O'Brien EC, Roe MT, Fraulo ES, et al. Rationale and design of the familial hypercholesterolemia foundation Cascade screening for awareness and detection of familial hypercholesterolemia registry. Am Heart J 2014;167:342–9.e17.

42. Cohen JC, Boerwinkle E, Mosley TH Jr, et al. Sequence variations in PCSK9, low LDL, and protection against coronary heart disease. N Engl J Med 2006;354:1264–72.

43. Dadu RT, Ballantyne CM. Lipid lowering with PCSK9 inhibitors. Nat Rev Cardiol 2014;11:563–75.

44. Choumerianou DM, Dedoussis GV. Familial hypercholesterolemia and response to statin therapy according to LDLR genetic background. Clin Chem Lab Med 2005;43:793–801.

45. Raal FJ, Honarpour N, Blom DJ, et al. Inhibition of PCSK9 with evolocumab in homozygous familial hypercholesterolaemia (TESLA Part B): a randomised, double-blind, placebo-controlled trial. Lancet 2014. [Epub ahead of print].

46. Shiffman D, Chasman DI, Zee RY, et al. A kinesin family member 6 variant is associated with coronary heart disease in the Women's Health Study. J Am Coll Cardiol 2008;51:444–8.

47. Morrison AC, Bare LA, Chambless LE, et al. Prediction of coronary heart disease risk using a genetic risk score: the Atherosclerosis Risk in Communities study. Am J Epidemiol 2007;166:28–35.

48. Iakoubova OA, Tong CH, Rowland CM, et al. Association of the Trp719Arg polymorphism in kinesin-like protein 6 with myocardial infarction and coronary heart disease in 2 prospective trials: the CARE and WOSCOPS trials. J Am Coll Cardiol 2008;51:435–43.

49. Ridker PM, MacFadyen JG, Glynn RJ, et al. Kinesin-like protein 6 (KIF6) polymorphism and the efficacy of rosuvastatin in primary prevention. Circ Cardiovasc Genet 2011;4:312–7.

50. Arsenault BJ, Boekholdt SM, Hovingh GK, et al. The 719Arg variant of KIF6 and cardiovascular outcomes in statin-treated, stable coronary patients of the Treating to New Targets and Incremental Decrease in End Points through Aggressive Lipid-lowering prospective studies. Circ Cardiovasc Genet 2012;5:51–7.

51. Search Collaborative Group. SLCO1B1 variants and statin-induced myopathy–a genomewide study. N Engl J Med 2008;359:789–99.

52. Ridker PM, Danielson E, Fonseca FA, et al. Rosuvastatin to prevent vascular events in men and women with elevated C-reactive protein. N Engl J Med 2008;359:2195–207.

53. Vasan RS. Biomarkers of cardiovascular disease: molecular basis and practical considerations. Circulation 2006;113:2335–62.

54. Samani NJ, Erdmann J, Hall AS, et al. Genomewide association analysis of coronary artery disease. N Engl J Med 2007;357:443–53.

55. McPherson R, Pertsemlidis A, Kavaslar N, et al. A common allele on chromosome 9 associated with coronary heart disease. Science 2007;316:1488–91.

56. Schunkert H, Gotz A, Braund P, et al. Repeated replication and a prospective meta-analysis of the association between chromosome 9p21.3 and coronary artery disease. Circulation 2008;117:1675–84.

57. Myocardial Infarction Genetics Consortium. Genome-wide association of early-onset myocardial infarction with single nucleotide polymorphisms and copy number variants. Nat Genet 2009;41:334–41.

58. Brautbar A, Ballantyne CM. Pharmacological strategies for lowering LDL cholesterol: statins and beyond. Nat Rev Cardiol 2011;8:253–65.

59. Paynter NP, Chasman DI, Buring JE, et al. Cardiovascular disease risk prediction with and without knowledge of genetic variation at chromosome 9p21.3. Ann Intern Med 2009;150:65–72.

60. Hegele RA, Ginsberg HN, Chapman MJ, et al. The polygenic nature of hypertriglyceridaemia: implications for definition, diagnosis, and management. Lancet Diabetes Endocrinol 2014;2:655–66.

61. Palacios L, Grandoso L, Cuevas N, et al. Molecular characterization of familial hypercholesterolemia in Spain. Atherosclerosis 2012;221:137–42.

62. Avogaro P, Bittolo Bon G, Cazzolato G. Presence of a modified low density lipoprotein in humans. Arteriosclerosis 1988;8:79–87.

63. Ballantyne CM, Houri J, Notarbartolo A, et al. Effect of ezetimibe coadministered with atorvastatin in 628 patients with primary hypercholesterolemia: a prospective, randomized, double-blind trial. Circulation 2003;107:2409–15.

64. Berry EM, Eisenberg S, Haratz D, et al. Effects of diets rich in monounsaturated fatty acids on plasma lipoproteins—the Jerusalem Nutrition Study: high MUFAs vs high PUFAs. Am J Clin Nutr 1991;53: 899–907.

# Lipid Management in Human Immunodeficiency Virus

Merle Myerson, MD, EdD, FACC, FNLA

## KEYWORDS

- HIV • Dyslipidemia • Cardiovascular risk factors • Antiretroviral therapy • Infectious diseases

## KEY POINTS

- Antiretroviral therapy has changed human immunodeficiency virus (HIV) from a fatal disease to a chronic disease whereby extended and productive life spans are possible.
- People living with HIV are at increased risk for cardiovascular disease partly because of the HIV itself, the use of antiretroviral therapy (ART), and because people are living to an age when cardiovascular disease is more prevalent.
- HIV produces metabolic abnormalities, including dyslipidemia, that are exacerbated by ART.
- Diagnosis and management of dyslipidemia for patients living with HIV are needed to help prevent manifest cardiovascular disease.
- There are no comprehensive guidelines for the treatment of dyslipidemia specific to this population. Existing guidelines for the general population are currently used with modification for use with patients living with HIV.

## INTRODUCTION

On June 5, 1981, the *Morbidity and Mortality Weekly Report* published by the Centers for Disease Control and Prevention provided the first report on young, gay men with a rare lung infection, *Pneumocystis carinii* pneumonia, as well as other abnormalities attributed to immune system deficiency.[1] By 1982, the disease had a name, Acquired Immune Deficiency Syndrome (AIDS). Two separate research groups, one led by Dr Robert Gallo of the National Institutes of Health (NIH) and Dr Luc Montagnier of the Pasteur Institute in France, independently reported that a retrovirus could be the cause of AIDS. The virus that each group identified was the same and in 1986 it was given the name *human immunodeficiency virus* (HIV). It was thought that the virus originated in nonhuman primates in West-Central Africa and jumped to humans in the early 1900s.

There was no cure or treatment of HIV, large numbers of those who became infected, mostly gay men, hemophiliacs, Haitians, and intravenous drug users, did not live. In 1987, the Food and Drug Administration (FDA) approved the first antiretroviral drug, zidovudine, which began a new era for those infected with HIV. Opportunistic infections and death were no longer inevitable, and longer and productive life spans were possible. HIV was becoming a chronic disease.

With the advent of antiretroviral therapy (ART) also came a new spectrum of diseases for patients living with HIV. These included diseases related to the metabolic changes brought about by the virus itself, side effects of ART, and that people infected

Disclosures: Research: LipoScience. Education grant: Kowa, Gilead, Abbvie, Amgen. Consultant: Kowa, Gilead.
Cardiovascular Disease Prevention Program & Lipid Clinic, Cardiology Section, Institute for Advanced Medicine (HIV), Mount Sinai St. Luke's, Mount Sinai Roosevelt, 1111 Amsterdam Avenue, New York, NY 10025, USA
*E-mail address:* myersonm@optonline.net

Cardiol Clin 33 (2015) 277–298
http://dx.doi.org/10.1016/j.ccl.2015.01.003
0733-8651/15/$ – see front matter © 2015 Elsevier Inc. All rights reserved.

with HIV were living to ages when other diseases, such as cardiovascular disease (CVD), were more prevalent.[2–4]

In response to this, the American Heart Association (AHA) convened a multidisciplinary State of the Science Conference in June of 2007: Initiative to Decrease Cardiovascular Risk and Increase Quality of Care for Patients Living with HIV/AIDS. This conference summarized existing knowledge and outlined key questions and areas where more information was needed to provide optimal care for this patient population.[5]

More recent epidemiologic studies have shown that people infected with HIV have an increased risk of CVD at all ages compared with the general population, which remains even after control of traditional risk factors.[2] This population also has higher rates of smoking and behavioral and social factors that increase the risk.[6,7] It is anticipated that CVD will be the leading cause of morbidity and mortality in this patient population making diagnosis and management of CVD risk factors, in particular dyslipidemia, essential to patient care.[2,3] It is important to note that this need is not yet universal, as access to the more basic needs of diagnosis and treatment with ART remain limited in areas such as Sub-Saharan Africa and many parts of Asia.

This review is intended to provide a brief overview of HIV and ART with a focus on how the virus and the treatment impact on cardiovascular risk, in particular dyslipidemia. Currently, there are no specific and comprehensive guidelines or risk stratification schemes for the management of dyslipidemia in patients infected with HIV; but existing recommendations as well as those for the general population are discussed with suggestions as to how they may be applied to this patient population. Recommendations for the clinician who is taking care of these patients are presented based on established guidelines, evidence from epidemiologic and clinical trials, as well as the clinical experience of this author. Issues for which there is little or no information available are noted to highlight the many gaps in our knowledge regarding cardiovascular care for patients living with HIV.

## BACKGROUND
### Human Immunodeficiency Virus

The virus infects cells in the immune system, specifically CD4[+] T cells, which are white blood cells. After entering the CD4[+] T cell, the viral RNA genome is converted (known as reverse transcription) into double-stranded DNA that becomes integrated into the cell nucleus and rapidly replicates. The virus has a high mutation rate making treatment and finding a vaccine challenging.[8,9]

### Human Immunodeficiency Virus and Risk for Cardiovascular Disease

Infection with HIV produces a cardiometabolic syndrome consisting of insulin resistance, lipodystrophy (fat maldistribution including increase in abdominal visceral fat), and abnormal lipids (elevated triglycerides and low high-density lipoprotein cholesterol [HDL-C]). Therapy with ART may exacerbate these abnormalities.[5,10,11] The mechanisms of these metabolic abnormalities are complex and interdependent with the impaired glucose metabolism and dyslipidemia partly due to abnormal fat distribution (especially abdominal fat) and inflammation.[12,13]

The role of inflammation in the pathogenesis of atherosclerosis is well known in the general population[14] and is thought to play a significant and unique role in the development of CVD and increased risk in patients infected with HIV.

In the Strategies for Management of Antiretroviral Therapy (SMART) study, patients with CD4 cell counts greater than 350 cells per microliter were randomized to either continuous or intermittent ART. The trial was stopped early as those in the intermittent group had greater opportunistic disease, death from any cause, and major CVD.[15] Follow-up analysis of stored samples from the SMART study showed that inflammatory and coagulation biomarkers, interleukin 6 and D-dimer levels were significantly increased in the intermittent compared with the continuous therapy group and that these levels were strongly related to all-cause mortality.[16] It was hypothesized that therapies that reduce the inflammation response to HIV may be relevant to the care for patients infected with HIV.[16]

Mangili and colleagues[17] examined the association of all-cause mortality in patients infected with HIV and carotid intima-media thickness (cIMT) and high-sensitivity C-reactive protein (hsCRP). The median follow-up time was 3 years; although ART regimens were similar in all, those who died (11.6%) had higher cIMT (>75th percentile) and higher hsCRP. The investigators conclude that abnormal cIMT and elevated hsCRP suggest that inflammation, subclinical atherosclerosis, and immune activation may identify those at higher risk.

Subramanian and colleagues[18] investigated arterial inflammation in 27 HIV-infected people without known cardiac disease. They used PET with [18]fluorine-2-deoxy-D-glucose, an imaging method that can measure inflammation in the arterial wall. All participants with HIV were on

ART with viral suppression and good CD4 count. Those with HIV had higher aortic inflammation compared with non-HIV controls matched for Framingham Risk Score. The study provided evidence that HIV is associated with a high degree of inflammation within the arterial wall and that patients infected with HIV have added CVD risk, beyond that estimated by traditional risk factors.

More research is needed to better define the role of inflammation in HIV and how this influences the risk for CVD. The NIH has initiated the REPRIEVE study, a multicenter, prospective, randomized clinical trial of HIV-infected individuals who are at low risk according to the "2013 ACC/AHA Guideline on the Treatment of Blood Cholesterol to Reduce Atherosclerotic Cardiovascular Risk in Adults."[19] Participants will be randomized to either statin therapy (pitavastatin) or placebo and followed to investigate how statins may reduce the risk for CVD through non-LDL lowering benefits including antiinflammatory properties. The study is sponsored by the National Heart, Lung, and Blood Institute with collaboration with the National Institute of Allergy and Infectious Diseases.[20]

### Antiretroviral Therapy

At present there is no cure for HIV. ART provides viral suppression but not elimination of the virus and allows the body to maintain higher CD4 counts and better immune function. With viral suppression there is reduced likelihood of transmission from an infected to an uninfected individual. The various classes of ART prevent viral replication in different ways and are used in combination. Newer drugs with higher potency, lower toxicity, better dosing, and fewer side effects now exist facilitating early and long-term treatment. Measurements of CD4 count and viral are used to monitor treatment progress. CD4 counts of 300 cells per microliter or greater were found to be associated with good immune function.[21] Healthy persons who are not infected with HIV generally have CD4 counts of 800 to 1200 cells per microliter. Viral suppression is achieved when plasma RNA levels are less than the detectable limits.[22]

There are various classes of ART, each interfering with a different step in the replication of the virus. These classes include entry inhibitors, fusion inhibitors, nucleoside/nucleotide reverse transcriptase inhibitors (NRTI), non-nucleoside reverse transcriptase inhibitors (NNRTI), integrase inhibitors, and protease inhibitors (PIs). Combination regimens are standard.

As noted earlier, infection with HIV confers metabolic changes that may be exacerbated by ART. PIs are the agents that produce the most adverse effects, but other categories, in particular non-nucleoside/nucleotide reverse transcriptase inhibitors may also influence lipids.[10,22–24]

### Lipid Changes with Human Immunodeficiency Virus Infection and Antiretroviral Therapy

Acute infection lowers low-density-lipoprotein cholesterol (LDL-C),[25] but levels may return to baseline after virologic suppression with ART.[26,27] Chronically, there is often a pattern of low HDL and elevated triglycerides (TG) that results from the metabolic abnormalities (insulin resistance, central adiposity, low HDL, and high TG) clustered in these patients[28,29] and often worsened by specific antiretrovirals, many of which are now less commonly prescribed.[23,30] The magnitude of these changes is also reflective of ethnicity, race, sex, lifestyle factors, and genomic traits.[31] As noted earlier, the PI and the NNRTI are the ART that most significantly influence lipid levels. **Tables 1** and **2** provide detail on the changes that are seen with use of medications in each of these classes of ART.

## GUIDELINES FOR THE MANAGEMENT OF DYSLIPIDEMIA IN PATIENTS INFECTED WITH HUMAN IMMUNODEFICIENCY VIRUS

There are currently no guidelines specifically for the diagnosis and management of dyslipidemia in patients infected with HIV. In 2003, The HIV Medical Association (HIVMA) of the Infectious Disease Society of American (IDSA) and AIDS Clinical Trials Group (ACTG)[32] recommended using the National Cholesterol Education Program Adult Treatment Panel III (NCEP ATP III), as did the 2013 HIVMA IDSA Primary Care Guidelines. Recommendations based on guidelines for the general population are presented here along with comments on how they may be applied to management of dyslipidemia in patients infected with HIV.[33]

### Risk Stratification and Scores

No validated risk score or stratification scheme currently exists for patients infected with HIV, although 2 groups have proposed scoring systems. The Data Collection on Adverse Effects of Anti-HIV Drugs (D:A:D) Study Group has developed a risk calculator that includes both traditional risk factors and exposure to individual antiretroviral drugs.[34] The Veterans Aging Cohort Study (VACS) was used to develop the VACS Index to predict overall mortality. The index includes age, CD4 count, viral load, hemoglobin, aspartate and alanine transaminase, platelets,

**Table 1**
**Lipid changes associated with PI use**

| | Lipids | | | |
|---|---|---|---|---|
| PI | Total Cholesterol | HDL-C | LDL-C | Triglycerides |
| Atazanavir | ↔ | ↔ | ↔ By 16% | ↓ By 12% |
| Atazanavir + ritonavir and Atazanavir/cobicistat | ↔ | ↔ | ↑ | ↑ |
| Darunavir + ritonavir | ↔ | ↔ | ↑ | ↑ |
| Fosamprenavir + ritonavir | ↑↑ | ↔ | ↑ | ↑↑ |
| Lopinavir/ritonavir (coformulated) | ↑↑ (Additional increase over ritonavir alone) | ↔ No change | ↑ No additional increase over ritonavir alone | ↑↑ No additional increase over ritonavir alone |
| Nelfinavir | ↑ | ↔ | ↑↑ | ↑ |
| Ritonavir (low dose for boosting) | ↑ By 10% | ↓ By 5% | ↑ By 16% | ↑↑ By 26% |
| Saquinavir + ritonavir | ↑↑ | ↔ | ↑ | ↑ |
| Tipranavir + ritonavir | ↑↑ | Not known | Not known | ↑↑↑ |

Key: ↑, some increase; ↑↑, moderate increase; ↑↑↑, large increase; ↓, some decrease; ↔, no significant change.
Boosting means use as a pharmacoenhancer with another drug.
From Myerson M, Malvestutto C, Aberg JA. Management of lipid disorders in patients living with HIV. J Clin Pharmacol 2015. [Epub ahead of print]; with permission.

creatinine, and hepatitis C status. The VACS Index has been used in studies predicting coronary heart disease (CHD) risk but has not been validated for this use.[35]

Use of the Framingham Risk Score, although not validated in patients with HIV, is endorsed by HIVMA of the IDSA[33] and the European AIDS Clinical Society (EACS)[36]; however, it is unclear if Framingham and other risk scores are appropriate for this patient population.

The Framingham Risk Score predicted risk accurately and was associated with abnormal early and late surrogate markers (cIMT) in a group of 334 adults infected with HIV.[37]

However, in other studies it did not predict well. In studies by Friis-Moller and colleagues[34] and Parra and colleagues,[38] the Framingham Risk Score underestimated the presence of subclinical atherosclerosis and manifest disease in HIV-infected patients. In another study, Law and colleagues[39] compared the number of myocardial infarctions observed among those infected with HIV in the D:A:D study with the number predicted by conventional risk factor equations. They found that the Framingham equation overpredicted rates in patients who did not receive ART and underpredicted rates in patients on ART. These studies suggest a need to develop risk equations specific

**Table 2**
**Lipid changes associated with NNRTI use**

| | Lipids | | | |
|---|---|---|---|---|
| NNRTI | Total Cholesterol | HDL-C | LDL-C | Triglycerides |
| Efavirenz | ↑ | ↑ | ↑ | ↑ |
| Etravirine | ↔ | ↔ | ↔ | ↔ |
| Nevirapine | ↑ | ↑↑ Larger increase with efavirenz | ↑ | ↑ Lower increase than with efavirenz |
| Rilpivrine | ↑ | Not known | ↑ Lower increase than with efavirenz | ↑ Lower increase than with efavirenz |

Key: ↑, some increase; ↑↑, moderate increase; ↑↑↑, large increase; ↓, some decrease; ↔, no significant change.
From Myerson M, Malvestutto C, Aberg JA. Management of lipid disorders in patients living with HIV. J Clin Pharmacol 2015. [Epub ahead of print]; with permission.

to people infected with HIV and perhaps account for the use of ART.

Zanni and colleagues[40] used computed tomography angiography (CTA) to see how the 2013 ACC/AHA guidelines would perform for people with HIV. One hundred eight HIV-infected patients without known CVD had CTA and classification of coronary atherosclerotic plaque morphology as with or without high-risk characteristics. Thirty-nine participants had high-risk morphology; however, statin therapy would not be recommended for 74% of these by the ACC/AHA guideline. The ACC/AHA guideline has been debated, and some groups in the United States have continued to recommend risk stratification similar to that in the NCEP ATP III guideline.[41–43]

Measures of subclinical atherosclerosis, including coronary artery calcium, hsCRP, and ultrasound measure of cIMT, have been studied in small numbers of patients with HIV.[44,45] In the Multicenter AIDS Cohort Study, participants who were infected with HIV and underwent coronary CTA had a greater prevalence of coronary artery calcium, of any plaque, and noncalcified plaque compared with participants who were not infected.[46] At this time, there is not enough information to consider these measures for use in this patient population.

The influence of CD4 count and viral load on risk has not been determined. Silverberg and colleagues[47] compared myocardial infarction (MI) rates for 22,081 HIV-positive subjects and 230,069 HIV-negative subjects from 1996 to 2009 in a cohort of patients from Kaiser Permanente California health plan members. HIV-positive subjects with recent or nadir CD4 counts of 500 or greater cells per microliter had similar rates compared with HIV-negative subjects. HIV-positive subjects with recent CD4 counts less than 200 cells per microliter had an adjusted relative risk (RR) of 1.76 (95% confidence interval [CI]: 1.31–2.37) for MI compared with HIV-negative subjects. HIV-positive subjects with a nadir CD4 count less than 200 cells per microliter had an adjusted RR of 1.74 (95% CI: 1.47–2.06). Viral load, prior ART use, and duration of PIs and NNRTIs were not associated with MIs.

## Lipid Targets for Patients Living With Human Immunodeficiency Virus

### Low-density lipoprotein cholesterol
Treatment of and targets for dyslipidemia for the general population have traditionally been focused on LDL-C and based on risk stratification with lower targets for those with greater risk.

Existing guidelines in Europe[48] and Canada[49] and by the International Atherosclerosis Society (IAS)[50] continue to have LDL-C targets based on risk scores (Systemic Coronary Risk Estimation in Europe, Framingham Risk Score in Canada, and Framingham Risk Score as a core estimate followed by recalibration for individual countries in the IAS) as had the NCEP ATP III guidelines.[51]

The 2013 ACC/AHA guideline[19] introduced a new risk calculator, the Pooled Cohort Risk Assessment Equations, that, along with 4 defined groups of patients, is used to determine who should be treated with a statin drug. Targets for LDL-C were eliminated. There are no recommendations for patients with HIV in this document.

In 2014, the National Lipid Association in the United States issued a statement recommending continued use of a Framingham-based risk stratification and outlining targets for both LDL-C and non–HDL-C. Risk categories are defined as very high, high, moderate, or low risk. Apolipoprotein B (apoB) is considered a secondary, optional target for therapy; LDL-particle number (LDL-P) is noted to be a risk indicator that may be considered for risk refinement.[52] There is no information provided for patients infected with HIV however the Association will be issuing a second part to these guidelines with a section for "Patients Living With Human Immunodeficiency Virus."

The more recent guidelines for management of dyslipidemia in the general population have introduced the concept of "residual risk."[51] Low-density lipoprotein cholesterol is highly associated with CVD, but does not reflect the total amount of atherosclerotic particles,[53–55] meaning all particles that have an apoB (very-low-density lipoprotein [VLDL], intermediate-density lipoprotein, LDL, and lipoprotein [a]). Measures of residual risk, including non–HDL-C (total cholesterol minus HDL-C), apoB, or LDL-P, better predict the risk for CVD than LDL-C with apoB and LDL-P performing better than non-HDL-C.[53,54] Certain populations of patients, such as those with diabetes, are thought to have discordance between LDL-C and these other measures, which may result in undertreatment or overtreatment.[53,56] This discordance has also been shown in patients infected with HIV with the LDL-C lower relative to the ApoB or LDL-P. Therefore, patients that may be at target according to LDL-C may have residual risk.[57,58] Although ApoB and LDL-P appear to better measure atherosclerotic particle burden, LDL-C remains the primary target for both the general and HIV populations.

Existing recommendations for patients infected with HIV include the EACS whereby a target of less than 155 mg/dL for total cholesterol and less than 80 mg/dL for LDL-C is identified.[36]

Recently issued guidelines by the HIVMA of the IDSA for the primary care of patients with HIV state that lipid testing and targets should be based on the NCEP ATP III guidelines with consideration for more stringent targets.[33] Metabolic syndrome is considered to be a risk factor in the NCEP ATP III; as this is prevalent in patients infected with HIV, clinicians should assess for metabolic syndrome and, if present, incorporate in the risk stratification and identification of target for LDL-C.[30]

### Triglycerides

The association between triglycerides and risk for CVD has been debated but an independent association with CVD has been established although less strong than that with LDL-C. High TG levels are often accompanied by other metabolic abnormalities such as insulin resistance, abdominal fat, hypertension, and low HDL-C making it harder to separate out the influence of elevated TG alone.[59]

Treatment of mildly or moderately elevated TG (<500 mg/dL) is not recommended by the European AIDS Clinical Society as there is no clear evidence of benefit in this population.[36] As in the general population, TG<500 mg/dL are often treated with lifestyle modification (weight loss, diet, exercise) with higher levels requiring medication to lessen the likelihood of pancreatitis.[59] The dyslipidemia in patients with HIV is characterized by mild-to-moderate TG elevation and low HDL-C felt to be caused by the HIV infection and metabolic disturbances resulting from ART such as impaired glucose tolerance, insulin resistance, visceral adiposity, and peripheral lipoatrophy.[60,61]

Triglycerides are commonly measured in the fasting state because they can vary greatly with food consumption. Non-fasting TG (known as "postprandial") is also felt to be important because patients are in the postprandial state for more hours than in the fasting state. In addition, TG remnant particles have been shown to be associated with CVD risk.[62] Less is known about postprandial measures and influence of ART in patients infected with HIV.[63,64]

As obtaining fasting TG may not always be feasible, a non-fasting value can be used for screening. A low-fat breakfast (less than 15 g of fat) should not raise TG above 200 mg/dL. If a value is greater than this, a fasting measure should be obtained.[59] Because fat content of breakfast may not be known and may vary considerably it is unclear how a non-fasting measure can be utilized, especially for patients with HIV who generally have higher TG levels.

### High-density lipoprotein cholesterol

Targets for HDL-C have been established (greater than 40 mg/dL for men and greater than 50 mg/dL for women)[51] however specific treatment for low HDL-C is not recommended for the general population and patients infected with HIV. The National Lipid Association issued a statement saying that although low HDL-C identifies patients at elevated risk for cardiovascular disease, and much investigation suggests that HDL may play a variety of anti-atherogenic roles, HDL-C is not a therapeutic target at the present time."[65] HDL-C levels may rise in response to viral suppression and treatment of diabetes, reduction of abdominal obesity, lowering TG, and physical activity. Niacin can raise HDL-C but is often poorly tolerated and may worsen the cluster of metabolic abnormalities including insulin resistance. Therefore, treatment aimed specifically for low HDL-C should not be recommended for patients infected with HIV.

## MANAGEMENT OF DYSLIPIDEMIA IN PATIENTS INFECTED WITH HUMAN IMMUNODEFICIENCY VIRUS

This section provides a guide for the evaluation and management of dyslipidemia in patients infected with HIV. **Box 1** outlines a risk stratification scheme and is based on existing guidelines and expert statements[51,52,66] as well as the opinion and clinical experience of the author of this review. This information is not intended to be a guideline but a recommendation based on existing schemes. HIV-specific information, such as viral load and CD4 count, are not considered. Ranges for apoB and LDL-P are included but not recommended in the routine management because of the added cost and less evidence that measurement will change outcomes. As noted earlier, metabolic syndrome is considered a risk factor, and it is important to assess for this in patients infected with HIV. The clinician "may increase risk one risk category based on clinical judgment."[51] Until specific risk predictors and scores are validated for patients with HIV, consideration for increasing one risk category may be reasonable.

**Table 3** lists targets for lipids and lipid biomarkers. Once again, this is not meant to be a guideline but rather a suggestion based on existing guidelines and recommendations.[51,52,66]

The NCEP ATP III recommends achieving LDL-C targets as a first priority unless TG is greater than 500 mg/dL at baseline, then the first priority is to lower TG to prevent pancreatitis. After TG is less than 500 mg/dL, reevaluate LDL-C for

**Box 1**
**CHD risk classification**

*Very high risk*

- High risk criteria (see below under "High risk")
- Plus one or more of the following: diabetes, active smoking, chronic kidney disease, abdominal aortic aneurysm, >20% Framingham Risk Score

*High risk* (one of the following)

- Known coronary heart disease or event, cerebrovascular disease or event, peripheral artery disease
- CHD risk equivalent: diabetes, chronic kidney disease, abdominal aortic aneurysm, >20% Framingham Risk Score

*Moderate high risk*

- Metabolic syndrome
- Two or more risk factors (men aged ≥45 years, women aged ≥55 years, HDL <40, active smoking, hypertension, family history of CHD in first-degree family member aged <55 years [men] or <65 years [women]) and 10%–20% 10-year Framingham Risk Score

*Moderate risk*

- Metabolic syndrome
- Two or more risk factors (men aged ≥45 years, women aged ≥55 years, HDL <40, active smoking, hypertension, family history of CHD in first-degree family member aged <55 years [men] or <65 years [women]) and 10%–20% 10-year Framingham Risk Score

*Low risk*

- Zero or one major risk factor

Note: May increase one risk category based on clinical judgment.
Note: If multiple risk factors are present (≥2), use the Framingham Risk Score to determine the 10-year risk of developing CHD.

appropriate management as indicated. For patients with TG greater than or equal to 200 mg/dL after the LDL target is reached, a secondary target is to achieve a non–HDL-C approximately 30 mg/dL more than the LDL-C target.

The 2014 National Lipid Association recommendations identify targets for LDL-C as well as non-HDL-C. For LDL-C this is <100 mg/dL for all groups except those at very high risk where it is <70 mg/dL; targets for non-HDL-C are 30 mg/dL higher than the LDL-C target. These are lower than previous guidelines and may not be easily achieved in all patients, particularly those infected with HIV.[52]

**Table 3**
**Targets for LDL-C, non–HDL-C, apoB, LDL-P[51,52,66]**

| Risk Category | LDL-C (mg/dL) | Non–HDL-C (mg/dL) | apoB (mg/dL) | LDL-P (nmol/L) |
|---|---|---|---|---|
| Very high | <70 | <100 | <80 | <1000 |
| High | <100 (Optional <70) | <130 (Optional <100) | <80 | <1000 |
| Moderate high | <100 | <130 | 80–119 | 1000–1559 |
| Moderate | <130 | <160 | 80–119 | 1000–1559 |
| Low | <130 | <160 | ≤120 | ≤1600 |

*From* Kellick KA, Bottorff M, Toth PP. A Clinician's Guide to Statin Drug-Drug Interactions. Journal of Clinical Lipidology 2014;8:S30–46; with permission.

## When to Use Measures of Residual Risk

Measures other than LDL-C are currently being used to provide a more complete determination of atherosclerotic particle burden, including non–HDL-C, apoB, and LDL-P. Practical considerations limit the use of apoB and LDL-P measurements as not all laboratories are equipped to measure these and insurance coverage for these measurements is not universal. Non–HDL-C is calculated from the basic lipid panel and is recommended as a measure of residual risk for patients infected with HIV.

## History and Physical Examination

The history and physical examination can provide useful information to assess the risk for CVD and the presence of dyslipidemia. **Box 2** outlines a history and examination that include aspects specific for patients infected with HIV. The measures listed do not constitute an established guideline but reflect what is known from existing guidelines, research (both randomized clinical trials and observational studies), as well as the clinical experience of the author.

---

**Box 2**
**History and physical examination**

*History*

1. Men aged 45 years or older and women aged 55 years or older

2. Personal history of CVD: coronary artery disease, cerebrovascular disease, peripheral artery disease, abdominal aortic aneurysm

3. History of lipid abnormalities before diagnosis of HIV, at time of diagnosis or after treatment with antiretrovirals

4. Family history of premature CHD: first-degree male relative less than 55 years old or first-degree female relative less than 65 years old

5. Diet history including who buys and prepares food, whether patients are institutionalized or living without a kitchen area

6. Exercise and physical activity history

7. Family history of dyslipidemia: elevated LDL-C or triglycerides

8. Cigarette smoking (personal history, living with people who smoke, exposure to secondhand smoke)

9. History of symptoms: angina, anginal equivalents

10. Hormone history: menopausal status, use of oral contraceptives, hormone replacement therapy, testosterone therapy, hormone therapy for gender reassignment

11. Determination of diabetes mellitus and metabolic syndrome

12. Medication history, including ART, psychiatric medications, hepatitis B or C medications, methadone, anabolic steroids, immunosuppression medications (cyclosporine), selective estrogen receptor modulators

13. Hypertension and use of blood pressure–lowering medications

14. Substance use: illicit drugs, alcohol

15. Comorbidities that can increase LDL-C: hypothyroidism, renal disease, obstructive liver disease, anorexia nervosa, Cushing syndrome, polycystic ovarian syndrome

*Physical Examination*

1. Height, weight, body mass index, waist circumference, blood pressure

2. Evidence of hypothyroidism

3. Distal pulses and auscultation for bruit over arterial beds

4. Physical stigmata of elevated LDL-C: tendon xanthomas, xanthelasmas, and elevated triglycerides: eruptive xanthomas

5. Presence of lipohypertrophy and/or lipoatrophy

## Laboratory Evaluation

The core of the lipid examination consists of fasting total cholesterol, calculated LDL-C, HDL-C, and triglycerides. Non–HDL-C can be calculated (total cholesterol– HDL-C). When triglycerides are greater than 400 mg/dL, the calculation for LDL-C is inaccurate. Direct measurement of LDL-C is not recommended as not all laboratories are able to adequately perform this test and even under ideal conditions, the laboratory coefficient of deviation is often quite large.[67] A recommended panel of laboratory tests for initial evaluation is presented in **Box 3**.

## Therapeutic Lifestyle Modification

Therapeutic lifestyle changes are advised for all patients regardless of their level of risk. These changes are outlined in **Box 4**.[51] Caring for patients living with HIV has many unique and challenging aspects. Access to healthy food choices and options for exercise and physical activity can be limited by availability, knowledge, or finances. Prevalence of smoking is higher than the general population as is alcohol and illicit drug use and

---

**Box 3**
**Initial laboratory evaluation**

1. Fasting lipid profile

2. Calculate non–HDL-cholesterol (apoB and LDL-P not routinely recommended)

3. Lipoprotein (a) (a lipid particle that is heavily influenced by genetics, is structurally similar to plasminogen, and is independently predictive of risk) Consider measurement in patients with premature CVD, family history of premature CVD, or familial hypercholesterolemia

4. At present there is no clear indication for measurement of hsCRP or inflammatory factors

5. Thyroid-stimulating hormone: evaluate for thyroid disease

6. Aspartate transaminase and alanine transaminase: baseline testing before starting lipid medication and evaluation for obstructive liver disease

7. Serum creatinine kinase

8. Serum creatinine and calculation of glomerular filtration rate

9. Urinalysis

10. Uric acid if history of gout

11. Fasting glucose and/or hemoglobin A1c

---

**Box 4**
**Therapeutic lifestyle modification**

1. Diet: reduce intake of saturated fats to less than 7% of total calories and intake of cholesterol to less than 200 mg/d

2. Weight reduction if indicated

3. Increased physical activity

4. Cessation of smoking

---

addiction. To address this, more medical centers now have comprehensive HIV clinics with nutrition counselors and smoking cessation programs. Educational materials can be provided to patients that reflect language and cultural aspects of the local patient population.

## Medications

### Statins

The statin drugs (HMG-Co-A Reductase Inhibitors) are the most widely used medications for treatment of elevated LDL-C. They also can raise HDL-C and lower Triglycerides but these effects are relatively modest. Research has shown that they have benefits in addition to lowering LDL-C that include improvement in endothelial function, reduced inflammation, and decreased platelet aggregation.[68] There has not been extensive research on how statins are metabolized in patients infected with HIV and their benefit on clinical outcomes.

**Efficacy** Pravastatin was the main statin option for HIV-infected patients in early studies because of the favorable safety profile and limited interactions with ART. In 2005, the ACTG 5087 trial reported a comparison of pravastatin 40 mg/d to fenofibrate 200 mg/d for the treatment of mixed dyslipidemia in 174 HIV-infected patients. At week 12, changes in LDL/HDL/TG were +13/+4/−118 mg/dL for fenofibrate therapy and −30/0/−27 mg/dL for pravastatin therapy. A total of 136 subjects who were not at the NCEP goals were then given both drugs. By week 48, 10% of the combination drug group was at the NCEP goals. Although combination therapy with fenofibrate and pravastatin improved lipid parameters, it was unlikely to achieve all NCEP targets.[69]

Rosuvastatin has been shown to produce greater reduction in cholesterol. Eighty-five patients on ART were randomized to treatment with rosuvastatin (10 mg daily), pravastatin (20 mg daily), or atorvastatin (10 mg daily). At 1 year, there was a mean decrease in total cholesterol of 25.2% with rosuvastatin, 19.8% with atorvastatin, and

17.6% with pravastatin.[70] Rosuvastatin 10 mg daily produced a significantly larger reduction in LDL-C than pravastatin in the ANRS 126 study in HIV-infected patients taking ritonavir-boosted PIs.[71]

Pitavastatin is the newest FDA-approved statin, although it had been used in Japan for many years. Pitavastatin has been studied in patients with HIV. The INTREPID study was a phase 4, multicenter randomized, double-blind, double-dummy superiority study comparing pitavastatin 4 mg with pravastatin 40 mg in adults aged 18 to 70 years on stable ART with a viral load less than 200 copies per milliliter and CD4 count greater than 200 cells per cubic microliter. This study demonstrated that pitavastatin 4 mg was superior to pravastatin 40 mg in LDL-C and non–HDL-C reduction at 52 weeks in HIV-infected patients with dyslipidemia.[72] In a post hoc analysis of the INTREPID trial, at 12 weeks, pitavastatin significantly reduced LDL-C (31.6%), apoB (23.8%), and non–HDL-C (26.8%) more than pravastatin in men aged 45 years or older. In women aged 55 years or older, pitavastatin also showed significant reductions in these measures (LDL-C 29.5%, apoB 20.4%, and non–HDL-C 29.1%); but this did not reach significance when compared with pravastatin because of small numbers.[73] In an additional analysis of the INTREPID study, there were no significant effects on glucose homeostasis.[74]

**Drug-drug interactions between antiretroviral therapy and statins** Table 4 provides a summary of the interactions between ART and statin drugs.[31,75] Lovastatin and simvastatin are contraindicated with PI because they have extensive first-pass metabolism by cytochrome P450 3A isoenzymes (CYP3A4) in the liver. Atorvastatin undergoes less first-pass metabolism by CYP3A4, and doses up to 40 mg daily can be used with PI. Fluvastatin (metabolized primarily by cytochrome P450 2C9 isoenzyme [CYP2C9]) and pravastatin, pitavastatin, and rosuvastatin (minimally metabolized by the CYP450 enzymes)[75–77] can be used with PI.

The HIV produces an inflammatory state that can affect the metabolism, distribution, and elimination of many drugs.[78,79] There may also be host and pharmacogenomic factors influencing the interaction of statin drugs with ART. However, these have not been characterized; the information provided in the FDA-approved package insert should be used for guidance.

**Statin use with antiretroviral therapy pharmacokinetic enhancers** Some of the ART may be administered with pharmacokinetic enhancers often referred to as *boosters*. These drugs enhance the effectiveness of a medication. Ritonavir is a potent inhibitor of CYP3A4 and is primarily used as a pharmacokinetic enhancer for other PIs. Ritonavir should be used with caution in patients taking PIs.[80] Cobicistat is another potent CYP3A4 inhibitor and used as an enhancer for the integrase inhibitor elvitegravir. Because several statins also depend on CYP3A4 for metabolic clearance, the coadministration of cobicistat with simvastatin and lovastatin can result in markedly elevated plasma levels of statins and is contraindicated. Atorvastatin can be used with cobicistat but must be started at the lowest dosage (10 mg daily) and titrated up carefully while monitoring for safety.[81]

**Treatment of patients coinfected with hepatitis C** As coinfection with hepatitis C virus (HCV) is common in HIV-infected patients, care should also be taken when HCV antiviral medication is used with statins. Table 5 lists these interactions.

**Other classes of antiretroviral therapy** Prescribing statins with classes of ART other than PI or NNRTI are generally safe as there are few if any significant drug interactions. The integrase inhibitor elvitegravir must be prescribed with cobicistat, which has interactions as noted earlier.

**Side effects of statin drugs** There are no specific guidelines for patients infected with HIV; but because patients are generally on other medications with potential side effects and interactions in addition to other comorbidities, caution is advised. The following sections provide information on the common side effects of statins; please also refer to the articles on statins and side effects in this volume of *Cardiology Clinics*.

**Liver side effects** As ART can influence liver function, and prevalence of hepatitis and alcohol abuse are also greater, consideration for monitoring liver function is recommended. The protocol in **Box 5** is from the National Lipid Association's "An Assessment by the Statin Liver Safety Task Force: 2014 Update"[82]:

**Muscle** Muscle soreness, or statin myopathy, is a frequent complaint by patients taking statin medications. Serum creatine kinase (CK) may or may not be elevated in those with symptoms. Rhabdomyolysis is an uncommon but serious condition with marked elevations in CK and acute renal failure.

Baseline measurement and routine monitoring of CK is not advised for the general population unless a patient has renal dysfunction, complaints of muscle soreness, or other clinical indications. Patients infected with HIV often have other indications, including medications, medical conditions, and substance abuse, that can increase the risk of myopathy (alcohol, cocaine, opioids, ART, fibrates, infectious and immune disorders, hypothyroidism) and would merit monitoring in patients, especially those with symptoms.[83] In addition, observational studies have shown that African Americans have higher and often elevated baseline CK levels compared with other ethnic groups.[84] The clinical significance of this is unclear, and a threshold for the safety of statin therapy has not been identified. **Box 6** summarizes monitoring for muscle and CK side effects.

**Neurologic** Statin use has been associated with neurologic side effects, and a 2012 FDA communication described postmarketing statin adverse event reports in patients older than 50 years who experienced memory loss or impairment that was reversible with cessation of statin therapy. This finding has not been fully supported by clinical or observational studies,[77] and larger and better-designed studies are needed to clarify the effect of statins on cognition. Patients infected with HIV often have neurocognitive changes; although the introduction of ART has reduced the prevalence of more severe forms,[85] statin use remains an area of concern with regard to neurologic side effects.

**Diabetes and insulin resistance** The 2012 FDA statement also noted an increased incidence of diabetes associated with statin use[77]; however, it is unclear if these patients would have progressed to manifest diabetes regardless of statin use.[86] It is thought that the cardiovascular benefits of statins outweigh these small increased risks.[77]

It is unclear if patients with HIV have increased risk for developing diabetes as insulin resistance is more prevalent among these patients. Initial information from the INTREPID study did not show clinically relevant changes in glucose homeostasis with the use of Pitavastatin in this patient population.[74] **Box 7** outlines recommendations for monitoring blood glucose for patients on statin drugs.

### Nonstatin drugs for the treatment of dyslipidemia

**Intestine absorption inhibitors** The intestine absorption inhibitor drug ezetimibe does not utilize the cytochrome P450 system and does not interact with ART.[87]

Ezetimibe lowers LDL-C, but research has not been conclusive regarding the overall cardiovascular benefits. The recent IMPROVE-IT (ImProved Reduction of Outcomes: Vytorin Efficacy International Trial) study enrolled patients with ST-elevation MI, unstable angina, or non–ST-elevation MI and randomized them to simvastatin alone or simvastatin in combination with ezetimibe. At 7 years, 32% of the group on combination therapy experienced a primary end point (cardiovascular death, MI, stroke, rehospitalization for unstable angina, or coronary revascularization) compared with 34% in the simvastatin-only group.[88]

Studies in patients infected with HIV have shown favorable changes in lipids. In a randomized study of 20 HIV-infected patients, ezetimibe monotherapy reduced LDL-C by 20%, which was similar to that of fluvastatin 80 mg.[89] When used as an add-on to maximally tolerated lipid-lowering therapy, ezetimibe achieved incremental lipid reductions in a retrospective analysis of 33 HIV-infected patients. They were prescribed ezetimibe 10 mg/d in addition to current therapy; the mean TC, LDL-C, and TG were reduced by an additional 21%, 35%, and 34% from baseline, respectively. Mean HDL-C also increased by 8%.[90] A crossover study of 44 HIV-infected adults on stable ART with LDL-C greater than 130 mg/dL were randomized to receive ezetimibe 10 mg daily or placebo on top of their statin therapy. There was a median decrease in LDL-C of 20.8% with ezetimibe versus 0.7% with placebo. No significant changes were noted in HDL-C or TG.[91]

**Niacin (Nicotinic acid)** Niacin has a variety of effects on lipid metabolism. It lowers LDL-C by inhibiting the hepatic production of VLDL and consequently LDL. It increases HDL-C by reducing lipid transfer from HDL to VLDL and delaying HDL clearance[92] and lowers TG by 15% to 20% when used in higher dosages (2000 mg daily).[93] Niacin has been associated with an increase in serum glucose and insulin resistance, but studies have not confirmed clinically significant increases in hemoglobin A1c.[94,95] Niacin use is also associated with worsening of gout.

Use of niacin is limited by side effects, primarily flushing but also itching and headache. The flushing can be minimized by taking aspirin 30 minutes before administering medication. Limited research is available but the dose of aspirin that is felt to be effective is 325 mg. Some over-the-counter preparations of niacin are marketed as no flush but are not regulated and have no free nicotinic acid and, therefore, are ineffective in treating

**Table 4**
Statin interactions with antiretroviral medication

| Drug | PI | Effect on PI or Concomitant Drug Concentrations | Recommendation |
|---|---|---|---|
| Atorvastatin | ATV/r | ↑ atorvastatin possible | Titrate atorvastatin dose carefully and use lowest dose necessary |
| | ATV | | |
| | DRV/r | DRV/r + atorvastatin 10 mg similar to atorvastatin 40 mg administered alone; | Titrate atorvastatin dose carefully and use the lowest necessary dose. Do not exceed 20 mg atorvastatin daily |
| | FPV/r | FPV ± RTV ↑ atorvastatin AUC 130% to 153%; | |
| | FPV | | |
| | SQV/r | SQV/r ↑ atorvastatin AUC 79% | |
| | LPV/r | LPV/r ↑ atorvastatin AUC 488% | Use with caution and use the lowest atorvastatin dose necessary |
| | TPV/r | ↑ atorvastatin AUC 836% | DO NOT COADMINISTER |
| Lovastatin | All PIs | Significant ↑ lovastatin expected | Contraindicated. Do not coadminister |
| Pitavastatin | All PIs | ATV ↑ pitavastatin AUC 31% and $C_{max}$ ↑ 60% | No dose adjustment necessary |
| | | ATV: no significant effect | |
| | | LPV/r ↓ pitavastatin AUC 20% | |
| | | LPV: no significant effect | |
| Pravastatin | DRV/r | Pravastatin AUC ↑ 81% | Use lowest possible starting dose of pravastatin with careful monitoring |
| | LPV/r | Pravastatin AUC ↑ 33% | No dose adjustment necessary |
| | SQV/r | Pravastatin AUC ↓ 47% to 50% | No dose adjustment necessary |
| Rosuvastatin | ATV/r | ATV/r ↑ rosuvastatin AUC 3-fold and | Titrate rosuvastatin dose carefully and use the lowest necessary dose. Do not exceed 10 mg rosuvastatin daily |
| | LPV/r | $C_{max}$ ↑ 7-fold | |
| | | LPV/r ↑ rosuvastatin AUC 108% and $C_{max}$ ↑ 366% | |
| | DRV/r | Rosuvastatin AUC ↑ 48% and $C_{max}$ ↑ 139% | Titrate rosuvastatin dose carefully and use the lowest necessary dose while monitoring for toxicities |
| | FPV ± RTV | No significant effect on rosuvastatin | No dosage adjustment necessary |
| | SQV/r | No data available | Titrate rosuvastatin dose carefully and use the lowest necessary dose while monitoring for toxicities |
| | TPV/r | Rosuvastatin AUC ↑ 26% and $C_{max}$ ↑ 123% | No dose adjustment necessary |
| Simvastatin | All PIs | Significant ↑ simvastatin level; | CONTRAINDICATED, do not coadminister |
| | | SQV/r 400 mg/400 mg BID | |
| | | ↑ simvastatin AUC 3059% | |

| Concomitant Drug Class/Name | NNRTI | Effect on NNRTI or Concomitant Drug Concentrations | Recommendations |
|---|---|---|---|
| Fluvastatin | ETR | ↑ fluvastatin possible | ↑ fluvastatin possible |
| Lovastatin | EFV | Simvastatin AUC ↓ 68% | Adjust simvastatin dose according to lipid responses, not to exceed the maximum recommended dose. If EFV used with RTV-boosted PI, simvastatin and lovastatin should be avoided |
| Simvastatin | ETR | ↓ Lovastatin possible | Adjust lovastatin or simvastatin dose according to lipid responses, not to exceed the maximum recommended dose. If ETR or NVP used with RTV-boosted PI, simvastatin and lovastatin should be avoided |
| | NVP | ↓ Simvastatin possible | No recommendation |
| Pitavastatin | EFV, ETR, NVP, RPV | No data | |
| Pravastatin, rosuvastatin | EFV | Pravastatin AUC ↓ 44% rosuvastatin: no data | Adjust statin dose according to lipid responses, not to exceed the maximum recommended dose. |
| | ETR | No significant effect expected | No dosage adjustment necessary |

*Abbreviations:* ABC, abacavir; APV, amprenavir; ATV/r, ritonavir-boosted atazanavir; AUC, area under the curve; $C_{max}$, maximum drug concentration; DRV/r, ritonavir-boosted darunavir; EFV, efavirenz; ETR, etravirine; FPV/r, ritonavir-boosted fosamprenavir; LPV/r, ritonavir-boosted lopinavir; NFV, nelfinavir; NNRTI, non-nucleoside reverse transcriptase inhibitor; NVP, nevirapine; RAL, raltegravir; RPV, rilpivirine; RTV, ritonavir; SQV/r, ritonavir-boosted saquinavir; T20, enfuvirtide; TDF, tenofovir disoproxil fumarate; TPV/r, ritonavir-boosted tipranavir.

*Adapted from* Kellick KA, Bottorff M, Toth PP. A clinician's guide to satin drug-drug interactions. J Clin Lipidol 2014;8:S30–46; with permission.

**Table 5**
**Statin use with hepatitis C antiviral medications**

| HCV Antiviral/Class | Interaction | Notes |
|---|---|---|
| Boceprevir (NS3/4A PI) | Potentially toxic with statins | No longer routinely used[76] |
| Telaprevir (NS3/4A PI) | Potentially toxic with statins | No longer routinely used[76] |
| Simeprevir (NS3/4A PI) | Rosuvastatin: initiate at 5 mg, do not exceed 10 mg<br>Atorvastatin: initiate at 10 mg, do not exceed 40 mg<br>Simvastatin: keep at lowest dose possible<br>Pitavastatin, pravastatin, lovastatin: no data | [75,80] |
| Sofosbuvir (NS5B polymerase inhibitor) | No contraindications for statin use | [80,120–122] |
| Ledipasvir (NS5A polymerase inhibitor) | Rosuvastatin: use not recommended<br>No reports for other statins | Is coadministered with sofosbuvir |

dyslipidemia. Other over-the-counter formulations of sustained-release over-the counter niacin preparations been associated with an increased risk of hepatotoxicity.[96]

The role of niacin in preventing CVD morbidity and mortality is uncertain. Early clinical studies suggested that niacin had a mortality benefit when used in the secondary prevention of CHD compared with other nonstatin drugs,[97] but recent

**Box 5**
**Monitoring liver side effects of statins**

- Conduct baseline testing of aspartate transaminase (AST) and alanine transaminase (ALT) and, if normal, begin statin therapy. Repeat AST and ALT testing in 1 month.

- If baseline or follow-up AST and ALT levels are elevated but less than 3 times the upper limit of normal, check bilirubin. If it is normal or patients have nonalcoholic fatty liver disease or Gilbert syndrome, statin therapy can be initiated or continued with follow-up measurement of AST, ALT, and bilirubin. Otherwise, a workup for the cause of liver tests should be undertaken.

- If baseline or follow-up AST and ALT levels are greater than 3 times the upper limit of normal, statin therapy should not be initiated or continued until further workup is performed.

**Box 6**
**Monitoring muscle and CK side effects of statins**

- Mild elevations in CK ($\leq$3 times the upper limit of normal) in the absence of symptoms → continue statin therapy with monitoring

- Higher CK (>3 times the upper limit of normal), symptoms, renal insufficiency, dark-colored urine → stop statin and proceed with further evaluation

- Muscle soreness and normal CK options

  o Hold the statin and see if symptoms resolve, and then rechallenge to see if symptoms return.

  o Hold the statin; if symptoms resolve, rechallenge with a lower dose of the same statin or another statin.

  o There is no strong evidence that one statin over another produces fewer symptoms, but small studies have suggested that pitavastatin may be better tolerated.

  o Consider alternate-day dosing: Statins with longer half-lives (atorvastatin, rosuvastatin, and pitavastatin) can be effective in less-than-daily dosing.

*Data from* Rosenson RS, Baker SK, Jacobson TA, et al. An assessment by the Statin Muscle Safety Task Force: 2014 update. J Clin Lipidol 2014;8(3 Suppl):S58–71; and Duggan ST. Pitavastatin: a review of its use in the management of hypercholesterolaemia or mixed dyslipidaemia. Drugs 2012;72(4):565–84.

- Assess patients for risk of developing diabetes before starting a statin.

- Monitor blood glucose and hemoglobin A1c.

- Continue to emphasize lifestyle modifications to prevent diabetes.

- In general, statin therapy should be continued as benefits are felt to outweigh risks.

studies have found no additional benefit compared with statin use alone.[98] The Heart Protection Study (HPS)-2 THRIVE trial enrolled participants who had CVD, but there were no entry criteria for lipid levels. There was no reduction in the risk of major vascular events and an increase in the risk of serious adverse events when a niacin/laropiprant combination was added to a statin despite lowering LDL-C (10 mg/dL) and triglycerides (33 mg/dL) and increasing HDL-C (6 mg/dL). Laropiprant is an antagonist of prostaglandin D2 receptor DP1 that helps reduce the side effect of flushing with niacin.[99]

Niacin has been tested in patients infected with HIV. Niacin 1500 mg daily was well tolerated in 23 participants, lowering non–HL-C and TG and increasing HDL-C. Increases in glucose and insulin resistance were transient.[100] Fourteen participants taking 2000 mg of niacin daily had significant reductions in TG and non–HDL-C. Seven were glucose intolerant; this was a new finding for 3 of the 7.[101] In the open-label ACTG A5148 trial, extended-release niacin was used in escalating doses for up to 44 weeks to treat hypertriglyceridemia and resulted in a median decrease in TG of 38%.[100]

Niacin is not a potent LDL-C–lowering medication, and treatment of hypertriglyceridemia requires high doses. Guidelines do not suggest specific treatment of low HDL with niacin or other lipid medications other than treating metabolic abnormalities that influence HDL levels. Together with the side effects, niacin is not thought to be an ideal medication for patients with HIV.

**Bile acid sequestrants** Bile acid sequestrants bind bile acids in the intestine and prevent reabsorption of cholesterol. They were the first lipid-lowering medications developed. Original formulations were colestipol and cholestyramine however a newer drug, colesevelam is now available in both tablet form (6 large pills) or an oral suspension that can be dissolved in water and other liquids.[102]

Drugs in this class are less potent than statins in reducing LDL-C and have gastrointestinal side effects and may interfere with the absorption of other medications. These drugs have not been evaluated in HIV-infected patients and there is concern about reducing absorption of ART. Bile acid sequestrants can also raise TG, especially when baseline levels are elevated.

## Treatment of Hypertriglyceridemia

Hypertriglyceridemia with a low HDL-C pattern is prevalent among those infected with HIV. First-line treatment of moderately elevated TG (<500 mg/dL) is lifestyle modification including weight loss in overweight or obese patients, aerobic exercise, avoidance of concentrated sugars, and strict glycemic control in diabetic patients. For markedly elevated TG (greater than 500 mg/dL), prevention of pancreatitis requires medication along with lifestyle modification and treatment of possible secondary causes of hypertriglyceridemia.

Because values for TG vary considerably, it is helpful to have several fasting measures to determine the need for medication. Statins have a modest effect on TG; fibrate and fish oil are indicated for lowering TG with high-dose niacin as an option, if tolerated.

### Fibrates

Gemfibrozil is an older fibrate and, in patients with HIV, has been shown to have only modest additional efficacy over a low-saturated-fat diet in reducing TG for those with TG greater than 266 and taking PIs.[103] PI induction of glucuronidation of gemfibrozil may explain the lower-than-expected efficacy of gemfibrozil in these patients. Gemfibrozil may increase serum concentrations of statins through inhibition of drug transporters, such as ornithine aminotransferase, and increase the risk of rhabdomyolysis.[104] Gemfibrozil has more interactions than newer fibrates and is dosed twice daily, a consideration for patients taking multiple medications. Unlike the newer fibrates, it does not have to be adjusted for patients with chronic kidney disease.[103] Gemfibrozil should be used with caution in patients with HIV.

Fenofibrate lacks significant interactions with ART and is the most commonly prescribed fibrate for HIV-infected patients for the treatment of hypertriglyceridemia. Fenofibrate is eliminated by the kidneys and should be dose adjusted in patients with reduced renal function or on other nephrotoxic drugs.[105]

In a study of 635 HIV-infected patients on PI-based ART with TG greater than 300 mg/dL, patients were treated with bezafibrate, gemfibrozil, or fenofibrate. All fibrates showed a similar and significant efficacy.[106] In a prospective study, fenofibrate 200 mg daily was given to 20 HIV-infected patients on ART with baseline TG greater than 400 mg/dL despite diet and exercise. Triglycerides were reduced 54% after 24 weeks.[107] In the ACTG 5087 study, there was a reduction in TG of 35% versus 13% ($P$<.001) for patients on fenofibrate 200 mg/d versus pravastatin 40 mg/d.[69]

### Fish oil

Long-chain omega-3 polyunsaturated fatty acids are present in cold-water fish and can lower TG[108] and reduce CVD events in the general population.[59] Two purified forms of ethyl esterized n-3 fatty acids, docosahexaenoic acid (DHA) (all-cis-4,7,10,13, 16,19-docosahexaenoic acid) and eicosapentaenoic acid (EPA) (all-cis-5,8,11,14,17-eicosapentaenoic acid), are commonly used in combination (DHA/EPA). Lower doses (1 g daily) are recommended for the prevention of CVD.[108] Higher doses of DHA and EPA (4 g daily) reduce TG levels by 22% to 33% compared with placebo.[109] Comparisons between studies are difficult because of the different concentrations of EPA and DHA used in each trial.

Most studies of patients infected with HIV suggest a moderate reduction (about 25%) in TG levels when compared with diet and exercise alone or placebo.[110,111] One study found no significant decrease in TG with salmon oil; but there were study limitations, including low doses of EPA and DHA and confounding caused by the high prevalence of concomitant lipid-lowering therapy use.[112]

In a recent study, HIV-infected patients on ART with baseline TG between 300 and 1000 mg/dL taking fibrates or niacin (but not taking statins) were randomized to receive either fish oil or placebo. A 27% reduction compared with a 13% increase in TG was observed for fish oil and placebo, respectively.[113] In the ACTG A5186 study, 100 patients were randomized to receive fish oil (EPA + DHA 4.86 g/d) or fenofibrate 160 mg/d. The fish oil group reduced TG by 46%, whereas the fenofibrate group achieved a 58% reduction at 8 weeks.[114] A recent retrospective observational cohort study compared the effectiveness of multiple treatment interventions to reduce TG in 493 HIV-infected patients with a mean TG of 347 mg/dL at baseline. Fibrate use resulted in larger TG reductions than fish oil.[115]

Fish oil is particularly useful in the treatment of hypertriglyceridemia in patients infected with HIV due to the lack of interactions with ART and other medications although the size and number (4) of capsules in a standard daily dose may reduce adherence. If the prescription formulation is not covered by insurance, a patient can be instructed to take the equivalent of approximately 4 g daily equally divided between DHA and EPA supplemental (non-prescription) formulation.

### Niacin

Niacin in higher dosages (2000 mg daily) can lower triglycerides in the range of 30% to 45%,[59] but side effects often limit adherence.

## Other Issues Related to Drug Therapy

### Cost of drugs and coverage

This patient population often has straight Medicaid or a managed Medicaid plan with a limited formulary or only AIDS Drug Assistance Program (ADAP), which may not offer coverage for lipid medications. Authorizations and appeals can be time consuming but may result in coverage for a medication, so providers are encouraged to submit requests if prescriptions are initially declined.

### Combination with other nonstatin drugs

If one medication does not bring patient to or near target or for patients who need treatment for both elevated LDL-C and TG combination drug therapy should be used. Patients with very high (>500 mg/dL) TG should have treatment for this first and when at or near target, should be reevaluated to determine need for LDL-C lowering. Second or third medications should be started at lower doses and titrated one at a time. There is an increased risk for elevation of liver enzymes with combinations of statins, fibrates, and niacin and routine monitoring should be considered.

## Familial Hypercholesterolemia

Familial hypercholesterolemia (FH) is a term representing a group of genetic defects that result in markedly elevated levels of LDL-C.[116] More detail on FH can be found elsewhere in this issue. At present there is no information specific to FH in patients infected with HIV, and the prevalence is unknown.

New and more potent drugs have been approved by the FDA for treatment of homozygous FH but have not been tested in patients infected with HIV. The medications are mipomersen, an antisense nucleotide that inhibits apoB synthesis and lomitapide, a microsomal triglyceride transfer protein inhibitor. Lomitapide levels are increased with CYP3A4 inhibitors and could not be used with PIs. Another class of drug is currently in Phase III trials and inhibits PCSK9. The PCSK9 promotes LDL receptor degradation within hepatocytes. There is also apheresis, a procedure similar to hemodialysis which removes LDL-C for those with

FH or markedly elevated LDL-C who are unable to have levels lowered by medication.[117]

## Switching Antiretroviral Therapy

Many ART influence lipids levels; however, changing an ART regimen to less offensive drugs may also present problems. At the time of evaluation for dyslipidemia, many patients have already undergone genotype and phenotype evaluation for ART and have been stable on a virologic effective regimen that is tolerated. Because virologic suppression is a priority, it is reasonable to treat the lipid abnormalities on an established ART regimen. Switching regimens may not significantly improve lipids and may also result in virologic failure. Switching can be considered for patients with marked lipid abnormalities, who are at very high risk, or who are unable to attain a reasonable response with therapy. This change should be done in consultation with the provider who is managing the patients' ART.[118,119]

## Monitoring and Follow-up

According to the European guidelines, recommendations for follow-up after beginning therapy "stem from consensus rather than evidence-based guidelines" and that "response to therapy can be assessed at 6–8 weeks from initiation or dose increases for statins, but response to fibrates and lifestyle may take longer."[48]

For most patients, maximum LDL and triglyceride lowering is evident by 6 weeks after starting therapy. If patients are not at the goal, titrate to higher doses or add a second drug and recheck lipid levels in another 6 weeks. If a patient is already on combination therapy, only one drug should be titrated at a time. Monitoring of liver function tests, CK, glucose, and symptoms (such as muscle soreness) are as discussed earlier and should be performed when indicated.

It is important to understand that attainment of the targets for LDL-C and TG may not be reached. Care for patients living with HIV is complex, with side effects of medications, problems with adherence to a multidrug regimen, and comorbidities that impact on lipids. Reviewing all medical conditions and medications with the patients' other providers can help to identify priorities for patients. Viral suppression is generally considered foremost, although treatment of other conditions may also merit priority.

Patients with known CVD or at very high risk should aim to have LDL-C reach the goal. If goal attainment is not possible, there remains an incremental benefit to lowering LDL-C even if the goal cannot be reached. A triglyceride goal of less than 150 mg/dL may not be attainable, but attempts to lower this (with both lifestyle and medication) should be made. When levels are extremely high (>500 mg/dL), lowering to prevent pancreatitis is a priority.

## SUMMARY

This review has provided background on HIV and how both the virus and therapy impact on CVD and risk factors, in particular dyslipidemia. With HIV becoming a more chronic disease and patients are living to ages where CVD is more prevalent, it will become important to diagnose and treat risk factors. In addition, primary care providers for these patients should receive training in identifying those at risk and managing risk factors as well as understanding when to refer to cardiovascular and lipid specialists.

Epidemiologic studies and clinical trials are needed to establish specific and comprehensive guidelines for this patient population. Until we have the results of studies conducted in persons with HIV infection, we must rely on guidelines for non-HIV patients with extrapolation to HIV-infected patients to guide us in helping patients who are living with HIV.

## REFERENCES

1. Morbidity and Mortality Weekly Report. Pneumocystitis Pneumonia—Los Angeles June 5, 1981;30(21): 1–3.
2. Triant VA, Lee H, Hadigan C, et al. Increased acute myocardial infarction rates and cardiovascular risk factors among patients with human immunodeficiency virus disease. J Clin Endocrinol Metab 2007;92(7):2506–12.
3. Smith CJ, Ryom L, Weber R, et al. Trends in underlying causes of death in people with HIV from 1999 to 2011 (D:A:D): a multicohort collaboration. Lancet 2014;384(9939):241–8.
4. Esser S, Gelbrich G, Brockmeyer N, et al. Prevalence of cardiovascular diseases in HIV-infected outpatients: results from a prospective, multicenter cohort study. Clin Res Cardiol 2013;102(3):203–13.
5. Grinspoon SK, Grunfeld C, Kotler DP, et al. State of the science conference: initiative to decrease cardiovascular risk and increase quality of care for patients living with HIV/AIDS: executive summary. Circulation 2008;118(2):198–210.
6. Myerson M, Poltavskiy E, Armstrong EJ, et al. Prevalence, treatment, and control of dyslipidemia and hypertension in 4278 HIV outpatients. J Acquir Immune Defic Syndr 2014;66(4):370–7.
7. Petoumenos K, Worm S, Reiss P, et al. Rates of cardiovascular disease following smoking cessation in

patients with HIV infection: results from the D:A:D study(*). HIV Med 2011;12(7):412–21.

8. Taylor BS, Hammer SM. The challenge of HIV-1 subtype diversity. N Engl J Med 2008;359(18):1965–6.

9. Ackerman M, Alter G. Mapping the journey to an HIV vaccine. N Engl J Med 2013;369(4):389–91.

10. Galescu O, Bhangoo A, Ten S. Insulin resistance, lipodystrophy and cardiometabolic syndrome in HIV/AIDS. Rev Endocr Metab Disord 2013;14(2):133–40.

11. Reyskens KM, Essop MF. The maladaptive effects of HIV protease inhibitors (lopinavir/ritonavir) on the rat heart. Int J Cardiol 2013;168(3):3047–9.

12. Magkos F, Mantzoros CS. Body fat redistribution and metabolic abnormalities in HIV-infected patients on highly active antiretroviral therapy: novel insights into pathophysiology and emerging opportunities for treatment. Metabolism 2011;60(6):749–53.

13. Brown TT, Tassiopoulos K, Bosch RJ, et al. Association between systemic inflammation and incident diabetes in HIV-infected patients after initiation of antiretroviral therapy. Diabetes Care 2010;33(10):2244–9.

14. Libby P, Ridker P. Inflammation and atherothrombosis: from population biology and bench research to clinical practice. J Am Coll Cardiol 2006;48(9, Supplement A):A33–46.

15. El-Sadr WM, Lundgren J, Neaton JD, et al. CD4+ count-guided interruption of antiretroviral treatment. N Engl J Med 2006;355(22):2283–96.

16. Kuller LH, Tracy R, Belloso W, et al. Inflammatory and coagulation biomarkers and mortality in patients with HIV infection. PLoS Med 2008;5(10):e203.

17. Mangili A, Polak JF, Quach LA, et al. Markers of atherosclerosis and inflammation and mortality in patients with HIV infection. Atherosclerosis 2011;214(2):468–73.

18. Subramanian S, Tawakol A, Burdo TH, et al. Arterial inflammation in patients with HIV. JAMA 2012;308(4):379–86.

19. Stone NJ, Robinson J, Lichtenstein AH, et al. 2013 ACC/AHA guideline on the treatment of blood cholesterol to reduce atherosclerotic cardiovascular risk in adults: a report of the American College of Cardiology/American Heart Association task force on practice guidelines. J Am Coll Cardiol 2013;63(25 Pt B):2889–934.

20. Available at: http://reprievetrial.org/. Accessed March 5, 2015.

21. Gale HB, Gitterman SR, Hoffman HJ, et al. Is frequent CD4+ T-lymphocyte count monitoring necessary for persons with counts >=300 cells/muL and HIV-1 suppression? Clin Infect Dis 2013;56(9):1340–3.

22. Gunthard HF, Aberg JA, Eron JJ, et al. Antiretroviral treatment of adult HIV infection: 2014 recommendations of the International Antiviral Society-USA Panel. JAMA 2014;312(4):410–25.

23. Friis-Moller N, Reiss P, Sabin CA, et al. Class of antiretroviral drugs and the risk of myocardial infarction. N Engl J Med 2007;356(17):1723–35.

24. Reyskens KM, Fisher TL, Schisler JC, et al. Cardiometabolic effects of HIV protease inhibitors (lopinavir/ritonavir). PLoS One 2013;8(9):e73347.

25. Stein JH, Komarow L, Cotter BR, et al. Lipoprotein changes in HIV-infected antiretroviral-naive individuals after starting antiretroviral therapy: ACTG Study A5152s Stein: lipoprotein changes on antiretroviral therapy. J Clin Lipidol 2008;2(6):464–71.

26. Riddler SA, Li X, Chu H, et al. Longitudinal changes in serum lipids among HIV-infected men on highly active antiretroviral therapy. HIV Med 2007;8(5):280–7.

27. Riddler SA, Smit E, Cole SR, et al. Impact of HIV infection and HAART on serum lipids in men. JAMA 2003;289(22):2978–82.

28. Jarrett OD, Wanke CA, Ruthazer R, et al. Metabolic syndrome predicts all-cause mortality in persons with human immunodeficiency virus. AIDS Patient Care STDS 2013;27(5):266–71.

29. Alencastro PR, Fuchs SC, Wolff FH, et al. Independent predictors of metabolic syndrome in HIV-infected patients. AIDS Patient Care STDS 2011;25(11):627–34.

30. Martin Lde S, Pasquier E, Roudaut N, et al. Metabolic syndrome: a major risk factor for atherosclerosis in HIV-infected patients (SHIVA study). Presse Med 2008;37(4 Pt 1):579–84.

31. Malvestutto CD, Aberg JA. Management of dyslipidemia in HIV-infected patients. Clin Lipidol 2011;6(4):447–62.

32. Dube MP, Stein JH, Aberg JA, et al. Guidelines for the evaluation and management of dyslipidemia in human immunodeficiency virus (HIV)-infected adults receiving antiretroviral therapy: recommendations of the HIV Medical Association of the Infectious Disease Society of America and the Adult AIDS Clinical Trials Group. Clin Infect Dis 2003;37(5):613–27.

33. Aberg JA, Gallant JE, Ghanem KG, et al. Primary care guidelines for the management of persons infected with HIV: 2013 update by the HIV medicine association of the Infectious Diseases Society of America. Clin Infect Dis 2014;58(1):e1–34.

34. Friis-Moller N, Thiebaut R, Reiss P, et al. Predicting the risk of cardiovascular disease in HIV-infected patients: the data collection on adverse effects of anti-HIV drugs study. Eur J Cardiovasc Prev Rehabil 2010;17(5):491–501.

35. Justice AC, Freiberg MS, Tracy R, et al. Does an index composed of clinical data reflect effects of inflammation, coagulation, and monocyte activation on mortality among those aging with HIV? Clin Infect Dis 2012;54(7):984–94.

36. Lundgren JD, Battegay M, Behrens G, et al. European AIDS Clinical Society (EACS) guidelines on the prevention and management of metabolic diseases in HIV. HIV Med 2008;9(2):72–81.

37. Falcone EL, Mangili A, Skinner S, et al. Framingham risk score and early markers of atherosclerosis in a cohort of adults infected with HIV. Antivir Ther 2011;16(1):1–8.

38. Parra S, Coll B, Aragones G, et al. Nonconcordance between subclinical atherosclerosis and the calculated Framingham risk score in HIV-infected patients: relationships with serum markers of oxidation and inflammation. HIV Med 2010;11(4):225–31.

39. Law MG, Friis-Moller N, El-Sadr WM, et al. The use of the Framingham equation to predict myocardial infarctions in HIV-infected patients: comparison with observed events in the D:A:D Study. HIV Med 2006;7(4):218–30.

40. Zanni MV, Fitch KV, Feldpausch M, et al. 2013 American College of Cardiology/American Heart Association and 2004 Adult Treatment Panel III cholesterol guidelines applied to HIV-infected patients with/without subclinical high-risk coronary plaque. AIDS 2014;28(14):2061–70.

41. Ginsberg HN. The 2013 ACC/AHA guidelines on the treatment of blood cholesterol: questions, questions, questions. Circ Res 2014;114(5):761–4.

42. Martin SS, Blumenthal RS. Concepts and controversies: the 2013 American College of Cardiology/American Heart Association risk assessment and cholesterol treatment guidelines. Ann Intern Med 2014;160(5):356–8.

43. Ridker PM, Cook NR. Statins: new American guidelines for prevention of cardiovascular disease. Lancet 2013;382(9907):1762–5.

44. Hulten E, Mitchell J, Scally J, et al. HIV positivity, protease inhibitor exposure and subclinical atherosclerosis: a systematic review and meta-analysis of observational studies. Heart 2009;95(22):1826–35.

45. Hsu R, K P, J L, et al. Independent predictors of carotid intimal thickness differ between HIV+ and HIV- patients with respect to traditional cardiac risk factors, risk calculators, lipid subfractions, and inflammatory markers. Paper presented at: 7th International AIDS Conference on HIV Pathogenesis, Treatment, and Prevention. Kuala Lumpur, Malaysia, July 3, 2013.

46. Post WS, Budoff M, Kingsley L, et al. Associations between HIV infection and subclinical coronary atherosclerosis. Ann Intern Med 2014;160(7):458–67.

47. Silverberg MJ, Leyden WA, Xu L, et al. Immunodeficiency and risk of myocardial infarction among HIV-positive individuals with access to care. J Acquir Immune Defic Syndr 2014;65(2):160–6.

48. Catapano AL, Chapman J, Wiklund O, et al. The new joint EAS/ESC guidelines for the management of dyslipidaemias. Atherosclerosis 2011;217(1):1.

49. Anderson TJ, Gregoire J, Hegele RA, et al. 2012 update of the Canadian Cardiovascular Society guidelines for the diagnosis and treatment of dyslipidemia for the prevention of cardiovascular disease in the adult. Can J Cardiol 2013;29(2): 151–67.

50. Expert Dyslipidemia Panel of the International Atherosclerosis Society Panel members. An International Atherosclerosis Society position paper: global recommendations for the management of dyslipidemia–full report. J Clin Lipidol 2014;8(1): 29–60.

51. Third Report of the National Cholesterol Education Program (NCEP) Expert Panel on Detection. Evaluation, and treatment of high blood cholesterol in adults (adult treatment panel III) final report. Circulation 2002;106(25):3143–421.

52. Jacobson TA, Ito MK, Maki KC, et al. National Lipid Association recommendations for patient-centered management of dyslipidemia: part 1-executive summary. J Clin Lipidol 2014;8(5):473–88.

53. Otvos JD, Mora S, Shalaurova I, et al. Clinical implications of discordance between low-density lipoprotein cholesterol and particle number. J Clin Lipidol 2011;5(2):105–13.

54. Cromwell WC, Otvos JD, Keyes MJ, et al. LDL particle number and risk of future cardiovascular disease in the Framingham offspring study - implications for LDL management. J Clin Lipidol 2007; 1(6):583–92.

55. Manickam P, Rathod A, Panaich S, et al. Comparative prognostic utility of conventional and novel lipid parameters for cardiovascular disease risk prediction: do novel lipid parameters offer an advantage? J Clin Lipidol 2011;5(2):82–90.

56. Malave H, Castro M, Burkle J, et al. Evaluation of low-density lipoprotein particle number distribution in patients with type 2 diabetes mellitus with low-density lipoprotein cholesterol <50 mg/dl and non-high-density lipoprotein cholesterol <80 mg/dl. Am J Cardiol 2012;110(5):662–5.

57. Myerson M, Lee R, Varela D, et al. Lipoprotein measurements in patients infected with HIV: is cholesterol content of HDL and LDL discordant with particle number? J Clin Lipidol 2014;8(3): 332–3.

58. Swanson B, Sha BE, Keithley JK, et al. Lipoprotein particle profiles by nuclear magnetic resonance spectroscopy in medically-underserved HIV-infected persons. J Clin Lipidol 2009;3(6):379–84.

59. Miller M, Stone NJ, Ballantyne C, et al. Triglycerides and cardiovascular disease: a scientific statement from the American Heart Association. Circulation 2011;123(20):2292–333.

60. Bucher HC, Richter W, Glass TR, et al. Small dense lipoproteins, apolipoprotein B, and risk of coronary events in HIV-infected patients on antiretroviral

therapy: the Swiss HIV Cohort Study. J Acquir Immune Defic Syndr 2012;60(2):135–42.

61. Anastos K, Lu D, Shi Q, et al. Association of serum lipid levels with HIV serostatus, specific antiretroviral agents, and treatment regimens. J Acquir Immune Defic Syndr 2007;45(1):34–42.

62. Hegele RA, Ginsberg HN, Chapman MJ, et al. The polygenic nature of hypertriglyceridaemia: implications for definition, diagnosis, and management. Lancet Diabetes Endocrinol 2014;2(8): 655–66.

63. Stein JH, Merwood MA, Bellehumeur JB, et al. Postprandial lipoprotein changes in patients taking antiretroviral therapy for HIV infection. Arterioscler Thromb Vasc Biol 2005;25(2):399–405.

64. Anuurad E, Thomas-Geevarghese A, Devaraj S, et al. Increased lipoprotein remnant cholesterol levels in HIV-positive patients during antiretroviral therapy. Atherosclerosis 2008;198(1):192–7.

65. Toth PP, Barter PJ, Rosenson RS, et al. High-density lipoproteins: a consensus statement from the National Lipid Association. J Clin Lipidol 2013; 7(5):484–525.

66. Davidson MH, Ballantyne CM, Jacobson TA, et al. Clinical utility of inflammatory markers and advanced lipoprotein testing: advice from an expert panel of lipid specialists. J Clin Lipidol 2011;5(5):338–67.

67. Baruch L, Agarwal S, Gupta B, et al. Is directly measured low-density lipoprotein clinically equivalent to calculated low-density lipoprotein? J Clin Lipidol 2010;4(4):259–64.

68. Marzilli M. Pleiotropic effects of statins: evidence for benefits beyond LDL-cholesterol lowering. Am J Cardiovasc Drugs 2010;10(Suppl 1):3–9.

69. Aberg JA, Zackin RA, Brobst SW, et al. A randomized trial of the efficacy and safety of fenofibrate versus pravastatin in HIV-infected subjects with lipid abnormalities: AIDS Clinical Trials Group Study 5087. AIDS Res Hum Retroviruses 2005;21(9):757–67.

70. Calza L, Manfredi R, Colangeli V, et al. Two-year treatment with rosuvastatin reduces carotid intima-media thickness in HIV type 1-infected patients receiving highly active antiretroviral therapy with asymptomatic atherosclerosis and moderate cardiovascular risk. AIDS Res Hum Retroviruses 2013;29(3):547–56.

71. Aslangul E, Assoumou L, Bittar R, et al. Rosuvastatin versus pravastatin in dyslipidemic HIV-1-infected patients receiving protease inhibitors: a randomized trial. AIDS 2010;24(1):77–83.

72. Sponseller CA, Campbell SE, Thompson M, et al. Pitavastatin is superior to pravastatin for LDL-C lowering in patients with HIV. Conference on Retroviruses and Opportunistic Infections. Boston (MA), March 3–6, 2014.

73. Sponseller CA, Tanahashi M, Suganami H, et al. Pitavastatin 4 mg vs. pravastatin 40 mg in HIV: dyslipidemia: post-hoc analysis of the INTREPID trial based on the independent CHD risk factor of age. National Lipid Association Annual Scientific Sessions. Orlando (FL), May 1–4, 2014.

74. Aberg JA, Sponseller CA. Neutral Effects of pitavastatin 4 grams and pravastatin 40 mg on blood glucose levels over 12 weeks. Prespecified safety analysis from INTREPID. San Francisco (CA): ID Week Infectious Disease Society of America. October 2–6, 2013.

75. Kellick KA, Bottorff M, Toth PP, The National Lipid Association's Safety Task Force. A clinician's guide to statin drug-drug interactions. J Clin Lipidol 2014; 8(3 Suppl):S30–46.

76. Chauvin B, Drouot S, Barrail-Tran A, et al. Drug-drug interactions between HMG-CoA reductase inhibitors (statins) and antiviral protease inhibitors. Clin Pharm 2013;52(10):815–31.

77. FDA Drug Safety Communication: Important safety label changes to cholesterol-lowering statin drugs. February 28, 2012.

78. Morgan ET. Impact of infectious and inflammatory disease on cytochrome P450-mediated drug metabolism and pharmacokinetics. Clin Pharmacol Ther 2009;85(4):434–8.

79. Morgan ET, Goralski KB, Piquette-Miller M, et al. Regulation of drug-metabolizing enzymes and transporters in infection, inflammation, and cancer. Drug Metab Dispos 2008;36(2):205–16.

80. Kohli A, Shaffer A, Sherman A, et al. Treatment of hepatitis C: a systematic review. JAMA 2014; 312(6):631–40.

81. Bichoupan K, Dieterich DT, Martel-Laferriere V. HIV-hepatitis C virus co-infection in the era of direct-acting antivirals. Curr HIV/AIDS Rep 2014;11(3): 241–9.

82. Bays H, Cohen DE, Chalasani N, et al. An assessment by the statin liver safety task force: 2014 update. J Clin Lipidol 2014;8(3 Suppl):S47–57.

83. Rosenson RS, Baker SK, Jacobson TA, et al. An assessment by the statin muscle safety task force: 2014 update. J Clin Lipidol 2014;8(3 Suppl):S58–71.

84. Neal RC, Ferdinand KC, Ycas J, et al. Relationship of ethnic origin, gender, and age to blood creatine kinase levels. Am J Med 2009;122(1):73–8.

85. Chan P, Brew BJ. HIV associated neurocognitive disorders in the modern antiviral treatment era: prevalence, characteristics, biomarkers, and effects of treatment. Curr HIV/AIDS Rep 2014; 11(3):317–24.

86. Sattar N, Ginsberg HN, Ray KK. The use of statins in people at risk of developing diabetes mellitus: evidence and guidance for clinical practice. Atheroscler Suppl 2014;15(1):1–15.

87. Sweeney ME, Johnson RR. Ezetimibe: an update on the mechanism of action, pharmacokinetics and recent clinical trials. Expert Opin Drug Metab Toxicol 2007;3(3):441–50.

88. Cannon C. Improved reduction of outcomes: Vytorin efficacy International Trial American Heart Association. Chicago (IL): American Heart Association Scientific Sessions. November 15–19, 2014.

89. Coll B, Aragones G, Parra S, et al. Ezetimibe effectively decreases LDL-cholesterol in HIV-infected patients. AIDS 2006;20(12):1675–7.

90. Bennett MT, Johns KW, Bondy GP. Ezetimibe is effective when added to maximally tolerated lipid lowering therapy in patients with HIV. Lipids Health Dis 2007;6:15.

91. Chow D, Chen H, Glesby MJ, et al. Short-term ezetimibe is well tolerated and effective in combination with statin therapy to treat elevated LDL cholesterol in HIV-infected patients. AIDS 2009; 23(16):2133–41.

92. Digby JE, Ruparelia N, Choudhury RP. Niacin in cardiovascular disease: recent preclinical and clinical developments. Arterioscler Thromb Vasc Biol 2012;32(3):582–8.

93. Brunzell JD. Clinical practice. Hypertriglyceridemia. N Engl J Med 2007;357(10):1009–17.

94. Rajanna V, Campbell KB, Leimberger J, et al. Elevation of fasting morning glucose relative to hemoglobin A1c in normoglycemic patients treated with niacin and with statins. J Clin Lipidol 2012; 6(2):168–73.

95. Guyton JR, Bays HE. Safety considerations with niacin therapy. Am J Cardiol 2007;99(6A):22C–31C.

96. Meyers CD, Carr MC, Park S, et al. Varying cost and free nicotinic acid content in over-the-counter niacin preparations for dyslipidemia. Ann Intern Med 2003;139(12):996–1002.

97. Canner PL, Berge KG, Wenger NK, et al. Fifteen year mortality in Coronary Drug Project patients: long-term benefit with niacin. J Am Coll Cardiol 1986;8(6):1245–55.

98. Boden WE, Probstfield JL, Anderson T, et al. Niacin in patients with low HDL cholesterol levels receiving intensive statin therapy. N Engl J Med 2011;365(24):2255–67.

99. Landray MJ, Haynes R, Hopewell JC, et al. Effects of extended-release niacin with laropiprant in high-risk patients. N Engl J Med 2014;371(3):203–12.

100. Dube MP, Wu JW, Aberg JA, et al. Safety and efficacy of extended-release niacin for the treatment of dyslipidaemia in patients with HIV infection: AIDS Clinical Trials Group Study A5148. Antivir Ther 2006;11(8):1081–9.

101. Gerber MT, Mondy KE, Yarasheski KE, et al. Niacin in HIV-infected individuals with hyperlipidemia receiving potent antiretroviral therapy. Clin Infect Dis 2004;39(3):419–25.

102. Available at: http://www.welchol.com. Accessed March 5, 2015.

103. Available at: http://www.pfizer.com/files/products/uspi_lopid.pdf.

104. Nakagomi-Hagihara R, Nakai D, Tokui T, et al. Gemfibrozil and its glucuronide inhibit the hepatic uptake of pravastatin mediated by OATP1B1. Xenobiotica 2007;37(5):474–86.

105. Attridge RL, Frei CR, Ryan L, et al. Fenofibrate-associated nephrotoxicity: a review of current evidence. Am J Health Syst Pharm 2013;70(14): 1219–25.

106. Calza L, Manfredi R, Chiodo F. Use of fibrates in the management of hyperlipidemia in HIV-infected patients receiving HAART. Infection 2002;30(1):26–31.

107. Palacios R, Santos J, Gonzalez M, et al. Efficacy and safety of fenofibrate for the treatment of hypertriglyceridemia associated with antiretroviral therapy. J Acquir Immune Defic Syndr 2002;31(2): 251–3.

108. Bays HE, Tighe AP, Sadovsky R, et al. Prescription omega-3 fatty acids and their lipid effects: physiologic mechanisms of action and clinical implications. Expert Rev Cardiovasc Ther 2008;6(3):391–409.

109. Isosapent ethyl (Vascepa) for severe hypertriglyceridemia. Med Lett Drugs Ther 2013;55:33–4.

110. Wohl DA, Tien HC, Busby M, et al. Randomized study of the safety and efficacy of fish oil (omega-3 fatty acid) supplementation with dietary and exercise counseling for the treatment of antiretroviral therapy-associated hypertriglyceridemia. Clin Infect Dis 2005;41(10):1498–504.

111. De Truchis P, Kirstetter M, Perier A, et al. Reduction in triglyceride level with N-3 polyunsaturated fatty acids in HIV-infected patients taking potent antiretroviral therapy: a randomized prospective study. J Acquir Immune Defic Syndr 2007;44(3): 278–85.

112. Baril JG, Kovacs CM, Trottier S, et al. Effectiveness and tolerability of oral administration of low-dose salmon oil to HIV patients with HAART-associated dyslipidemia. HIV Clin Trials 2007;8(6):400–11.

113. Peters BS, Wierzbicki AS, Moyle G, et al. The effect of a 12-week course of omega-3 polyunsaturated fatty acids on lipid parameters in hypertriglyceridemic adult HIV-infected patients undergoing HAART: a randomized, placebo-controlled pilot trial. Clin Ther 2012;34(1):67–76.

114. Gerber JG, Kitch DW, Fichtenbaum CJ, et al. Fish oil and fenofibrate for the treatment of hypertriglyceridemia in HIV-infected subjects on antiretroviral therapy: results of ACTG A5186. J Acquir Immune Defic Syndr 2008;47(4):459–66.

115. Munoz MA, Liu W, Delaney JA, et al. Comparative effectiveness of fish oil versus fenofibrate, gemfibrozil, and atorvastatin on lowering triglyceride levels among HIV-infected patients in routine

clinical care. J Acquir Immune Defic Syndr 2013; 64(3):254–60.

116. Goldberg AC, Hopkins PN, Toth PP, et al. Familial hypercholesterolemia: screening, diagnosis and management of pediatric and adult patients: clinical guidance from the National Lipid Association Expert Panel on Familial Hypercholesterolemia. J Clin Lipidol 2011;5(3 Suppl):S1–8.

117. Rader DJ, Kastelein JJP. Lomitapide and Mipomersen. Circulation 2014;129:1022.

118. Nguyen ST, Eaton SA, Bain AM, et al. Lipid-lowering efficacy and safety after switching to atazanavir-ritonavir-based highly active antiretroviral therapy in patients with human immunodeficiency virus. Pharmacotherapy 2008;28(3):323–30.

119. Bain AM, White EA, Rutherford WS, et al. A multimodal, evidence-based approach to achieve lipid targets in the treatment of antiretroviral-associated dyslipidemia: case report and review of the literature. Pharmacotherapy 2008;28(7):932–8.

120. Available at: http://hcp.sovaldi.com/important-safety-information. Accessed November 29, 2014.

121. Available at: http://www.pegasys.com/hcp/treatment/chronic-hcv/safety. Accessed November 29, 2014.

122. Available at: http://www.moderiba.com/hcp. Accessed November 29, 2014.

# Managing Residual Risk After Myocardial Infarction Among Individuals with Low Cholesterol Levels

CrossMark

Lisandro D. Colantonio, MD, MSc[a],*,
Vera Bittner, MD, MSPH, FNLA[b]

## KEYWORDS

- Myocardial infarction • Disease management • Secondary prevention • Lipid-lowering medications
- Statins • Ezetimibe

## KEY POINTS

- About half of individuals with an acute myocardial infarction (MI) have a low-density lipoprotein cholesterol (LDL-C) level of less than 100 mg/dL.
- Management of individuals with MI and low LDL-C should include cardiac rehabilitation, lifestyle changes, evidence-based post-MI pharmacologic treatment, and adequate control of concomitant coronary risk factors.
- All individuals with a prior MI are recommended to take high-intensity statins (moderate intensity for those ≥75 years of age).
- Ezetimibe can be used as adjunctive lipid-lowering therapy among individuals with an MI and low LDL-C, particularly if they have inadequate response or intolerance to recommended intensity of statins.
- Little evidence exists to support the use of lipid-lowering medications other than ezetimibe in combination with statins among individuals with a prior MI.

## INTRODUCTION

Despite substantial improvements in the last 50 years, coronary heart disease (CHD) remains an important cause of morbidity and mortality in the United States and globally.[1] Lipid-lowering medications, particularly statins, have been a core element of primary and secondary prevention of CHD over the past decades. In 2001, the Third Report of the National Cholesterol Education Program, Expert Panel on Detection, Evaluation, and Treatment of High Blood Cholesterol in Adults (ATP-III) recommended a low-density lipoprotein cholesterol (LDL-C) of less than 100 mg/dL as a therapeutic target in high-risk individuals.[2] An optional therapeutic target of an LDL-C of less than 70 mg/dL was suggested later for very high-risk patients, including those with acute coronary syndrome (ACS) and an LDL-C of less than 100 mg/dL at the time of the event.[3] An increasing number of patients present with LDL-C levels below these targets, but remain at risk for a recurrent event. In this article,

Disclosures: V. Bittner has received research support from NIH grant R01 HL080477, Amgen, AstraZeneca, Bayer Healthcare, Janssen Pharmaceuticals, Pfizer, Sanofi Aventis. She has participated in advisory panels for Amgen and Eli Lilly.

[a] Department of Epidemiology, University of Alabama at Birmingham, 1530 3rd Avenue South, RPHB 217C, Birmingham, AL 35294, USA; [b] Division of Cardiovascular Disease, Department of Medicine, University of Alabama at Birmingham, 701 19th Street South, LHRB 310, Birmingham, AL 35294, USA
* Corresponding author.
E-mail address: lcolantonio@uab.edu

we review the current evidence and guidelines on the post-acute event management of individuals with myocardial infarction (MI) and LDL-C of less than 100 mg/dL.

## EPIDEMIOLOGY AND SIGNIFICANCE

Cholesterol levels have declined in the United States as awareness of cholesterol as a CHD risk factor and use of statins have increased.[4] As a consequence, the population presenting with MI in the current era is enriched by individuals with low LDL-C. Using data from the Get With The Guidelines program, Sachdeva and colleagues[5] reported that about one-half of individuals hospitalized for MI in 2000 through 2006 had an LDL-C level of less than 100 mg/dL, and 17.6% had an LDL-C of less than 70 mg/dL.

Individuals with an acute MI have an increased risk for recurrent coronary events and death. About 11% of all men and 22% of all women 45 to 64 years of age with a first MI will have a recurrent event or fatal CHD within 5 years (**Fig. 1**).[1] Overall, 14.8% of individuals with a history of atherosclerotic disease will have an MI, stroke,

revascularization, or cardiovascular death within 1 year.[6] These figures highlight the importance of considering residual risk among individuals with CHD, including those with low LDL-C levels.

Several factors are associated with risk for a recurrent MI or death in addition to blood cholesterol levels (**Box 1**). A formal appraisal of this residual risk could be performed using the Framingham risk prediction equations for subsequent coronary events, the CRUSADE long-term risk score, or the GRACE prediction tool.[7–9] However, these prediction models have not been incorporated into current guidelines and their applicability to individuals on "optimal medical therapy" is unclear.

Lifestyle changes and evidence-based pharmacologic therapy can effectively reduce risk among individuals with CHD. However, several investigators have shown that prescription of evidence-based post-MI pharmacologic therapy (both in hospital and at discharge) remains inadequate and that adherence to such therapy in the outpatient setting is suboptimal.[10,11] For example, only about 27% of Medicare beneficiaries fill a prescription for high-intensity statins after discharge for an MI.[12]

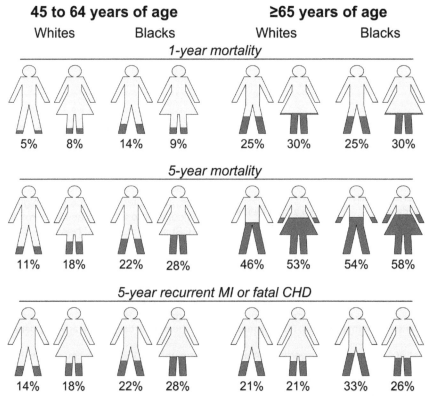

**Fig. 1.** Risk for all-cause mortality and recurrent myocardial infarction (MI) or coronary heart disease (CHD) death among individuals with a first MI. (*Data from* Go AS, Mozaffarian D, Roger VL, et al. Heart disease and stroke statistics 2014 update: a report from the American Heart Association. Circulation 2014;129:e231.)

**Box 1**
**Factors associated with residual risk for death or recurrent event in secondary prevention for MI**

Older age[7,55]

Male sex[55]

Social deprivation[56]

Increased body mass index[55]

Diabetes mellitus[7,55]

Hypertension[7,55]

Heart failure or high Killip class at the presentation of prior MI[9]

Smoking[7,55]

Elevated apolipoprotein B[55]

Reduced apolipoprotein A-I and HDL-C[42,55]

Chronic kidney disease, elevated urea nitrogen, and elevated creatinine[9,55,57]

Anhedonia, depressive mood, anxiety, stress, and type D personality[58–61]

*Abbreviations:* HDL-C, high-density lipoprotein cholesterol; MI, myocardial infarction.

## CURRENT GUIDELINES FOR POST-MYOCARDIAL INFARCTION MANAGEMENT AND SUPPORTING EVIDENCE

Current secondary prevention guidelines in the United States, UK, and Canada emphasize the importance of cardiac rehabilitation, lifestyle changes, and evidence-based post-MI pharmacologic therapy, as well as treatment for complications and other comorbidities in the management of individuals with established CHD.[13–16] Guidelines also emphasize the importance of a shared patient–provider decision-making process, in accordance with the principle of autonomy.

### Cardiac Rehabilitation and Lifestyle Changes

Current guidelines recommend referral to and participation in cardiac rehabilitation for all MI survivors.[13,14,16] This recommendation is based on prior clinical trials showing that exercise-based post-MI cardiac rehabilitation is associated with a lower risk for reinfarction (odds ratio [OR], 0.53; 95% CI, 0.38–0.76), cardiac mortality (OR, 0.64; 95% CI, 0.46–0.88), and all-cause mortality (OR, 0.74; 95% CI, 0.58–0.95) compared with no exercise.[17] An observational study of 1692 individuals with MI showed that those engaged in cardiac rehabilitation were less likely to discontinue prescribed medication, including statins (hazard ratio

[HR], 0.66; 95% CI, 0.45–0.92) and β-blockers (HR, 0.70; 95% CI, 0.49–0.98).[18]

Recommendations for lifestyle changes include increasing physical activity, adopting a healthier diet, weight management, and limited alcohol consumption (**Table 1**). Among smokers, smoking status should be assessed at every encounter and smoking cessation counseling should be provided. For those who express their desire to quit, proper support should be offered, including pharmacologic therapy. Current US guidelines also recommend avoiding exposure to air pollution and second-hand smoke.[13]

### Evidence-Based Post-Myocardial Infarction Pharmacologic Treatment

#### Antiplatelet therapy

Several studies have shown that antiplatelet therapy is effective in reducing the risk for vascular events after an MI.[19] Low-dose aspirin (75–150 mg/d) has been shown to be as effective as higher doses and similar to other antiplatelet drugs, and is considered the first choice in current guidelines.[13–15]

Dual antiplatelet therapy (DAPT) is more effective than aspirin alone among individuals with ACS, although the excess risk for bleeding needs to be counterbalanced. In a metaanalysis of 5 clinical trials comparing aspirin plus clopidogrel versus aspirin monotherapy for secondary prevention, DAPT was associated with a reduced risk for MI (OR, 0.82; 95% CI, 0.75–0.89), stroke (OR, 0.82; 95% CI, 0.73–0.93), and all-cause mortality (OR, 0.94; 95% CI, 0.89–0.99), but increased risk of major bleeding (OR, 1.26; 95% CI, 1.11–1.41).[20]

In the PLATO study, 18,624 individuals with ACS who received aspirin if tolerated were assigned randomly to ticagrelor or clopidogrel.[21] After 12 months follow-up, the risk for MI, stroke or cardiovascular death was lower among those who received ticagrelor (9.8%; HR, 0.84; 95% CI, 0.77–0.92) compared with those assigned to clopidogrel (11.7%), with a similar risk for major bleeding.

Indefinite antiplatelet therapy with aspirin is recommended for all MI survivors.[13,14] The 2013 NICE guidelines recommend DAPT with aspirin/ticagrelor for all individuals with ACS for up to 12 months.[14] The 2014 American College of Cardiology (ACC)/American Heart Association (AHA) guidelines recommend DAPT with aspirin plus either clopidogrel or ticagrelor for up to 12 months for the management of patients with non–ST-elevation ACS.[16] For those who received drug-eluting stents, DAPT could be extended for up to

**Table 1**
**Recommendations for lifestyle changes according to current guidelines**

| Guidelines | Recommendations |
|---|---|
| Increasing physical activity | |
| 2012 US guidelines[a,13] | Perform 30–60 min of moderate-intensity aerobic activity 5–7 days per week. |
| 2013 NICE guidelines (UK)[14] | Exercise 20–30 min a day to the point of slight breathlessness. |
| 2014 CCS guidelines (Canada)[15] | A total of 150 min of moderate to vigorous physical activity cumulated per week. |
| Adopting a healthier diet | |
| 2012 US guidelines[a,13] | Diet high in fresh fruits, whole grains, and vegetables, with low saturated fat (<7% total calories), cholesterol (<200 mg/dL per day) and trans fat (<1% total calories), and reduced sodium intake. |
| 2013 NICE guidelines (UK)[14] | Mediterranean-style diet. |
| Limited alcohol consumption | |
| 2012 US guidelines[a,13] | 1 drink per day for nonpregnant women and 1–2 drinks per day for men. |
| 2013 NICE guidelines (UK)[14] | No more than 21 and 14 units of alcohol per week for men and nonpregnant women, respectively. |

*Abbreviations:* CCS, Canadian Cardiovascular Society; NICE, National Institute of Health and Care Excellence.
[a] Guidelines from the American College of Cardiology Foundation, American Heart Association, American College of Physicians, American Association for Thoracic Surgery, Preventive Cardiovascular Nurses Association, Society for Cardiovascular Angiography, Society of Thoracic Surgeons.

30 months according to a recently published clinical trial.[22]

### Renin–angiotensin system inhibition

Angiotensin-converting enzyme (ACE) inhibitors reduce cardiovascular risk after MI regardless of the presence of left ventricular dysfunction (LVD).[23,24] In the HOPE study, 9297 individuals without heart failure (HF) but with history of MI, atherosclerotic disease or 2 or more risk factors, including diabetes, were randomly assigned to ramipril 10 mg/d or placebo.[23] After 5 years of follow-up, 14.4% of participants assigned to ramipril had an MI, stroke, or cardiovascular death compared with 17.8% in the control group (P<.001).

The ONTARGET study showed noninferiority of angiotensin-receptor blockade with telmisartan versus ACE inhibition with ramipril to prevent cardiovascular events among 25,620 individuals with atherosclerotic disease without HF.[25] After a median follow-up of 56 months, the risk for death from cardiovascular causes, MI, stroke, or hospitalization for HF among individuals assigned to ramipril or telmisartan was 16.5% and 16.7% (relative risk [RR], 1.01; 95% CI, 0.94–1.09), respectively. The RR associated with telmisartan monotherapy was statistically lower than the noninferiority boundary of 1.13 (P = .003) defined a

priori. In this study, combined therapy with telmisartan/ramipril was not superior to ramipril monotherapy (RR, 0.99; 95% CI, 0.92–1.07) and was associated with hypotensive symptoms, renal impairment, and hyperkalemia.

Current US guidelines recommend indefinite therapy with ACE inhibitors for individuals with CHD who have hypertension, diabetes, LVD (<40%), or stable chronic kidney disease and consider it reasonable for individuals with CHD and other vascular disease.[13,16] In contrast, UK and Canadian guidelines recommend ACE inhibition for all individuals with CHD.[14,15] Guidelines agree that angiotensin-receptor blockade should be offered to those with intolerance to ACE inhibitors.[13–15]

### β-Blocker therapy

β-Blockers have been a cornerstone in the management of individuals with CHD for decades. In the BHAT study, 3828 individuals with a recent MI (5–21 days after the event) were assigned randomly to propranolol or placebo.[26] After 25.1 months of follow-up, participants assigned to propranolol had a lower risk for all-cause mortality (7.2% vs 9.8%; P<.01), CHD mortality (6.2% vs 8.5%; P<.01), and sudden death (3.3% vs 4.6%; P<.05) compared with those who received placebo. Similar results were found in the Norwegian timolol study, in which β-blockade reduced the risk for sudden death (7.7% vs 13.9%, P<.001) and reinfarction (14.4% vs 20.1%; P<.001) versus placebo after 33 months of follow-up among 1884 individuals with a recent MI.[27]

Recent studies have questioned the role of β-blockers for secondary prevention in the era of revascularization and statin therapy. Bangalore and colleagues[28] conducted a metaanalysis of 60 randomized, controlled trials with more than 100 participants comparing β-blockers versus placebo, no treatment, or other active treatment among individuals with an MI. β-Blockers were associated with a lower risk for all-cause mortality (RR, 0.86; 95% CI, 0.79–0.94) in studies conducted in the pre-revascularization era (ie, studies with <50% of participants receiving revascularization or a combination of aspirin plus statins), but not in studies conducted in the revascularization era (RR, 0.98; 95% CI, 0.92–1.05). Although β-blockers were associated with a lower risk for recurrent MI in studies conducted in the revascularization era (RR, 0.72; 95% CI, 0.62–0.83), they were also associated with an increased risk for HF (RR 1.10; 95% CI, 1.05–1.16) and cardiogenic shock (RR, 1.29; 95% CI, 1.18–1.40).

In the CHARISMA study initiated in 2002, β-blocker users versus nonusers had lower risk for nonfatal MI, stroke, or cardiovascular death after propensity score adjustment when comparing individuals with a prior MI (7.1% vs 10.2%, respectively; HR, 0.69; 95% CI, 0.50–0.94) but not among those with atherosclerotic disease without MI (6.7% vs 6.2%; HR, 1.06; 95% CI, 0.82–1.38).[29] β-Blockade did not reduce all-cause mortality in either group.

Current guidelines recommend initiation of β-blockade within 24 hours in patients with ACS who do not have signs of acute HF or increased risk for cardiogenic shock or high-degree heart block.[16] β-Blockade is recommended to be continued for up to 3 years for individuals without LVD.[13] Among those with clinically stable LVD, β-blockade with carvedilol, metoprolol succinate, or bisoprolol is recommended to be continued indefinitely given its association with reduced mortality.[13,15]

### Statin therapy

Statin therapy after MI reduces major coronary events by 22% (95% CI, 16%–26%) per 1 mm/L (39 mg/dL) reduction in LDL-C.[30] Furthermore, data suggest that individuals with baseline low LDL-C benefit as well. In the Heart Protection Study, participants with a baseline LDL-C of less than 100 mg/dL who were randomly assigned to simvastatin 40 mg/d had a significantly lower risk

for nonfatal MI, CHD death, stroke, or revascularization compared with those who received placebo (16.4% vs 21.0%; P<.001).[31]

Several post–ATP-III clinical trials have shown that universal high-intensity statin therapy in secondary prevention is more effective than less intensive therapy, regardless of LDL-C levels.[32–34] In a meta-analysis using individual data from 5 clinical trials, participants assigned to high-intensity statin therapy had lower risk for nonfatal MI, stroke, coronary revascularization, or CHD death compared with those receiving less intensive therapy (4.5% vs 5.3% annually; RR, 0.85; 95% CI, 0.82–0.89).[35] The same association was observed among individuals with an LDL-C level of less than 77 mg/dL at baseline (4.6% vs 5.2% annual risk; RR, 0.71; 95% CI, 0.52–0.98).

Based on this evidence, the 2013 ACC/AHA treatment guidelines recommend high-intensity statin therapy (see definition in **Table 2**) after an MI for those under age 75 without contraindications, regardless of prior therapy or cholesterol levels at the time of the event.[36] For older individuals or those

**Table 2**
**High-, moderate- and low-intensity statins according to the 2013 ACC/AHA guideline on the treatment of blood cholesterol**

| Intensity | Generic Drug | Daily Dose (mg) |
|---|---|---|
| High-intensity (reduction in LDL-C ≥50% on average) | Atorvastatin | 40 or 80 |
| | Rosuvastatin | 20 or 40 |
| Moderate-intensity (reduction in LDL-C by ≥30% to <50% on average) | Atorvastatin | 10 or 20 |
| | Rosuvastatin | 5 or 10 |
| | Simvastatin | 20 or 40 |
| | Pravastatin | 40 or 80 |
| | Lovastatin | 40 |
| | Fluvastatin XL | 80 |
| | Fluvastatin | 40 twice a day |
| | Pitavastatin | 2 or 4 |
| Low-intensity (reduction in LDL-C by <30% on average) | Simvastatin | 10 |
| | Pravastatin | 10 or 20 |
| | Lovastatin | 20 |
| | Fluvastatin | 20 or 40 |
| | Pitavastatin | 1 |

Abbreviations: ACC, American College of Cardiology; AHA, American Heart Association; LDL-C, low-density lipoprotein cholesterol.

Data from Stone NJ, Robinson JG, Lichtenstein AH, et al. 2013 ACC/AHA guideline on the treatment of blood cholesterol to reduce atherosclerotic cardiovascular risk in adults: a report of the American College of Cardiology/American Heart Association Task Force on Practice Guidelines. Circulation 2014;129:S13.

with comorbidities preventing high-intensity statin therapy, moderate-intensity treatment is appropriate. According to the guidelines, it is reasonable to add a nonstatin lipid-lowering medication when recommended doses of statins cannot be achieved because of intolerance or if the reduction in LDL-C is less than expected (<50% or <30% vs untreated levels for high- and moderate-intensity therapy, respectively).

## Complications and Comorbidities

In addition to lifestyle changes and post-MI pharmacologic treatment, current guidelines emphasize investigation and treatment of complications and comorbidities that may increase cardiovascular risk, including coronary disease with indication for revascularization, diabetes, hypertension, LVD, HF, and chronic kidney disease.[13–16] In addition, US guidelines also recommend annual influenza and pneumococcal vaccination, and management of stress and depression.[13]

## MANAGING SERUM LIPIDS IN THE CONTEMPORARY ERA

Meta-analyses and subgroup analyses of individual statin trials suggest that individuals who achieve LDL-C levels well below 100 mg/dL have better outcomes than those who have higher on treatment LDL-C levels, giving rise to the notion that "lower is better."[35] Based on these results, addition of nonstatin lipid-lowering medications may be considered for individuals with a prior MI who are receiving appropriate statin therapy.

The IMPROVE-IT study presented in November 2014 at the AHA Scientific Sessions provides evidence to support the use of combined lipid-lowering therapy for secondary prevention.[37] In this study, 18,144 individuals with ACS and low LDL-C (≤125 mg/dL or ≤100 mg/dL if prior statin therapy; mean LDL-C, 95 mg/dL) were randomized to simvastatin/ezetimibe 40/10 mg/d or simvastatin 40 mg/d (with simvastatin uptitrated to 80 mg if required). After 7 years of follow-up, the simvastatin/ezetimibe group had a 2% absolute risk reduction (32.7% vs 34.7%, P = .02) in the primary endpoint of MI, unstable angina, coronary revascularization beyond 30 days, and stroke or cardiovascular death, corresponding with a number needed to treat of 50 participants to prevent 1 event. There were significant reductions in components of this endpoint, including MI, stroke, and combined MI, stroke, or cardiovascular death. However, there were no differences in all-cause or cardiovascular mortality.

Niacin and bile acid sequestrants are other lipid-lowering medications that can reduce LDL-C

modestly. Both niacin and bile acid sequestrants, separately or in combination, could be used among individuals with intolerance to statins.[13,36] However, there is limited evidence that adding these medications to recommended doses of statins reduces cardiovascular events.

Proprotein convertase subtilisin kexin type 9 (PCSK9) is a protein that downregulates LDL-C receptors in the liver and is responsible for maintaining serum LDL-C levels. Prior studies have shown that treatment with statin and ezetimibe increases the expression of PCSK9, which may reduce their effectiveness.[38] Recently developed PCSK9 inhibitors reduce LDL-C by about 40% to 70%.[39] These drugs could be used in the future among individuals with familial hypercholesterolemia or statin intolerance, or simply as an adjunct to statins. Several phase III trials are ongoing to assess the efficacy of PCSK9 inhibitors to reduce CHD risk (NCT01764633, NCT01975376, NCT01975389, NCT01663402).

## Other Lipid Targets

In addition to LDL-C, other lipid markers are associated with increased risk for recurrent events, including low high-density lipoprotein cholesterol (HDL-C) and high triglycerides.[40,41] Abnormal values for these lipid markers are common among individuals on statin therapy. For example, although 17.6% of patients with MI studied by Sachdeva and colleagues[5] had LDL-C of less than 70 mg/dL at the time of their hospitalization, only 1.4% had both LDL-C of less than 70 mg/dL and HDL-C of 60 mg/dL or higher. Importantly, on statin treatment levels of HDL-C and triglycerides were predictive of cardiovascular events in post hoc analyses of the TNT and PROVE IT-TIMI 22 studies, respectively.[42,43]

Older studies have suggested that fibrates can reduce coronary risk among those with low HDL-C or high triglycerides.[44] However, there are no trials to document incremental benefit from fibrates on statin background therapy. In particular, gemfibrozil use is not recommended in combination with statins because of increased risk for hepatotoxicity and rhabdomyolysis.[45] Two large trials (FIELD and ACCORD) failed to show a benefit of fenofibrate as monotherapy or when added to statins, respectively, among individuals with diabetes.[46,47]

Niacin also increases HDL-C and reduces triglycerides. However, 2 large clinical trials (AIM-HIGH and HPS2-THRIVE) failed to show a benefit when niacin was added to statin background therapy, including among individuals with low HDL-C.[48,49] Importantly, niacin therapy was

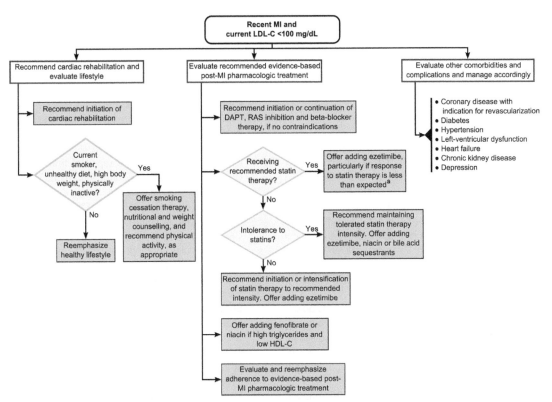

**Fig. 2.** Summary of evidence-based recommendations and guidelines for management of individuals with MI and LDL-C of less than 100 mg/dL. DAPT, dual antiplatelet therapy; HDL-C, high-density lipoprotein cholesterol; LDL-C, low-density lipoprotein cholesterol; MI, myocardial infarction; RAS, renin–angiotensin system. [a] Less than 50% or less than 30% versus untreated levels for high- and moderate-intensity statins, respectively.

associated with an increased risk for serious adverse events, including infections.[49,50]

Although trials have shown no effect of adding fibrate or niacin to statin background therapy overall, some subgroup analyses suggest that those with both low HDL-C and high triglycerides may have benefitted.[46,51] Prospective clinical trials are needed to confirm these findings.

Cholesteryl ester transfer protein (CETP) inhibitors substantially increase HDL-C while reducing LDL-C levels to varying degrees. Two outcomes studies with torcetrapib and dalcetrapib were stopped early because of increased risk for cardiovascular events and all-cause mortality or futility to show benefits for the primary outcome, respectively.[52,53] Trials with other CETP inhibitors are ongoing (NCT01252953, NCT01687998).

## SUMMARY

The 2013 ACC/AHA guideline on the treatment of blood cholesterol to reduce atherosclerotic cardiovascular risk in adults has introduced a new paradigm in the management of serum lipids among individuals with MI. All individuals less than 75 years of age with a prior MI are recommended to receive high-intensity statin therapy, regardless of LDL-C levels. A subsequent study suggests that ezetimibe could be considered as adjunctive therapy among individuals on statins. Efforts to further reduce CHD risk among those receiving high-intensity statin therapy with or without ezetimibe should focus on maintaining good adherence to their lipid-lowering regimen, attendance at cardiac rehabilitation, adoption of healthier lifestyles, use of evidence-based post-MI pharmacologic treatment, and achieving adequate control of concomitant cardiovascular risk factors such as hypertension or diabetes (**Fig. 2**).

The high "residual" risk for cardiovascular events among IMPROVE-IT participants on simvastatin/ezetimibe (32.7% after 7 years of follow-up), who had mean LDL-C, HDL-C, and triglycerides of 53, 49, and 126 mg/dL, respectively, suggests that much of this risk in contemporary post-ACS populations is mediated by factors other than dyslipidemia. Given the burden of atherosclerosis generally present at the time of an MI, even the best evidence-based therapy currently available is unlikely to completely eliminate this residual risk. Primordial and primary prevention hold the key to future population health. The recently outlined new paradigm of early atherosclerosis treatment to arrest the disease process should be tested in future trials.[54]

# REFERENCES

1. Go AS, Mozaffarian D, Roger VL, et al. Heart disease and stroke statistics–2014 update: a report from the American Heart Association. Circulation 2014;129:e28–292.

2. Expert Panel on Detection, Evaluation, and Treatment of High Blood Cholesterol in Adults. Executive summary of The Third Report of The National Cholesterol Education Program (NCEP) Expert Panel on Detection, Evaluation, and Treatment of High Blood Cholesterol in Adults (Adult Treatment Panel III). JAMA 2001;285:2486–97.

3. Smith SC Jr, Allen J, Blair SN, et al. AHA/ACC guidelines for secondary prevention for patients with coronary and other atherosclerotic vascular disease: 2006 update: endorsed by the National Heart, Lung, and Blood Institute. Circulation 2006;113:2363–72.

4. Carroll MD, Lacher DA, Sorlie PD, et al. Trends in serum lipids and lipoproteins of adults, 1960-2002. JAMA 2005;294:1773–81.

5. Sachdeva A, Cannon CP, Deedwania PC, et al. Lipid levels in patients hospitalized with coronary artery disease: an analysis of 136,905 hospitalizations in get with the guidelines. Am Heart J 2009;157:111–7.e2.

6. Steg PG, Bhatt DL, Wilson PW, et al. One-year cardiovascular event rates in outpatients with atherothrombosis. JAMA 2007;297:1197–206.

7. D'Agostino RB, Russell MW, Huse DM, et al. Primary and subsequent coronary risk appraisal: new results from the Framingham study. Am Heart J 2000;139:272–81.

8. Roe MT, Chen AY, Thomas L, et al. Predicting long-term mortality in older patients after non-ST-segment elevation myocardial infarction: the CRUSADE long-term mortality model and risk score. Am Heart J 2011;162:875–83.e1.

9. Fox KA, Dabbous OH, Goldberg RJ, et al. Prediction of risk of death and myocardial infarction in the six months after presentation with acute coronary syndrome: prospective multinational observational study (GRACE). BMJ 2006;333:1091.

10. Arnold SV, Spertus JA, Masoudi FA, et al. Beyond medication prescription as performance measures: optimal secondary prevention medication dosing after acute myocardial infarction. J Am Coll Cardiol 2013;62:1791–801.

11. Olomu AB, Stommel M, Holmes-Rovner MM, et al. Is quality improvement sustainable? Findings of the American College of Cardiology's Guidelines Applied in Practice. Int J Qual Health Care 2014;26:215–22.

12. Rosenson RS, Kent ST, Brown TM, et al. Underutilization of high intensity statin therapy following hospitalization for coronary heart disease. J Am Coll Cardiol 2015;65(3):270–7.

13. Fihn SD, Gardin JM, Abrams J, et al. 2012 ACCF/AHA/ACP/AATS/PCNA/SCAI/STS Guideline for the diagnosis and management of patients with stable ischemic heart disease: a report of the American College of Cardiology Foundation/American Heart Association Task Force on Practice Guidelines, and the American College of Physicians, American Association for Thoracic Surgery, Preventive Cardiovascular Nurses Association, Society for Cardiovascular Angiography and Interventions, and Society of Thoracic Surgeons. J Am Coll Cardiol 2012;60:e44–164.

14. National Institute for Health and Care Excellence. Secondary prevention in primary and secondary care for patients following a myocardial infarction. Clinical guideline 172. London: National Institute for Health and Care Excellence (NICE); 2013. Available at: http://www.gserve.nice.org.uk/ourguidance/reference.jsp?textonly=true.

15. Mancini GB, Gosselin G, Chow B, et al. Canadian Cardiovascular Society guidelines for the diagnosis and management of stable ischemic heart disease. Can J Cardiol 2014;30:837–49.

16. Amsterdam EA, Wenger NK, Brindis RG, et al. 2014 AHA/ACC guideline for the management of patients with non-ST-elevation acute coronary syndromes: A report of the American College of Cardiology/American Heart Association Task Force on Practice Guidelines. J Am Coll Cardiol 2014;64(24):e139–228.

17. Lawler PR, Filion KB, Eisenberg MJ. Efficacy of exercise-based cardiac rehabilitation post-myocardial infarction: a systematic review and meta-analysis of randomized controlled trials. Am Heart J 2011;162:571–84.e2.

18. Shah ND, Dunlay SM, Ting HH, et al. Long-term medication adherence after myocardial infarction: experience of a community. Am J Med 2009;122:961.e7–13.

19. Antithrombotic Trialists' Collaboration. Collaborative meta-analysis of randomised trials of antiplatelet therapy for prevention of death, myocardial infarction, and stroke in high risk patients. BMJ 2002;324:71–86.

20. Helton TJ, Bavry AA, Kumbhani DJ, et al. Incremental effect of clopidogrel on important outcomes in patients with cardiovascular disease: a meta-analysis of randomized trials. Am J Cardiovasc Drugs 2007;7:289–97.

21. Wallentin L, Becker RC, Budaj A, et al. Ticagrelor versus clopidogrel in patients with acute coronary syndromes. N Engl J Med 2009;361:1045–57.

22. Mauri L, Kereiakes DJ, Yeh RW, et al. Twelve or 30 months of dual antiplatelet therapy after drug-eluting stents. N Engl J Med 2014;371(23): 2155–66.

23. Yusuf S, Sleight P, Pogue J, et al. Effects of an angiotensin-converting-enzyme inhibitor, ramipril, on cardiovascular events in high-risk patients. The Heart Outcomes Prevention Evaluation Study Investigators. N Engl J Med 2000;342:145–53.

24. Fox KM. Efficacy of perindopril in reduction of cardiovascular events among patients with stable coronary artery disease: randomised, double-blind, placebo-controlled, multicentre trial (the EUROPA study). Lancet 2003;362:782–8.

25. Yusuf S, Teo KK, Pogue J, et al. Telmisartan, ramipril, or both in patients at high risk for vascular events. N Engl J Med 2008;358:1547–59.

26. A randomized trial of propranolol in patients with acute myocardial infarction. I. Mortality results. JAMA 1982;247:1707–14.

27. Timolol-induced reduction in mortality and reinfarction in patients surviving acute myocardial infarction. N Engl J Med 1981;304:801–7.

28. Bangalore S, Makani H, Radford M, et al. Clinical outcomes with beta-blockers for myocardial infarction: a meta-analysis of randomized trials. Am J Med 2014;127:939–53.

29. Bangalore S, Bhatt DL, Steg PG, et al. β-Blockers and cardiovascular events in patients with and without myocardial infarction: post hoc analysis from the CHARISMA trial. Circ Cardiovasc Qual Outcomes 2014;7(6):872–81.

30. Baigent C, Keech A, Kearney PM, et al. Efficacy and safety of cholesterol-lowering treatment: prospective meta-analysis of data from 90,056 participants in 14 randomised trials of statins. Lancet 2005;366:1267–78.

31. Heart Protection Study Collaborative Group. MRC/BHF Heart Protection Study of cholesterol lowering with simvastatin in 20,536 high-risk individuals: a randomised placebo-controlled trial. Lancet 2002; 360:7–22.

32. Cannon CP, Braunwald E, McCabe CH, et al. Intensive versus moderate lipid lowering with statins after acute coronary syndromes. N Engl J Med 2004;350: 1495–504.

33. Pedersen TR, Faergeman O, Kastelein JJ, et al. High-dose atorvastatin vs usual-dose simvastatin for secondary prevention after myocardial infarction: the IDEAL study: a randomized controlled trial. JAMA 2005;294:2437–45.

34. LaRosa JC, Grundy SM, Waters DD, et al. Intensive lipid lowering with atorvastatin in patients with stable coronary disease. N Engl J Med 2005;352: 1425–35.

35. Baigent C, Blackwell L, Emberson J, et al. Efficacy and safety of more intensive lowering of LDL cholesterol: a meta-analysis of data from 170,000 participants in 26 randomised trials. Lancet 2010;376:1670–81.

36. Stone NJ, Robinson JG, Lichtenstein AH, et al. 2013 ACC/AHA guideline on the treatment of blood cholesterol to reduce atherosclerotic cardiovascular risk in adults: a report of the American College of Cardiology/American Heart Association Task Force on Practice Guidelines. Circulation 2014; 129:S1–45.

37. IMPROVE-IT: Ezetimibe/simvastatin vs simvastatin monotherapy on CV outcomes after ACS. Cardiosource, American College of Cardiology, 2014. Available at: http://www.cardiosource.org/news-media/publications/cardiology-magazine/2014/11/improve-it-ezetimibe-simvastatin-vs-simvastatin-monotherapy-on-cv-outcomes-after-acs.aspx?WT.mc_id=Twitter. Accessed November 18, 2014.

38. Gouni-Berthold I, Berthold HK, Gylling H, et al. Effects of ezetimibe and/or simvastatin on LDL receptor protein expression and on LDL receptor and HMG-CoA reductase gene expression: a randomized trial in healthy men. Atherosclerosis 2008; 198:198–207.

39. Hochholzer W, Giugliano RP. Does it make sense to combine statins with other lipid-altering agents following AIM-HIGH, SHARP and ACCORD? Curr Atheroscler Rep 2013;15:290.

40. Nguyen SV, Nakamura T, Kugiyama K. High remnant lipoprotein predicts recurrent cardiovascular events on statin treatment after acute coronary syndrome. Circ J 2014;78:2492–500.

41. Sirimarco G, Labreuche J, Bruckert E, et al. Atherogenic dyslipidemia and residual cardiovascular risk in statin-treated patients. Stroke 2014;45:1429–36.

42. Barter P, Gotto AM, LaRosa JC, et al. HDL cholesterol, very low levels of LDL cholesterol, and cardiovascular events. N Engl J Med 2007;357:1301–10.

43. Miller M, Cannon CP, Murphy SA, et al. Impact of triglyceride levels beyond low-density lipoprotein cholesterol after acute coronary syndrome in the PROVE IT-TIMI 22 trial. J Am Coll Cardiol 2008;51: 724–30.

44. Jun M, Foote C, Lv J, et al. Effects of fibrates on cardiovascular outcomes: a systematic review and meta-analysis. Lancet 2010;375:1875–84.

45. Graham DJ, Staffa JA, Shatin D, et al. Incidence of hospitalized rhabdomyolysis in patients treated with lipid-lowering drugs. JAMA 2004;292:2585–90.

46. Ginsberg HN, Elam MB, Lovato LC, et al. Effects of combination lipid therapy in type 2 diabetes mellitus. N Engl J Med 2010;362:1563–74.

47. Tonkin A, Hunt D, Voysey M, et al. Effects of fenofibrate on cardiovascular events in patients with diabetes, with and without prior cardiovascular disease: the Fenofibrate Intervention and Event Lowering in Diabetes (FIELD) study. Am Heart J 2012;163:508–14.

48. Boden WE, Probstfield JL, Anderson T, et al. Niacin in patients with low HDL cholesterol levels receiving intensive statin therapy. N Engl J Med 2011;365: 2255–67.

49. Landray MJ, Haynes R, Hopewell JC, et al. Effects of extended-release niacin with laropiprant in high-risk patients. N Engl J Med 2014;371:203–12.

50. Anderson TJ, Boden WE, Desvigne-Nickens P, et al. Safety profile of extended-release niacin in the AIM-HIGH trial. N Engl J Med 2014;371:288–90.

51. Guyton JR, Slee AE, Anderson T, et al. Relationship of lipoproteins to cardiovascular events: the AIM-HIGH Trial (Atherothrombosis Intervention in Metabolic Syndrome With Low HDL/High Triglycerides and Impact on Global Health Outcomes). J Am Coll Cardiol 2013;62:1580–4.

52. Barter PJ, Caulfield M, Eriksson M, et al. Effects of torcetrapib in patients at high risk for coronary events. N Engl J Med 2007;357:2109–22.

53. Schwartz GG, Olsson AG, Abt M, et al. Effects of dalcetrapib in patients with a recent acute coronary syndrome. N Engl J Med 2012;367:2089–99.

54. Robinson JG, Gidding SS. Curing atherosclerosis should be the next major cardiovascular prevention goal. J Am Coll Cardiol 2014;63:2779–85.

55. Mora S, Wenger NK, Demicco DA, et al. Determinants of residual risk in secondary prevention patients treated with high- versus low-dose statin therapy: the Treating to New Targets (TNT) study. Circulation 2012;125:1979–87.

56. Buckley BS, Simpson CR, McLernon DJ, et al. Five year prognosis in patients with angina identified in primary care: incident cohort study. BMJ 2009;339: b3058.

57. Weiner DE, Tighiouart H, Stark PC, et al. Kidney disease as a risk factor for recurrent cardiovascular disease and mortality. Am J Kidney Dis 2004;44: 198–206.

58. Davidson KW, Burg MM, Kronish IM, et al. Association of anhedonia with recurrent major adverse cardiac events and mortality 1 year after acute coronary syndrome. Arch Gen Psychiatry 2010;67: 480–8.

59. Denollet J, Pedersen SS, Vrints CJ, et al. Usefulness of type D personality in predicting five-year cardiac events above and beyond concurrent symptoms of stress in patients with coronary heart disease. Am J Cardiol 2006;97:970–3.

60. Rosengren A, Hawken S, Ounpuu S, et al. Association of psychosocial risk factors with risk of acute myocardial infarction in 11119 cases and 13648 controls from 52 countries (the INTERHEART study): case-control study. Lancet 2004;364:953–62.

61. Ye S, Muntner P, Shimbo D, et al. Behavioral mechanisms, elevated depressive symptoms, and the risk for myocardial infarction or death in individuals with coronary heart disease: the REGARDS (Reason for Geographic and Racial Differences in Stroke) study. J Am Coll Cardiol 2013;61:622–30.

# Management of Hypertriglyceridemia for Prevention of Atherosclerotic Cardiovascular Disease

Eliot A. Brinton, MD, FAHA, FNLA

## KEYWORDS

- Hypertriglyceridemia • Atherosclerosis • Cardiovascular disease • Triglycerides

## KEY POINTS

- Mendelian randomization data strongly suggest that hypertriglyceridemia (HTG) causes atherosclerotic cardiovascular disease (ASCVD), and so triglyceride (TG) level–lowering treatment in HTG is now more strongly recommended to address the residual ASCVD risk than has been the case in (generally earlier) published guidelines.
- Fibrates are the best-established agents for TG level lowering and are generally used as first-line treatment of TG levels greater than 500 mg/dL.
- In addition to better ASCVD evidence, potential advantages of omega-3 compared with fenofibrate include that it is a natural product, it lacks any associated myopathy, and it might provide antiinflammatory, mood, cognitive, or other benefits.
- Statins are the best-established agents for ASCVD prevention, and so are usually used as first-line treatment of TG levels less than 500 mg/dL.

## EPIDEMIOLOGY AND PATHOPHYSIOLOGY OF HYPERTRIGLYCERIDEMIA

About 40 million US adults have hypertriglyceridemia (HTG), defined as a fasting triglyceride (TG) level more than 200 mg/dL. Of these, about 36 million have a TG level of 200 to 500 mg/dL and about 4 million have a TG level greater than 500 mg/dL.[1] Thus, moderate HTG is common, and very high TG level (>500 mg/dL) is more common than numerically similar cholesterol level increases. Further, the prevalence of HTG has increased several-fold over the past few decades.[2,3] This increase is coincident with, and most likely largely driven by, increasing obesity.[4] Although there is some controversy regarding categorization of HTG, most categories have a reasonable consensus, as noted in **Table 1**.

Increase of plasma TG level is related to an excess of one or more of the 3 main types of TG-rich lipoproteins: (1) chylomicrons, (2) very-low-density lipoprotein (VLDL), or (3) intermediate-density lipoprotein (IDL). In the case of chylomicronemia, TG levels usually exceed about 800 mg/dL and may be 10,000 mg/dL or higher.[5] The underlying cause is decreased lipolysis of TG in plasma caused by decreased (or absent) activity of lipoprotein lipase (LPL) in the vascular endothelium. Decreased TG lipolysis also tends to increase the TG content of VLDL and all other TG-rich lipoproteins, but decreased lipolysis has the greatest effect on chylomicrons because they have the greatest TG content. Because the TG/cholesterol ratio in chylomicrons is generally about 10:1, the plasma TG level is usually close to 10-fold higher than the plasma cholesterol level. Nevertheless, the total cholesterol level can

Atherometabolic Research, Utah Foundation for Biomedical Research, 419 Wakara Way, Suite 211, Salt Lake City, UT 84108, USA

*E-mail address:* eliot.brinton@utah.edu

Cardiol Clin 33 (2015) 309–323
http://dx.doi.org/10.1016/j.ccl.2015.02.007
0733-8651/15/$ – see front matter

**Table 1**
**Categorization of HTG**

| TG Range (mg/dL) | NCEP ATP-III 2004[1] | AHA Statement 2011[2] | Disease Risk | FDA Approval |
|---|---|---|---|---|
| <100 | Desirable | Optimal | None | No apparent interest |
| <150 | | Normal | Dyslipidemia | |
| 150–199 | Borderline high | Borderline | More dyslipidemia | |
| 200–499 | High | High | ↑CVD | Approve if ↓CVD likely |
| ≥500 | Very high | Very high | ↑CVD and ↑pancreatitis (especially ↑if >2000 mg/dL) | Approve if reasonable safety |

*Abbreviations:* AHA, American Heart Association; CVD, cardiovascular disease; FDA, US Food and Drug Administration; NCEP ATP-III, Third Adult Treatment Panel of the National Cholesterol Education Program.

far exceed 200 mg/dL in severe chylomicronemia, and so clinicians must always remember to look for severe HTG as a possible hidden cause of hypercholesterolemia.[6] Familial chylomicronemia classically is caused by homozygous deficiency of LPL but is more commonly caused by a combination of other genetic factors, such as absence or severe functional defects in the function of LPL-related factors, such as apolipoproteins C-II, C-III, and V; lipase maturation factor-1; and angiopoietinlike proteins 3, 4, and 8.[5,7] Environmental factors such as central obesity, insulin resistance, and diabetes mellitus can also play important contributory roles in decreasing LPL activity sufficient to cause chylomicronemia, with or without identifiable genetic abnormalities.[5]

In increased VLDL levels, by far the most common type of moderate HTG, the primary cause seems to be hepatic overproduction of VLDL. Two terms for increased VLDL levels are found in the scientific literature but do not seem to be clinically useful. Familial combined hyperlipoproteinemia (FCHL) is a term that has been used for moderate HTG presenting with or without increased cholesterol levels (or even as high cholesterol with normal TG), depending on environmental factors.[8] Familial HTG (FHTG) has been said always to present without hypercholesterolemia and to carry no increased risk of atherosclerotic cardiovascular disease (ASCVD),[9] whereas FCHL was said to increase ASCVD considerably.[8] However, subsequent research has not clearly sustained the original proposed distinctions between FCHL and FHTG, so there is little clinical impetus at present for distinguishing between them. A family history of ASCVD and the presence of hypercholesterolemia added to hypertriglyceridemia increase ASCVD risk, but pure HTG also carries excess risk, even in the absence of a clearly positive family history. Thus, efforts to make the distinction between FCHL and FHTG are probably not clinically beneficial, and treatment should

instead be directed according to lipid levels and other standard risk factors.

Increased IDL levels seem to be caused primarily by reduced hepatic clearance of IDL particles caused by impaired binding to the apolipoprotein (apo) B/E receptor. Although IDL levels should be increased with any loss of apo B/E receptor activity, such as familial hypercholesterolemia (which primarily involves decreased low-density lipoprotein [LDL] clearance), in some cases IDL clearance is selectively impaired. This condition is familial dysbetalipoproteinemia (sometimes referred to as type III disease), which is well documented to carry a high risk of ASCVD, beyond that expected from the moderately increased plasma TG levels.[10] It has been thought that dysbetalipoproteinemia is rare, occurring in only 1 in 10,000 in the general population and it has also been thought to require apo E2 homozygosity plus another, as yet unspecified metabolic defect.[10] However, recent studies have shown that apo E2 homozygosity is present only in a small minority of cases and that familial dysbetalipoproteinemia may affect as many as 1 in 200 of the general population.[11,12] However, it is difficult to diagnose dysbetalipoproteinemia. Suspicion of the existence of this disorder should be increased in the presence of roughly equally increased TG and TG levels, both within the range of 150 to 500 mg/dL, in an adult man or postmenopausal woman (uncommon in other demographics), especially if an ASCVD event has already occurred. Presence of palmar xanthomas (orange-yellow color in the palmar creases) is pathognomonic but often absent. The diagnoses can be made by one of several special tests: (1) confirming VLDL cholesterol (VLDL-C) enrichment (documented as a VLDL-C/plasma TG ratio >0.3 by beta-quantification), (2) a broad beta band on lipoprotein electrophoresis, (3) increased IDL levels by density gradient ultracentrifugation or nuclear magnetic resonance, or (4) an increased remnant lipoprotein cholesterol level by direct assay.[11,12]

## HYPERTRIGLYCERIDEMIA VERSUS ATHEROSCLEROTIC CARDIOVASCULAR DISEASE: ASSOCIATION AND POTENTIAL CAUSATION

Atherosclerosis is characterized by an accumulation of cholesterol in the artery wall, whereas TG does not accumulate. Further, the relationship between HTG and ASCVD is greatly diminished, and in some settings eliminated, by adjustment for other dyslipidemias (especially low high-density lipoprotein cholesterol [HDL-C] level and increased non–HDL-C level).[13] These two facts are often taken to imply that there is no meaningful causal association between HTG and ASCVD and that patients with HTG need no special consideration in management of ASCVD risk. However, results from many recent studies contain many types of data pointing to a strong and likely causal association. In general populations, TG levels are strong predictors of ASCVD risk. For example, one study found a 32% and 76% increased risk of cardiovascular disease (CVD) in men and women, respectively, for each 88-mg/dL increase in TG independent of HDL-C levels.[14] A large meta-analysis of 29 studies with 262,525 subjects found that HTG related to a 72% increase in CVD risk, even after correction for HDL-C.[15] Further, a more recent and even larger meta-analysis (330,566 subjects in 61 studies) reported a 22% increase in ASCVD for every 88-mg/dL increase in TG.[16] Other data show a curvilinear increase in risk across a range of TG level increases, above a TG level of 200 mg/dL and becoming especially pronounced above 500 mg/dL (**Fig. 1**).[10] Of greater clinical

relevance, HTG predicts residual ASCVD risk in the setting of aggressive statin-based low-density lipoprotein cholesterol (LDL-C) level lowering,[17–19] even with just mild HTG (>150 mg/dL) and even after aggressive statin therapy achieving an LDL-C level of less than 70 mg/dL (**Fig. 2**).[18]

### Mechanisms of Accelerated Atherogenesis in Hypertriglyceridemia

First, and most directly, LPL expression by arterial endothelium and artery wall macrophages lipolyze TG from TG-rich lipoproteins, producing free-fatty-acids (FFAs) both on the surface and inside the artery wall. These are proinflammatory, proatherogenic, and procoagulant.[20] (see also Ref.[21]) Second, several types of TG-rich lipoproteins are directly atherogenic[22,23] and their presence in excess is most readily signaled by high plasma TG levels. These atherogenic TG-rich lipoproteins are generally called remnants because they have had their TG content reduced by lipolysis by LPL in the plasma compartment. In addition, they lose some TG and become cholesterol enriched by action of cholesteryl-ester transfer protein (CETP), as noted later. One proatherogenic effect of these remnants is that they cause senescence of endothelial precursor cells, which lose their ability to maintain vascular endothelial integrity.[24] Also, remnants stimulate a key early step in atherogenesis by promoting their uptake by artery wall macrophages, which then become foam cells.[25] The increased atherogenicity seen with remnants is thought to operate especially during the postprandial period (during which chylomicrons and also VLDL undergo rapid TG lipolysis), which is associated with increases in endothelial microparticles (which are atherogenic),[26] in inflammatory

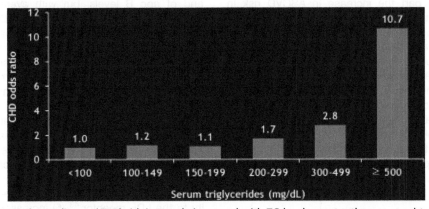

**Fig. 1.** Coronary heart disease (CHD) risk is greatly increased with TG levels greater than or equal to 500 mg/dL. TG is associated with premature familiar CHD independent of HDL-C. TG odds ratio adjusted for HDL-C; n = 653. N = 1029 controls. (*Adapted from* Hopkins PN, Wu LL, Hunt SC, et al. Plasma triglycerides and type III hyperlipidemia are independently associated with premature familial coronary artery disease. J Am Coll Cardiol 2005;45(7):1003–12; with permission.)

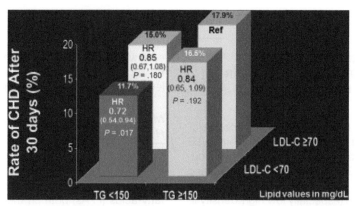

**Fig. 2.** TG level greater than 150 mg/DL increases CHD risk even when LDL-C level is less than 70 mg/DL on a statin (Pravastatin or Atorvastatin Evaluation and Infection Therapy—Thrombolysis in Myocardial Infarction 22 [PROVE IT-TIMI 22] PROVE IT-TIMI 22 subanalysis). CHD = death, myocardial infarction, and recurrent acute coronary syndrome. HR, hazard ratio. (*Adapted from* Miller M, Cannon CP, Murphy SA, et al. Impact of triglyceride levels beyond low-density lipoprotein cholesterol after acute coronary syndrome in the PROVE IT-TIMI 22 trial. J Am Coll Cardiol 2008;51(7):724–30; with permission.)

cytokines (also atherogenic),[27] and in apoptosis of artery wall cells (reflecting and possibly contributing to atherogenesis[28]; see also Ref.[21] for review). Importantly, the association of plasma apolipoprotein B48 levels (reflecting postprandial lipoproteins) with the presence of carotid plaque in diabetes mellitus type 2 (DM2),[29] and the strong and graded association between nonfasting TG levels and increasing ASCVD risk,[30] constitute epidemiologic data strongly supportive of the basic-science evidence for postprandial atherogenesis noted earlier.

In addition, apo C-III, which is associated with HTG by inhibiting LPL activity, also seems to be directly atherogenic by means of proinflammatory effects of activation of vascular endothelial binding to inflammatory cells,[31] and other mechanisms. (see Ref.[32] for review) Apo C-III production seems to be increased by hyperglycemia,[33] possibly explaining in part the increase in ASCVD risk in poorly controlled DM2.

The atherogenicity of lipoprotein remnants (which are rich in both TG and cholesterol) is most clearly seen in the classic disorder of remnant excess, best termed dysbetalipoproteinemia, in which both plasma TG and cholesterol levels are increased comparably, and the risk of ASCVD is very increased (see Ref.[12] for a recent review). Cholesterol enrichment of TG-rich lipoprotein remnants (and thus enhancement of their atherogenicity) also is promoted in most other HTG states, as noted later, although apparently to a lesser degree.

### The Atherogenic Dyslipidemia

Another important mechanism linking HTG and ASCVD risk is the effect of HTG on lipoproteins beyond those rich in TG. Core-lipid exchange

among major lipoproteins is facilitated by CETP, which moves TG from TG-rich lipoproteins (VLDL, chylomicrons, and chylomicron remnants) to TG-poor lipoproteins (principally LDL and high-density lipoprotein [HDL]). CETP also mediates movement of cholesteryl-ester (CE) in the opposite direction. Movement of CE promotes cholesterol enrichment of remnants, which, as discussed earlier, seems to account for much of their atherogenicity (**Fig. 3**).

The core-lipid exchange process leads to TG enrichment of LDL and HDL. Because of rapid subsequent lipolysis of TG from these lipoproteins, primarily by hepatic lipase, the net effect of this TG transfer is decreased size and increased density of LDL and HDL (see **Fig. 3**).[6,34] The presence of smaller, denser (SD) LDL particles is often accompanied by increased plasma levels of non–HDL-C and of apo B levels, but with average to low LDL-C levels. Counterintuitively, SD LDL particles seem to be more atherogenic per particle than normal-sized LDL, and an excess of SD LDL is associated with increased ASCVD risk.[35–38] The increased atherogenicity seems to result from several mechanisms: (1) increased transport into the subendothelial space (because of smaller size),[39,40] (2) increased binding to arterial proteoglycans (perhaps caused by decreased sialic acid content),[41] (3) increased susceptibility to oxidative modification (perhaps caused by decreased vitamin E content),[42] (4) prolonged plasma residence time caused by decreased affinity to the LDL receptor,[43] (5) increased glycation even in the absence of diabetes mellitus,[44] and (6) an increased tendency to carry atherogenic apoproteins (such as apo C-III).[45] Meanwhile, the presence of SD HDL particles is associated with

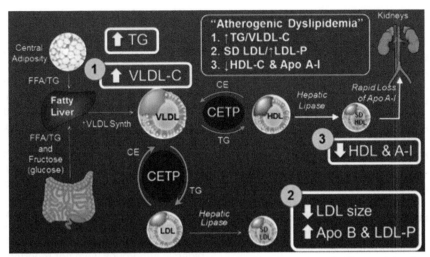

**Fig. 3.** Causes and atherogenic consequences of hypertriglyceridemia. Apo A-I, apolipoprotein A-I; Apo B, apolipoprotein B; CETP, cholesteryl-ster transfer protein; LDL-P, LDL particle concentration; SD, small, dense. (*Adapted from* Ginsberg HN. Insulin resistance and cardiovascular disease. J Clin Invest 2000;106(4):453–8.)

accelerated renal clearance of apo A-I (lost from HDL as it shrinks) and lower apo A-I levels,[46,47] likely diminishing the overall antiatherogenic function of HDL (see **Fig. 3**).

These 3 HTG-related lipoprotein changes (cholesterol enrichment of TG lipoproteins, SD LDL/increased non–HDL-C and apo B level, and low HDL-C level), constitute the atherogenic dyslipidemia characteristic of most patients with HTG, and can occur even at mildly increased TG levels. Also, it tends to be more pronounced in DM2 and other insulin-resistant states. This dyslipidemia responds poorly to statins and predicts much of the residual ASCVD risk seen with statin monotherapy in patients with HTG, whether the HTG is related to metabolic syndrome[48] or DM2.[19]

### Genetic Evidence for a Causal Role of Hypertriglyceridemia in Atherosclerotic Cardiovascular Disease

Concordant with the mechanisms discussed earlier linking HTG with increased atherosclerosis and ASCVD, mendelian randomization studies have recently provided strong evidence that the relationship between TG levels and ASCVD risk is causal. That is, several gene defects associated with moderate HTG are strongly associated with ASCVD.[49,50]

## EFFECTS OF TRIGLYCERIDE LEVEL–LOWERING MEDICATIONS ON ATHEROSCLEROTIC CARDIOVASCULAR DISEASE EVENTS: RANDOMIZED CLINICAL TRIALS

Although nearly all medication classes indicated and used for dyslipidemia reduce plasma TG levels (with the notable exception of the bile-acid sequestrants), only fibrates, niacin, and omega-3 are considered to be TG level–lowering drugs. The degree and mechanisms of lipid effects of these agents are of clinical importance, but have been reviewed elsewhere for fibrates,[51] niacin,[52] and omega-3[53] and so are not discussed in this article. Instead, this article reviews a clinically more important issue: their overall risk/benefit ratio (primarily regarding evidence for their ability to reduce the risk of ASCVD events) and the application of those data with regard to priority for clinical use.

Although niacin and omega-3 are available as dietary supplements as well as by prescription, this article focuses on the prescription formulations. This focus is because only prescription products are specifically formulated, reviewed, and regulated for the treatment of disease, and also because randomized clinical trial (RCT) data regarding ASCVD events for these agents are available primarily for the prescription versions.

### Randomized Clinical Trials of Fenofibrate

The most recent and most impactful fenofibrate trial is the Action to Control Cardiovascular Risk in Diabetes (ACCORD) trial of cardiovascular disease (ASCVD) effects of intensive glucose level–lowering treatment in patients with DM2, which included a major substudy called ACCORD-Lipid, which was recruited primarily for patients lacking extreme lipid levels.[54] All patients in ACCORD-Lipid were treated with open-label simvastatin then randomized to receive fenofibrate or matching placebo, on which they were followed for several years for ASCVD incidence. There was a modest trend toward an 8% decrease in ASCVD events with fenofibrate but this was far from being statistically significant.[54] However, there was an ASCVD benefit (statistically significant with an interaction $P$ value of .0567) in a prespecified subanalysis of subjects with both HTG (TG level >204 mg/dL) and low HDL-C level (<34 mg/dL) at baseline.[54,55] These same patients had substantially higher ASCVD risk than the others, compared within the placebo arm.[54,55] Thus, although ACCORD-Lipid had only a modest trend to benefit overall, it showed significant ASCVD risk reduction with fenofibrate in patients with the usual lipid indications for that agent. Further, the tolerability and safety of fenofibrate with a statin was excellent and there was no increase in myopathy or reported muscle symptoms,[54] despite a current US Food and Drug Administration (FDA) label warning against increased myopathy risk when fenofibrate is used with statins.

In addition to this finding in ACCORD-Lipid, other major RCTs of fibrates have shown a similar pattern of greater ASCVD benefit in patients with HTG and low HDL-C levels. The primary example is the Fenofibrate Intervention and Event Lowering in Diabetes (FIELD) trial, the only other major trial of fenofibrate effects on ASCVD.[56] As in ACCORD-Lipid, all patients had DM2 and there was little selection for dyslipidemia at baseline. All patients were randomized to receive fenofibrate or matching placebo, but in this study (conducted much sooner after initial availability of statins than was ACCORD) statins were not offered as a part of the study protocol. Nevertheless, statin drop-in therapy occurred, imbalanced in that 17% of placebo-treated subjects but only 8% of fenofibrate-treated subjects ($P<.0001$) received this incidental statin use, presumably because the primary care physicians were not blinded to lipid levels during the average 5-year study duration. Similar to ACCORD, there was a nonsignificant 11% trend toward decreased ASCVD among all fenofibrate-treated versus placebo-treated subjects.[56] In addition, similar to ACCORD-Lipid, in patients with HTG and low HDL-C levels there was both a much higher ASCVD risk, untreated, and also a statistically significant decrease in ASCVD with fenofibrate (which erased the excess risk).[57]

Note that this greater ASCVD benefit with fenofibrate in patients with HTG/low HDL-C levels has also been seen in the other major ASCVD trials with fibrates (bezafibrate and gemfibrozil).[58] Thus, fibrates in general and fenofibrate in particular seem to decrease risk of ASCVD events in patients with HTG, especially if they have the usual concomitant low HDL-C levels.

## Randomized Clinical Trials of Omega-3

Several recent RCTs of prescription ethyl ester omega-3 oil have focused on ASCVD effects, but they used different doses of different agents and found divergent results. The more recent trials used either a prescription formulation of an 85% pure mixture of eicosapentaenoic acid (EPA) with docosahexaenoic acid (DHA), or a comparable nonprescription formulation. One of these was the Risk and Prevention Trial, in which 12,505 subjects were selected for high risk for ASCVD (visible coronary artery disease and/or multiple risk factors) but not selected for HTG or low HDL-C level.[59] The intervention was low-dose (1 g/d) prescription EPA plus DHA (vs 1 g/d olive oil placebo) and there was no ASCVD benefit. Data from dyslipidemic subgroups were not reported.

A similar recent omega-3 trial was Outcome Reduction with Initial Glargine Intervention (ORIGIN), in which 12,536 patients considered to have prediabetes or recent-onset diabetes were randomized to receive the same low dose (1 g/d) of the same prescription EPA plus DHA fish oil as in the Risk and Prevention Trial versus placebo (along with insulin vs control in a 2 × 2 factorial design).[60] No decrease in ASCVD was noted with omega-3 (and no effect of insulin, or interaction between them) but again subjects were not selected for HTG or other dyslipidemia, and dyslipidemic subgroups were not reported.[60] Surprisingly, both the Risk and Prevention Trial and ORIGIN tended to show decreases in TG levels, despite only using very low doses of EPA plus DHA in patients without HTG. The primary focus of these studies and their most robust finding was the lack of ASCVD benefit from low-dose prescription EPA plus DHA.

Another, smaller RCT of omega-3 treatment (N = 4203) focused primarily on prevention of retinal disease but also tracked ASCVD events. It used a nonprescription formulation of EPA plus DHA similar to that used in the ORIGIN and Risk and Prevention Trial and at a comparable dose (in a 2 × 2 factorial design with xanthophylls), and also found no ASCVD benefit.[61]

The earliest of the contemporary ASCVD end point trials of omega-3 was the Japan EPA Lipid Intervention Study (JELIS).[62] In contrast with the others, JELIS studied a higher total dose (1.8 g/d) of omega-3 and used a pure EPA product (icosapent ethyl), such that the EPA dose was 3-fold to 4-fold higher than that of the other recent omega-3 RCTs. More than 18,000 Japanese study subjects were selected for either having had a prior ASCVD event (about one-fifth of subjects) or for having multiple risk factors but no prior event. They were further selected for a total cholesterol level more than 250 mg/dL. During a run-in period, all subjects were given a statin (doses per usual Japanese protocol) to bring their LDL-C levels within Japanese guidelines, with dose uptitration as needed.[62] The baseline LDL-C level of 182 mg/dL was reduced about 25% and subjects were then randomized to the study drug or control arm in an open-label fashion, again as per usual Japanese protocol. All end point adjudication and evaluations were blinded,[62] so the validity of the results of this prospective, open-label, blinded end point evaluation trial is considered roughly comparable with that of a standard double-blind trial. The baseline TG level of about 150 mg/dL was reduced by just 9% with EPA versus about a 3% decrease in the control, and there were no further changes in LDL-C or HDL-C levels. Despite these modest lipid effects, there was a statistically significant 19% reduction in ASCVD events, comparable in both primary and secondary prevention patients.[62] Importantly, safety and tolerability were excellent such that the risk/benefit ratio was favorable. Thus, icosapent ethyl in JELIS was the first agent to show clear RCT evidence of ASCVD benefit as a nonstatin added to a statin, despite current dogma that ezetimibe in the Improved Reduction of Outcomes: Vytorin Efficacy International Trial (IMPROVE-IT) was the first to do so.[63] Further, note that a prespecified subanalysis of 957 subjects in JELIS with HTG levels (>150 mg/dL) and low HDL-C levels (<40 mg/dL) at baseline showed a 53% decrease in ASCVD events versus control.[64] Thus, it seems that intermediate doses of a pure EPA omega-3 can reduce ASCVD when added to statin therapy, especially if the usual lipid indications (mainly HTG) are present.

### Randomized Clinical Trials of Niacin

Many RCTs have shown decreased ASCVD with niacin but niacin was generally studied in monotherapy and not separately as a statin adjunct.[65] Two recent RCTs have now suggested that niacin may not reduce ASCVD when added to a statin; however, important design problems and some positive subgroup results make this conclusion tenuous. The first recent RCT with niacin was Atherothrombosis Intervention in Metabolic Syndrome with Low HDL/High Triglycerides: Impact on Global Health Outcomes (AIM-HIGH).[66] Despite appearances to the contrary, AIM-HIGH was not a valid test of the effects of niacin on ASCVD. First, the greater LDL-C level lowering with niacin was largely counterbalanced by greater uptitration of statin dose and increased frequency of ezetimibe use in the control arm. Further, in order to maintain the study blind despite the expected frequent flushing in the treatment arm, the control arm was given low-dose niacin in every placebo tablet, further reducing lipid differences between study arms.[66] Thus, AIM-HIGH was an active comparator study of higher-dose (1500–2000 mg/d) extended-release nicotinic acid (ERNA) plus standard-dose statin and infrequent ezetimibe versus low-dose (100–150 mg/d) immediate-release nicotinic acid plus higher-dose statin and more frequent ezetimibe use.[66] The negative overall results presumably were caused at least in part by this diluted treatment comparison and there was little evidence for harm with high-dose ERNA.[66] Importantly, a post-hoc subanalysis of subjects in AIM-HIGH having both HTG and low HDL-C levels showed a statistically significant 26% reduction in the primary ASCVD end point.[67]

This subgroup finding in AIM-HIGH was not only comparable with that of the subanalyses of the several recent RCTs using fibrates and EPA outlined earlier, but it was also reminiscent of a subanalysis of the largest prior RCT of ASCVD effects of niacin, the Coronary Drug Project (CDP), originally published in 1975.[68] Subjects in CDP were assessed for the presence or absence of the metabolic syndrome, defined by slightly modified criteria because body mass index greater than 28 kg/m$^2$ had to substitute for a waist circumference greater than 100 cm (40 inches; all subjects were men and waist had not been measured), and HDL-C levels were available only in 492 of the 3906 subjects.[69] These patients with metabolic syndrome, most of whom had TG levels greater than 150 mg/dL, saw a 78% decrease in nonfatal myocardial infarction with niacin versus only a 24% decrease in patients without the metabolic syndrome.[69] Although the subgroup data in AIM-HIGH and the CDP individually are weak, they are strengthened by their consistency with each other, and also by consistency with subgroup findings in 5 fibrate RCTs and 1 omega-3 RCT (JELIS). Thus, HTG subgroups from a total of 8 RCTs of TG level lowering showed ASCVD benefit.

The most recent niacin RCT, Heart Protection Study 2–Treatment of HDL to Reduce the Incidence of Vascular Events (HPS2-THRIVE), involved 25,673 subjects with prior ASCVD, more than one-third having the metabolic syndrome and an overlapping one-third having DM2.[70] All patients received excellent lipid control with statin monotherapy before randomization, with mean levels of LDL-C, 63 mg/dL; TG, 125 mg/dL; and HDL-C,

44 mg/dL. However, this meant that the RCT was conducted in patients generally lacking any lipid-related indication for niacin treatment. Another unfortunate design element was that niacin was always given with laropiprant, a prostaglandin blocker with unknown safety or ASCVD effects. The primary composite ASCVD end point was not reduced significantly in the overall study population and so niacin was considered to have been proved incapable of decreasing ASCVD (at least when added to a statin).[70] More than 3400 ASCVD events were included and median follow-up was 3.9 years, suggesting a definitive result. Further, an excess of incident DM2, bleeding, and infection was also seen with ERNA plus laropiprant.

However, several aspects of HPS2-THRIVE weaken the conclusion that niacin does not have a favorable risk/benefit ratio as a TG level–lowering medication in ASCVD prevention. First, among the 57% of subjects who were from Europe (virtually all of whom were white) there was a borderline statistically significant 9% decrease in ASCVD, whereas the 43% of subjects from China (all of eastern Asian descent) had a nonsignificant 2% increase (this result being of borderline significance even by the stringent interaction test).[70] Also of likely clinical importance, there was a strong and statistically significant effect of baseline lipids such that those with LDL-C level greater than 57 mg/dL (most of them) had significantly fewer ASCVD events. Although subjects with HTG and low HDL-C levels were reported not to have ASCVD benefit, the HTG cutoff used was only 150 mg/dL,[70] not the 200 mg/dL cutoff required to see benefit with ERNA plus statin in AIM-HIGH or with fenofibrate plus statin in ACCORD-Lipid. Of potential importance, the ASCVD effects were significantly different between whites and Asian people, being nearly significantly beneficial in the former. Also, the event curves appeared to spread toward greater niacin benefit as the study ended. In addition, with regard to safety, some of the adverse events, such as infection and bleeding, had not been seen in several decades of prior niacin RCTs,[65] or at least not to the degree noted in HPS2-THRIVE,[70] suggesting that they may have resulted from laropiprant. However, neither the adverse events nor the intriguing effects of baseline lipid on ASCVD benefit were reported by racial groups so that the risk/benefit ratio of ERNA plus laropiprant in the divergent white and Asian populations remains unexplored. Thus, although HPS2-THRIVE lessens the priority for niacin use in management of HTG, it leaves many critical questions unanswered, especially in light of the more positive niacin RCT results without laropiprant in patients with HTG.

### Summary of Completed Randomized Clinical Trials of Triglyceride Level Lowering Versus Atherosclerotic Cardiovascular Disease

Thus, ASCVD reduction has been shown in several contemporary RCTs (and 1 older trial) of 3 classes of TG level–lowering drugs in patients who entered the studies with HTG and low HDL-C levels. Reliance on study subgroups is a major weakness, but this reliance is required mainly because of the consistent failure of clinical trialists to focus RCTs of TG level–lowering medications on patients who need TG lowering. The 2013 American College of Cardiology (ACC)/American Heart Association (AHA) cholesterol guidelines state that "nonstatin therapies, as compared with statin therapy, do not provide acceptable ASCVD risk reduction benefits compared to their potential for adverse effects in the routine prevention of ASCVD"[71] and "[there are] no data supporting the routine use of nonstatin drugs combined with statin therapy to further reduce ASCVD events."[71] Nevertheless, a large RCT showed that icosapent ethyl can safely decrease ASCVD risk beyond that of statin monotherapy, even without selecting for HTG,[62] and 1 RCT each with fenofibrate (ACCORD-Lipid; Ginsberg, HN. NEJM, e-published March 14, 2010[54]) and ERNA[67] showed reduced ASCVD in patient subgroups with baseline HTG and low HDL-C levels. Thus, it is reasonable to strongly consider use of icosapent ethyl (and perhaps other prescription omega-3) and also to consider fenofibrate and/or ERNA as statin adjuncts (or possibly as statin alternates in statin intolerance) for ASCVD prevention in patients with HTG.

### Ongoing Randomized Clinical Trials of Triglyceride Level Lowering Versus Atherosclerotic Cardiovascular Disease

Two RCTs of ASCVD effects of omega-3 treatment are now underway. The first is Reduction of Cardiovascular Events With EPA – Intervention Trial (REDUCE-IT, NCT01492361).[72] REDUCE-IT is studying icosapent ethyl, 2 g twice a day with meals, versus a matching mineral oil placebo with a composite of ASCVD events as the primary end point. It will involve about 8000 subjects selected for a prior cardiovascular event or otherwise at high ASCVD risk, and a plasma TG level of more than 150 mg/dL, and this is the first clinical end point RCT, with any agent, to use increased TG levels as a primary entry criterion. Recruitment is nearly complete, treatment will continue for about 4 to 6 years, and the trial is expected to be completed in about December 2017.[72]

The second omega-3 RCT is A Long-term Outcomes Study to Assess Statin Residual Risk

Reduction with Epanova in High Cardiovascular Risk Patients with Hypertriglyceridemia (STRENGTH).[73] Epanova, the newly approved carboxylic acid formulation of EPA and DHA, will be given once daily without reference to meals (at an as-yet unstated dose) versus a matching corn oil placebo and with an ASCVD event composite as the primary end point. It plans to involve 13,000 subjects and, like REDUCE-IT, subjects will be selected for high ASCVD risk and HTG. Recruitment is just beginning, treatment is expected to continue for 3 to 5 years, and the trial is expected to be completed in about June 2019.[73]

## TREATMENT RECOMMENDATIONS FOR HYPERTRIGLYCERIDEMIA
### Current Guidelines for Management of Hypertriglyceridemia

In 2004, an update of the Third Adult Treatment Panel (ATP-III) of the National Cholesterol Education Program (NCEP) carefully reviewed the issue of HTG and reiterated prior advice that fibrates and niacin could be considered for use with or without statin therapy in patients with high TG and/or low HDL-C levels.[74] The National Heart, Lung and Blood Institute (NHLBI) subsequently sponsored a major effort to review new scientific data and to replace ATP-III. However, the range of evidence ordinarily considered in guideline writing was sharply curtailed to allow only a few RCTs of the highest quality, and the scope was limited to hypercholesterolemia. At the end of the 5-year review process, the NHLBI stated that the work would be published simply as an evidentiary review, to serve as the basis for a multiparty effort to create new lipid guidelines.[75] Instead of following this course, as recommended by the sponsor of the writing, the ACC and the AHA chose to publish the review rapidly, just a couple of months later, as a finished guideline,[76] without seeking any further substantive scientific input. Because the 2013 ACC/AHA guidelines focused only on cholesterol and did not review HTG or address its management, they referred physicians to the 2011 AHA statement on HTG management.[6] The 2011 AHA statement is useful as a comprehensive review of causes and dietary and lifestyle treatments of HTG. In sharp contrast with the 2004 ATP-III update, it does not focus on pharmacotherapy or even mention the possible use of TG level–lowering medications for ASCVD prevention with fasting TG levels less than 500 mg/dL. However, the European Atherosclerosis Society also published guidance on management of HTG,[77] just 3 weeks before the 2011 AHA statement. The European guidelines recommend continued consideration of TG level–lowering agents for TG levels remaining in the range of 200 to 500 mg/dL despite statin therapy, just as had the ATP-III update.[74] As noted earlier, the approach recommended by the Europeans seems justified in light of current RCT and mechanistic data.

Dosing of fenofibrate is complicated in that there are 6 different brand names and 8 different formulations currently available in the United States alone, each with its own unique dose (**Table 2**). This situation is further complicated because each of these is available in a one-third dose for renal insufficiency. However, aside from considerations of pill/capsule size, insurance formulary, and price and availability, they all seem to be clinically equivalent. One of these formulations is fenofibric acid, the active metabolite of fenofibrate, which has yet another (seventh) brand name. It is chemically distinct but clinically indistinguishable because impaired conversion from fenofibrate to fenofibric acid has never been described. The sole advantage of fenofibric acid offers is that its FDA label does not warn against concurrent statin use.

Dosing of prescription omega-3 is generally 4 g/d, best given as 2 g twice daily with meals, except the new FFA formulation, which has better bioavailability and so can be given without food and at 2 g/d (albeit with less efficacy). Compared with EPA, DHA can depress LDL-receptor activity[78] and increase LDL-C levels,[79] so icosapent ethyl, being DHA-free, probably has more favorable effects on LDL-C levels than other omega-3

| Table 2 | | |
| --- | --- | --- |
| **Available fenofibrate doses** | | |
| Regular Dose (mg/d) | Reduced Dose[a] (mg/d) | Brand Name |
| 200 | 67[b] | Lofibra |
| 160 | 54/50 | Lofibra/Triglide |
| 150 | 50 | Lipofen |
| 145 | 48 | Tricor |
| 135 | 45 | Trilipix[c] |
| 130 | 43 | Antara |
| 120 | 40 | Fenoglide |
| 90 | 30 | Antara |

See FDA-approved prescribing information for further details.
[a] Primarily for renal or geriatric patients.
[b] Also available at 134 mg.
[c] Fenofibric acid (see text).
*Data from* Fenofibrate Interchange. Available at: http://www.drugs.com/fenofibrate.html. Accessed January 5, 2015.

preparations that contain DHA (the other prescription ethyl ester and FFA formulations, as well as all dietary supplements).

Dosing of ERNA is between 500 and 2000 mg per day, generally best tolerated at bedtime and with 325 mg of aspirin to reduce flushing. In patients with little or no flushing, immediate-release niacin can be tried, twice or 3 times daily up to 3 or 4 g/d. ERNA or sustained-release niacin should not be given more than once daily. Niacinamide, nicotinamide, and inositol hexaniacinate should be avoided because they have no lipid benefit.

### Diet and Lifestyle Treatment of Hypertriglyceridemia

All of the guidelines and statements discussed earlier mention diet and lifestyle treatment, and HTG is the dyslipidemia most responsive to non-pharmacologic treatments. The 2011 AHA statement on TG provides an excellent review of this subject,[6] the main principles of which are summarized here and in **Table 3**:

1. Sugar intake should be restricted. Most sugars, especially fructose, stimulate hepatic synthesis of FFAs and thus FFA and TG accumulation in the liver. This accumulation drives VLDL production and increases plasma TG level in the mild to moderate range ($\sim$100–500 mg/dL). Fructose is prevalent in the Western diet, being about half the content of sucrose (white or brown sugar), of high-fructose corn syrup, and also of honey, and being more than half

the content of the sugar in fruit juice and certain other sweeteners, like agave. Thus, restriction of sugar-sweetened beverages, other added sugars, and fruit juice (but not fruit) is usually helpful to reduce TG levels. Nonsugar carbohydrate (starch) has a weak TG level–raising effect, mainly if low in fiber, so restricting total carbohydrates may slightly reduce TG levels.

2. Increase dietary fiber intake. Fiber has a modest effect to blunt TG level increase with sugar and other carbohydrates.

3. Fat intake may need to be restricted. Dietary fat drives chylomicron production and restricting dietary fat is the most effective way to reduce TG levels of more than about 800 mg/dL. Saturated fats are slightly more likely to lead to HTG than unsaturated fats, but fatty fish has a paradoxic effect of lowering TG levels because of the several favorable effects of omega-3 oil on TG metabolism.

4. Physical activity should be increased. Increased exercise tends to reduce TG levels, likely because of increased muscle TG oxidation as a fuel source, improved glucose and insulin metabolism (including increased LPL activity/TG lipolysis), and decreased hepatic TG and FFA content.

5. Weight loss should be encouraged. Whether by decreasing total calories or increasing activity, negative caloric balance reduces TG levels, likely related to improvement in insulin resistance and decreased hepatic TG and FFA content.

6. Restriction of alcohol intake may be beneficial. Ethanol increases TG levels in many patients at any level of intake, and so a trial of decreased consumption is warranted for plasma TG levels of more than about 200 mg/dL in patients who consume more than about 2 servings per week. Tobacco and marijuana have minor TG level–raising effects that are generally not of clinical importance.

### Treatment of Secondary Factors in Hypertriglyceridemia

The treatment of secondary factors that promote HTG is always worth consideration in the clinical management of HTG. They are well outlined in the 2011 AHA statement[6] and are summarized here and in **Table 4**:

1. Diabetes mellitus should be prevented or controlled. DM2 and diabetes mellitus type 1 (DM1) contribute to HTG via hyperglycemia and insulin resistance (in the case of DM2). Treatment of hyperglycemia and prevention of DM2 reduce TG levels.

**Table 3**
**Diet and lifestyle treatments for hypertriglyceridemia**

| Intervention | Useful in TG Range | Strength of Effect |
|---|---|---|
| ↓ Sugar intake (especially fructose) | Mainly <800 mg/dL | Moderate |
| ↑ Fiber intake | Mainly <800 mg/dL | Weak |
| ↓ Fat intake | Only >800 mg/dL | Strong |
| ↑ Physical activity | Any TG level | Moderate |
| Weight loss | Any TG level | Moderate |
| ↓ Ethanol intake | Any TG level | Weak to moderate |

*Adapted from* Miller M, Stone NJ, Ballantyne C, et al. Triglycerides and cardiovascular disease: a scientific statement from the American Heart Association. Circulation 2011;123:2292–333.

**Table 4**
**Secondary causes of hypertriglyceridemia to treat to reduce TG levels**

| Cause | Comment |
| --- | --- |
| Hyperglycemia | Control glucose/prevent DM if possible, reduce insulin resistance |
| Insulin resistance | ↓ Calories and adiposity, ↑ exercise, consider insulin sensitizer medications |
| Hypothyroidism | Screen and treat if present |
| Proteinuria and renal insufficiency | Screen and treat if possible |
| Endogenous hypercortisolism | Consider screening, treat if present |
| Medications | Reduce dose or discontinue if clinically appropriate |
| Oral contraceptives | Variable effect |
| Oral estrogen replacement | Variable effect |
| Retinoic acid derivatives | Large effect |
| Systemic glucocorticoids | Large effect |
| Certain antiretroviral medications | Large effect |
| Certain antipsychotic medications | Modest effect |
| Most β-blockers | Weak effect |
| Thiazide diuretics | Weak effect |

Abbreviation: DM, diabetes mellitus.
*Adapted from* Miller M, Stone NJ, Ballantyne C, et al. Triglycerides and cardiovascular disease: a scientific statement from the American Heart Association. Circulation 2011;123:2292–333.

2. Reduce insulin resistance. Decreasing calories, increasing physical activity, and decreasing weight all seem to work by this mechanism. Treating or preventing DM2 with medications that reduce insulin resistance (such as thiazolidinediones or biguanides) may confer extra TG level–lowering benefit.
3. Screen for hypothyroidism and treat it if present. All patients with HTG should have their serum thyroid stimulating hormone (TSH) levels checked. If the TSH level is increased, levothyroxine replacement lowers TG levels (and is beneficial for many other reasons).
4. Proteinuria and renal insufficiency should be screened for and treated if possible. Both increase TG levels if left uncontrolled.
5. Endogenous hypercortisolism should be considered and treated if present. Although rare, it substantially increases plasma TG level and should always be considered in patients with HTG.
6. Medications that increase TG levels should be decreased or discontinued if possible, including:
   a. Oral contraceptives (primarily the estrogen component)
   b. Oral postmenopausal estrogen replacement
   c. Retinoic acid derivatives
   d. Systemic glucocorticoids
   e. Some antiretroviral medications
   f. Some antipsychotic medications
   g. Most β-blockers (generally only a weak effect)
   h. Thiazide diuretics (generally only a weak effect)

## Pharmacotherapy Treatment Recommendations Adjunctive to Current Guidelines

Mendelian randomization data strongly suggest that HTG causes ASCVD, and so TG level–lowering treatment in HTG is now more strongly recommended to address the residual ASCVD risk than has been the case in (generally earlier) published guidelines.[5]

Fibrates are the best-established agents for TG level lowering and are generally used first line for TG levels greater than 500 mg/dL. Fenofibrate is almost always preferred to gemfibrozil because it is far less likely to cause myopathy with concurrent statin use. Two exceptions are patients with severe renal insufficiency not taking a statin or likely to do so in the future, and patients taking fluvastatin, which has no adverse interaction with gemfibrozil.

There are 3 FDA-approved prescription omega-3 products: (1) an ethyl ester mix of EPA and DHA, (2) an ethyl ester pure EPA (icosapent ethyl), and (3) a carboxylic acid mix of EPA and DHA. They are much more expensive to manufacture than fenofibrate and so even the generic ethyl ester

EPA/DHA mix may incur higher out-of-pocket cost, even when covered by insurance. Omega-3 (at least icosapent ethyl in JELIS[62]) has been better proved to reduce ASCVD risk as a statin adjunct, and for this reason the class can be strongly considered for first-line use. Also, prescription omega-3 is generally as effective as fenofibrate for TG level lowering and is usually as well tolerated. In addition to better ASCVD evidence, other potential advantages of omega-3 compared with fenofibrate include that it is a natural product, it lacks any associated myopathy, and it might provide antiinflammatory, mood, cognitive, or other benefits, although none of these benefits is in the product label or has been established in an RCT. In light of the positive ASCVD results in JELIS[62] it is unfortunate that no current official lipid guidelines mention this class. Whether the preparation does or does not contain DHA, omega-3 is useful for treatment of HTG, and can be used as first or second line, ahead of or behind fibrates (generally in combination with them).

Niacin is usually reserved for third-line use because it is less well tolerated, may cause or worsen diabetes, and is generally harder to use. Statins are a crucial consideration for management of HTG in addition to the traditional TG level–lowering medications noted earlier. Statins are the best-established agents for ASCVD prevention, and so are usually used as first line for TG levels less than 500 mg/dL. Because they have lesser TG level–lowering efficacy than fibrates and omega-3, statins are generally not used as first line in patients with a fasting TG levels more than 500 mg/dL.

## REFERENCES

1. Maki KC, Bays HE, Dicklin MR. Treatment options for the management of hypertriglyceridemia: strategies based on the best-available evidence. J Clin Lipidol 2012;6:413–26.
2. Ford ES, Li C, Zhao G, et al. Hypertriglyceridemia and its pharmacologic treatment among US adults. Arch Intern Med 2009;169:572–8.
3. Christian JB, Bourgeois N, Snipes R, et al. Prevalence of severe (500 to 2,000 mg/dl) hypertriglyceridemia in United States adults. Am J Cardiol 2011; 107:891–7.
4. Roger VL, Go AS, Lloyd-Jones DM, et al. Heart disease and stroke statistics–2011 update: a report from the American Heart Association. Circulation 2011;123:e18–209.
5. Hegele RA, Ginsberg HN, Chapman MJ, et al. The polygenic nature of hypertriglyceridaemia: implications for definition, diagnosis, and management. Lancet Diabetes Endocrinol 2014;2:655–66.
6. Miller M, Stone NJ, Ballantyne C, et al. Triglycerides and cardiovascular disease: a scientific statement from the American Heart Association. Circulation 2011;123:2292–333.
7. Kersten S. Physiological regulation of lipoprotein lipase. Biochim Biophys Acta 2014;1841:919–33.
8. Glueck CJ, Fallat R, Buncher CR, et al. Familial combined hyperlipoproteinemia: studies in 91 adults and 95 children from 33 kindreds. Metabolism 1973;23: 1403–28.
9. Glueck CJ, Tsang R, Fallat R, et al. Familial hypertriglyceridemia: studies in 130 children and 45 siblings of 36 index cases. Metabolism 1973;22:1287–309.
10. Hopkins PN, Wu LL, Hunt SC, et al. Plasma triglycerides and type III hyperlipidemia are independently associated with premature familial coronary artery disease. J Am Coll Cardiol 2005;45:1003–12.
11. Hopkins PN, Nanjee MN, Wu LL, et al. Altered composition of triglyceride-rich lipoproteins and coronary artery disease in a large case-control study. Atherosclerosis 2009;207:559–66.
12. Hopkins PN, Brinton EA, Nanjee MN. Hyperlipoproteinemia type 3: the forgotten phenotype. Curr Atheroscler Rep 2014;16:440.
13. Sarwar N, Sandhu MS, Ricketts SL, et al. Triglyceride-mediated pathways and coronary disease: collaborative analysis of 101 studies. Lancet 2010; 375:1634–9.
14. Austin MA, Hokanson JE, Edwards KL. Hypertriglyceridemia as a cardiovascular risk factor. Am J Cardiol 1998;81:7B–12B.
15. Sarwar N, Danesh J, Eiriksdottir G, et al. Triglycerides and the risk of coronary heart disease: 10,158 incident cases among 262,525 participants in 29 western prospective studies. Circulation 2007;115: 450–8.
16. Liu J, Zeng FF, Liu ZM, et al. Effects of blood triglycerides on cardiovascular and all-cause mortality: a systematic review and meta-analysis of 61 prospective studies. Lipids Health Dis 2013;12:159.
17. Sacks FM, Alaupovic P, Moye LA, et al. VLDL, apolipoproteins B, CIII, and E, and risk of recurrent coronary events in the Cholesterol and Recurrent Events (CARE) trial. Circulation 2000;102:1886–92.
18. Miller M, Cannon CP, Murphy SA, et al. Impact of triglyceride levels beyond low-density lipoprotein cholesterol after acute coronary syndrome in the PROVE IT-TIMI 22 trial. J Am Coll Cardiol 2008;51: 724–30.
19. Drexel H, Aczel S, Marte T, et al. Factors predicting cardiovascular events in statin-treated diabetic and non-diabetic patients with coronary atherosclerosis. Atherosclerosis 2010;208:484–9.
20. Wang L, Gill R, Pedersen TL, et al. Triglyceride-rich lipoprotein lipolysis releases neutral and oxidized FFAs that induce endothelial cell inflammation. J Lipid Res 2009;50:204–13.

21. Goldberg IJ, Eckel RH, McPherson R. Triglycerides and heart disease: still a hypothesis? Arterioscler Thromb Vasc Biol 2011;31:1716–25.

22. Ginsberg HN. New perspectives on atherogenesis: role of abnormal triglyceride-rich lipoprotein metabolism. Circulation 2002;106:2137–42.

23. Schlaich MP, Grassi G, Lambert GW, et al. European Society of Hypertension Working Group on Obesity Obesity-induced hypertension and target organ damage: current knowledge and future directions. J Hypertens 2009;27:207–11.

24. Liu L, Wen T, Zheng XY, et al. Remnant-like particles accelerate endothelial progenitor cells senescence and induce cellular dysfunction via an oxidative mechanism. Atherosclerosis 2009;202:405–14.

25. Mahley RW, Innerarity TL, Rall SC Jr, et al. Lipoproteins of special significance in atherosclerosis. Insights provided by studies of type III hyperlipoproteinemia. Ann N Y Acad Sci 1985;454:209–21.

26. Ferreira AC, Peter AA, Mendez AJ, et al. Postprandial hypertriglyceridemia increases circulating levels of endothelial cell microparticles. Circulation 2004; 110:3599–603.

27. Norata GD, Grigore L, Raselli S, et al. Post-prandial endothelial dysfunction in hypertriglyceridemic subjects: molecular mechanisms and gene expression studies. Atherosclerosis 2007;193:321–7.

28. Shin HK, Kim YK, Kim KY, et al. Remnant lipoprotein particles induce apoptosis in endothelial cells by NAD(P)H oxidase-mediated production of superoxide and cytokines via lectin-like oxidized low-density lipoprotein receptor-1 activation: prevention by cilostazol. Circulation 2004;109:1022–8.

29. Tanimura K, Nakajima Y, Nagao M, et al. Association of serum apolipoprotein B48 level with the presence of carotid plaque in type 2 diabetes mellitus. Diabetes Res Clin Pract 2008;81:338–44.

30. Langsted A, Freiberg JJ, Tybjaerg-Hansen A, et al. Nonfasting cholesterol and triglycerides and association with risk of myocardial infarction and total mortality: the Copenhagen City Heart Study with 31 years of follow-up. J Intern Med 2011;270:65–75.

31. Zheng C, Azcutia V, Aikawa E, et al. Statins suppress apolipoprotein CIII-induced vascular endothelial cell activation and monocyte adhesion. Eur Heart J 2013;34:615–24.

32. Ginsberg HN, Brown WV. Apolipoprotein CIII: 42 years old and even more interesting. Arterioscler Thromb Vasc Biol 2011;31:471–3.

33. Caron S, Verrijken A, Mertens I, et al. Transcriptional activation of apolipoprotein CIII expression by glucose may contribute to diabetic dyslipidemia. Arterioscler Thromb Vasc Biol 2011;31:513–9.

34. Ginsberg HN. Insulin resistance and cardiovascular disease. J Clin Invest 2000;106:453–8.

35. Lamarche B, Tchernof A, Moorjani S, et al. Small, dense low-density lipoprotein particles as a predictor of the risk of ischemic heart disease in men. Prospective results from the Québec Cardiovascular Study. Circulation 1997;95:69–75.

36. St-Pierre AC, Ruel IL, Cantin B, et al. Comparison of various electrophoretic characteristics of LDL particles and their relationship to the risk of ischemic heart disease. Circulation 2001;104:2295–9.

37. Hirano T, Ito Y, Koba S, et al. Clinical significance of small dense low-density lipoprotein cholesterol levels determined by the simple precipitation method. Arterioscler Thromb Vasc Biol 2004;24:558–63.

38. Rizzo M, Kotur-Stevuljevic J, Berneis K, et al. Atherogenic dyslipidemia and oxidative stress: a new look. Transl Res 2009;153:217–23.

39. Packard C, Caslake M, Shepherd J. The role of small, dense low density lipoprotein (LDL): a new look. Int J Cardiol 2000;74(Suppl 1):S17–22.

40. Berneis KK, Krauss RM. Metabolic origins and clinical significance of LDL heterogeneity. J Lipid Res 2002;43:1363–79.

41. Anber V, Griffin BA, McConnell M, et al. Influence of plasma lipid and LDL-subfraction profile on the interaction between low density lipoprotein with human arterial wall proteoglycans. Atherosclerosis 1996; 124:261–71.

42. Goulinet S, Chapman MJ. Plasma LDL and HDL subspecies are heterogenous in particle content of tocopherols and oxygenated and hydrocarbon carotenoids. Relevance to oxidative resistance and atherogenesis. Arterioscler Thromb Vasc Biol 1997; 17:786–96.

43. Nigon F, Lesnik P, Rouis M, et al. Discrete subspecies of human low density lipoproteins are heterogeneous in their interaction with the cellular LDL receptor. J Lipid Res 1991;32:1741–53.

44. Younis N, Charlton-Menys V, Sharma R, et al. Glycation of LDL in non-diabetic people: Small dense LDL is preferentially glycated both in vivo and in vitro. Atherosclerosis 2009;202:162–8.

45. Zheng C, Khoo C, Furtado J, et al. Apolipoprotein C-III and the metabolic basis for hypertriglyceridemia and the dense low-density lipoprotein phenotype. Circulation 2010;121:1722–34.

46. Brinton EA, Eisenberg S, Breslow JL. Increased apo A-I and apo A-II fractional catabolic rate in patients with low high density lipoprotein-cholesterol levels with or without hypertriglyceridemia. J Clin Invest 1991;87:536–44.

47. Brinton EA, Eisenberg S, Breslow JL. Human HDL cholesterol levels are determined by apoA-I fractional catabolic rate, which correlates inversely with estimates of HDL particle size. Effects of gender, hepatic and lipoprotein lipases, triglyceride and insulin levels, and body fat distribution. Arterioscler Thromb 1994;14:707–20.

48. Rizzo M, Spinas GA, Cesur M, et al. Atherogenic lipoprotein phenotype and LDL size and subclasses

in drug-naive patients with early rheumatoid arthritis. Atherosclerosis 2009;207:502–6.

49. Do R, Willer CJ, Schmidt EM, et al. Common variants associated with plasma triglycerides and risk for coronary artery disease. Nat Genet 2013;45:1345–52.

50. Jørgensen AB, Frikke-Schmidt R, Nordestgaard BG, et al. Loss-of-function mutations in APOC3 and risk of ischemic vascular disease. N Engl J Med 2014; 371:32–41.

51. Chapman M. Fibrates: therapeutic review. Br J Diabetes Vasc Dis 2006;6:11–20.

52. Kamanna VS, Kashyap ML. Nicotinic acid (niacin) receptor agonists: will they be useful therapeutic agents? Am J Cardiol 2007;100:S53–61.

53. McKenney JM, Sica D. Role of prescription omega-3 fatty acids in the treatment of hypertriglyceridemia. Pharmacotherapy 2007;27:715–28.

54. Ginsberg HN, Elam MB, Lovato LC, et al. Effects of combination lipid therapy in type 2 diabetes mellitus. N Engl J Med 2010;362:1563–74.

55. Ginsberg HN. The ACCORD (Action to Control Cardiovascular Risk in Diabetes) Lipid trial: what we learn from subgroup analyses. Diabetes Care 2011;34(Suppl 2):S107–8.

56. Keech A, Simes RJ, Barter P, et al. Effects of long-term fenofibrate therapy on cardiovascular events in 9795 people with type 2 diabetes mellitus (the FIELD study): randomised controlled trial. Lancet 2005;366:1849–61.

57. Scott R, O'Brien R, Fulcher G, et al. Effects of fenofibrate treatment on cardiovascular disease risk in 9,795 individuals with type 2 diabetes and various components of the metabolic syndrome: the Fenofibrate Intervention and Event Lowering in Diabetes (FIELD) study. Diabetes Care 2009;32:493–8.

58. Sacks FM, Carey VJ, Fruchart JC. Combination lipid therapy in type 2 diabetes. N Engl J Med 2010;363: 692–4 [author reply: 694–5].

59. Risk, Prevention Study Collaborative Group, Roncaglioni MC, Tombesi M, et al. n-3 fatty acids in patients with multiple cardiovascular risk factors. N Engl J Med 2013;368:1800–8.

60. ORIGIN Trial Investigators, Bosch J, Gerstein HC, et al. n-3 fatty acids and cardiovascular outcomes in patients with dysglycemia. N Engl J Med 2012; 367:309–18.

61. Writing Group for the AREDS2 Research Group, Bonds DE, Harrington M, et al. Effect of long-chain omega-3 fatty acids and lutein + zeaxanthin supplements on cardiovascular outcomes: results of the Age-related Eye Disease Study 2 (AREDS2) randomized clinical trial. JAMA Intern Med 2014;174:763–71.

62. Yokoyama M, Origasa H, Matsuzaki M, et al. Effects of eicosapentaenoic acid on major coronary events in hypercholesterolaemic patients (JELIS): a randomised open-label, blinded endpoint analysis. Lancet 2007;369:1090–8.

63. Cannon C. Improved Reduction of Outcomes: Vytorin Efficacy International Trial (IMPROVE-IT). Chicago: AHA Scientific Sessions; 2014.

64. Saito Y, Yokoyama M, Origasa H, et al. Effects of EPA on coronary artery disease in hypercholesterolemic patients with multiple risk factors: sub-analysis of primary prevention cases from the Japan EPA Lipid Intervention Study (JELIS). Atherosclerosis 2008; 200:135–40.

65. Bruckert E, Labreuche J, Amarenco P. Meta-analysis of the effect of nicotinic acid alone or in combination on cardiovascular events and atherosclerosis. Atherosclerosis 2010;210:353–61.

66. Boden WE, Probstfield JL, Anderson T, et al. Niacin in patients with low HDL cholesterol levels receiving intensive statin therapy. N Engl J Med 2011;365: 2255–67.

67. Guyton JR, Slee AE, Anderson T, et al. Relationship of lipoproteins to cardiovascular events: The AIM-HIGH trial (atherothrombosis intervention in metabolic syndrome with low HDL/high triglycerides and impact on global health outcomes). J Am Coll Cardiol 2013;62:1580–4.

68. Group TCDPWR. Clofibrate and niacin in coronary heart disease. JAMA 1975;231:360–81.

69. Canner PL, Furberg CD, McGovern ME. Benefits of niacin in patients with versus without the metabolic syndrome and healed myocardial infarction (from the coronary drug project). Am J Cardiol 2006;97: 477–9.

70. HPS2-THRIVE Collaborative Group, Landray MJ, Haynes R, Hopewell JC, et al. Effects of extended-release niacin with laropiprant in high-risk patients. N Engl J Med 2014;371:203–12.

71. Stone NJ, Robinson JG, Lichtenstein AH, et al. 2013 ACC/AHA guideline on the treatment of blood cholesterol to reduce atherosclerotic cardiovascular risk in adults: a report of the American College of Cardiology/American Heart Association Task Force on Practice Guidelines. Circulation 2014;129:S1–45.

72. Reduction of Cardiovascular Events with EPA - Intervention Trial (REDUCE-IT). Available at: https://clinicaltrials.gov/ct2/show/NCT01492361?term=reduce-it&rank=1. Accessed January 6, 2015.

73. Outcomes Study to Assess STatin Residual Risk Reduction with EpaNova in HiGh Cardiovascular Risk PatienTs with Hypertriglyceridemia (STRENGTH). Available at: https://clinicaltrials.gov/ct2/show/NCT02104817?term=epanova&rank=4. Accessed January 6, 2015.

74. Grundy SM, Cleeman JI, Merz CN, et al. Implications of recent clinical trials for the national cholesterol education program adult treatment panel III guidelines. Circulation 2004;110:227–39.

75. Gibbons GH, Shurin SB, Mensah GA, et al. Refocusing the agenda on cardiovascular guidelines: an announcement from the National Heart, Lung,

and Blood Institute. J Am Coll Cardiol 2013;62: 1396–8.

76. Stone N, Robinson J, Lichtenstein, et al. 2013 ACC/ AHA guideline on the treatment of blood cholesterol to reduce atherosclerotic cardiovascular risk in adults: a report of the American College of Cardiology/American Heart Association Task Force on Practice Guidelines. Circulation 2013;1–84.

77. Chapman MJ, Ginsberg HN, Amarenco P, et al. Triglyceride-rich lipoproteins and high-density lipoprotein cholesterol in patients at high risk of cardiovascular disease: evidence and guidance for management. Eur Heart J 2011; 32:1345–61.

78. Ishida T, Ohta M, Nakakuki M, et al. Distinct regulation of plasma LDL cholesterol by eicosapentaenoic acid and docosahexaenoic acid in high fat diet-fed hamsters: participation of cholesterol ester transfer protein and LDL receptor. Prostaglandins Leukot Essent Fatty Acids 2013;88:281–8.

79. Wei MY, Jacobson TA. Effects of eicosapentaenoic acid versus docosahexaenoic acid on serum lipids: a systematic review and meta-analysis. Curr Atheroscler Rep 2011;13:474–83.

# Dyslipidemia in Special Ethnic Populations

Jia Pu, PhD[a],*, Robert Romanelli, PhD[a], Beinan Zhao, MS[a], Kristen M.J. Azar, RN, MSN, MPH[a], Katherine G. Hastings, BA[b], Vani Nimbal, MPH[a], Stephen P. Fortmann, MD[c], Latha P. Palaniappan, MD, MS[b]

## KEYWORDS

- Dyslipidemia • Racial/ethnic differences • Prevalence • Mortality • Treatment
- Lifestyle modification

## KEY POINTS

- Among racial/ethnic groups, Asian Indians, Filipinos and Hispanics are at greater risk for dyslipidemia, which is consistent with the higher coronary heart disease (CHD) mortality rates.
- Compared with other racial/ethnic groups, statins may have a higher efficacy for Asians. Studies suggest lower starting dosage in Asians, but the data are mixed.
- Genetic differences in statin metabolism can in part explain this racial/ethnic difference in statin sensitivity and adverse effects.
- Lifestyle modification is recommended as part of dyslipidemia control and management; African Americans and Hispanics have more sedentary behavior and a less favorable diet profile.

## INTRODUCTION

Dyslipidemia, including high levels of low-density lipoprotein cholesterol (LDL-C; ≥130 mg/dL), total cholesterol (≥200 mg/dL), and triglycerides (TG; ≥150 mg/dL), or low levels of high-density lipoprotein cholesterol (HDL-C; <40 [men] and <50 [women] mg/dL), is among the leading risk factors for coronary heart disease (CHD) and stroke.[1] A report of the National Health and Nutrition Examination Survey (NHANES) from 2003 to 2006 estimated that 53% (105.3 million) US adults have at least one lipid abnormality: 27% (53.5 million) have high LDL-C, 23% (46.4 million) have low HDL-C, and 30% (58.9 million) have high TG. In addition, 21% (42.0 million) of US adults have mixed dyslipidemia, defined as the presence of high LDL-C combined with at least one other lipid abnormality.[2]

Significant heterogeneity in patterns of dyslipidemia prevalence, its relation to CHD and stroke mortality rates, and response to lipid-lowering agents has been observed across racial/ethnic groups.[3] These differences in dyslipidemia provide important information that may in part explain the variation in cardiovascular disease (CVD) burden observed across racial/ethnic subgroups. Better understanding of dyslipidemia in special racial/ethnic populations is needed to guide prevention, screening, and treatment efforts.

## PREVALENCE OF DYSLIPIDEMIA SUBTYPES AMONG SPECIAL RACIAL/ETHNIC GROUPS

The NHANES is the primary data source for national prevalence rates of dyslipidemia in the United States, sampling mainly non-Hispanic whites (whites), non-Hispanic blacks (blacks),

Conflicts of Interest: All authors declare they have no conflicts of interest.
[a] Palo Alto Medical Foundation Research Institute, Ames Building, 795 El Camino Real, Palo Alto, CA 94301, USA; [b] Stanford University School of Medicine, 1265 Welch Road, Stanford, CA 94305, USA; [c] Kaiser Permanente Center for Health Research, 3800 North Interstate Avenue, Portland, OR 97227, USA
* Corresponding author.
*E-mail address:* puj@pamfri.org

Cardiol Clin 33 (2015) 325–333
http://dx.doi.org/10.1016/j.ccl.2015.01.005
0733-8651/15/$ – see front matter © 2015 Elsevier Inc. All rights reserved.

and Mexican Americans. The NHANES has very limited samples from the Asian subgroups.[4] Other data sources, such as primary care settings and observational studies, contribute to a comprehensive picture of racial/ethnic differences in dyslipidemia by providing important information about races and ethnicities that are less represented in the NHANES. One should be aware that the prevalence of dyslipidemia varies by data source. The observed differences in the prevalence rates of dyslipidemia between studies can be attributable to factors such as study design, sampling methods, time period, geographic variation, and participants' characteristics.

### Low-Density Lipoprotein Cholesterol

NHANES data in 2013 showed that the prevalence rate of high LDL-C was highest among Mexican men (40%) and women (30%), followed by non-Hispanic black men (33%) and women (31%). Non-Hispanic white men (30%) and women (29%) had the lowest prevalence of high LDL-C among the 3 racial/ethnic groups.[5]

Similarly, data from a clinic-based cohort in northern California from 2008 to 2011 showed that 63% of black men and 57% of black women had high LDL-C, which were slightly higher than the prevalence rates among non-Hispanic white men (62%) and women (53%).[3] Further, Mexican American men (66%) and women (57%) also had higher prevalence of high LDL-C compared with non-Hispanic whites.[3] Filipino men (73%) and women (63%) had the highest prevalence rates of high LDL-C among Asian subgroups, non-Hispanic whites, non-Hispanic blacks, and Hispanics.[3]

Several other studies provide further estimates for variation in prevalence among race/ethnic minority subgroups. Data from the Hispanic Community Health Study (HCHS)/Study of Latinos (SOL), an observational study in San Diego, Chicago, New York City, and Miami, showed variations among Hispanic subgroups with particularly high prevalence of dyslipidemia among Central American men (55%) and Puerto Rican women (41%).[6] The Study of Health Assessment and Health Risk in Ethnic groups (SHARE) investigated the prevalence of CHD risk factors for a multiethnic cohort from 3 Canadian cities. They found that South Asians, mainly Asian Indians, had an increased prevalence of higher total and LDL cholesterol compared with Europeans and Chinese.[7]

### High-Density Lipoprotein Cholesterol

NHANES data in 2013 showed that 20% of black men and 10% of black women had low HDL-C, defined as less than 40 mg/dL in both men and women, which were lower than the prevalence rates among non-Hispanic white men (33%) and women (12%).[5] NHANES data also showed Mexican American men (34%) and women (15%) had higher prevalence of low HDL-C compared with non-Hispanic whites.[5] According to NHANES data from 2011 to 2012, 25% of Asian American men and 5% of Asian American women had low HDL-C.[8]

Although NHANES data showed Asian Americans had the lowest prevalence of low HDL-C as an aggregated group, data from a clinic-based cohort with disaggregated Asian ethnic groups in northern California between 2008 and 2011 found that Asian Indian men (53%) and women (55%) had the highest prevalence of low HDL-C among Asian American subgroups; their prevalence was also higher than Mexican American men (48%) and women (51%), non-Hispanic black men (34%) and women (40%), and non-Hispanic white men (36%) and women (31%).[3] Similarly, data from the SHARE study showed South Asians including Asian Indians had an increased prevalence of low HDL-C compared with Europeans and Chinese.[7]

### Triglycerides

NHANES data from 1999 through 2008 showed 35% of Mexican Americans had high TG, followed by 33% among non-Hispanic whites, and 16% among non-Hispanic blacks.[9] Data from a clinic-based cohort in northern California from 2008 to 2011 found that Filipino men (60%) and Mexican women (45%) had the highest prevalence of high TG, compared with Mexican men (56%) and Filipino women (42%), Asian Indian men (55%) and women (37%), non-Hispanic white men (43%) and women (28%), and non-Hispanic black men (30%), and women (18%).[3] Data from the SHARE study showed South Asians had the highest prevalence of high TG among South Asians, Chinese, and Europeans.[7]

Potential explanations for racial/ethnic differences in dyslipidemia prevalence have been explored by several studies. In the Multi-Ethnic Study of Atherosclerosis (MESA), researchers found that ethnic disparities were substantially attenuated by adjusting for access to health care.[10] The racial/ethnic differences could also be related to lifestyle, genetic, and cultural differences associated with total and LDL-C concentrations.[11] For example, the predilection of South Asians to have lower HDL-C levels has been attributed to the higher prevalence of insulin resistance and related metabolic abnormalities, which may be the consequence of a combination of genetic predisposition, physical inactivity, and a high carbohydrate diet.[12–14]

## DYSLIPIDEMIA-RELATED MORTALITY IN SPECIAL RACIAL/ETHNIC GROUPS

Dyslipidemia often results in an increased risk of premature atherosclerosis, a major risk factor for CHD.[15] CHD is the leading cause of mortality for both men and women in the United States and worldwide, with increasing evidence of gender and racial/ethnic minority disparities in CHD morbidity and mortality.[16–19] Despite declines in CHD death rates over the past decades, CHD contributes to more than one-third of all deaths for those over the age of 35 years.[20]

Differences in mortality rate from CHD have been found across races/ethnicities. In the United States, CHD mortality rates are highest in blacks, intermediate in whites and Hispanics, and lowest in some Asian subgroups.[15,21,22] These CHD rates are paralleled with observed racial/ethnic disparities in dyslipidemia prevalence, with higher CHD rates seen in Hispanics and blacks, potentially owing to limited health care access and other less favorable behavioral factors seen in these groups.[10]

Meanwhile, although traditionally known as the "model minority," disproportionate mortality burden owing to CHD and stroke has been shown among certain Asian subgroups, such as Asian Indians, Filipinos, and Japanese.[23,24] Of note, the landmark Ni-Hon-San study showed increased CHD mortality rates and decreased stroke rates among Japanese-American men compared with rates in Japan, suggesting a differential disease impact of acculturation to Westernized lifestyles.[25] A recent study found higher proportional mortality owing to CHD among Asian Indians, especially in younger age groups, compared with all other racial/ethnic groups.[17] Increased burden from CHD mortality has been well-documented in both native and immigrant Asian Indian populations.[7,26,27] This observation is consistent with the higher prevalence rates of dyslipidemia (especially low HDL-C) in Asian Indians compared with other Asian subgroups and non-Hispanic whites in the United States.[3,7,28]

Environmental and social factors (eg, acculturation, socioeconomic status, diet) have been known to increase CHD mortality risk.[29,30] Cultural diets high in fat, increasing the risk for dyslipidemia, are also of concern.[31] Differences in susceptibility to CHD may also have a genetic basis, although this has not been determined adequately yet. Thus, it is critical for clinicians to modify lipid management appropriately among these rapidly growing populations.

## TREATMENT OF DYSLIPIDEMIA
### Overview

There are several US Food and Drug Administration (FDA)-approved 3-hydroxy-3-methyl-glutaryl-coenzyme A reductase inhibitors (statins) and a variety of nonstatin therapies available for the treatment of dyslipidemia, including bile acids sequestrants, cholesterol absorption inhibitors, fibrates, niacin, and omega-3 fatty acids. Statins are the most widely prescribed treatment for dyslipidemia, and one of the most commonly prescribed drugs in the United States.[32] In the most recent national cholesterol treatment guidelines, published in November 2013 by the American College of Cardiology (ACC)/American Heart Association (AHA),[1] the Expert Panel determined from robust clinical trial data that statins have the most acceptable CVD risk reduction benefit and side effect profile, and that the addition of nonstatin therapy does not seem to provide further benefit in reducing CVD. Clinical trials on which cholesterol treatment guidelines are based have often underrepresented racial/ethnic minority groups. Accordingly, our knowledge of optimal statin treatment regimens, and the effectiveness, tolerability, and safety of these regimens in clinical practice, is limited across diverse racial/ethnic populations.

### Racial/Ethnic Differences in Risk Stratification

The most recent ACC/AHA guidelines expand the criteria for patients who would benefit from statin treatment, and more than 80% of newly eligible patients are expected to have no prior CVD.[33] Therefore, they would be assessed for optimal statin treatment based on the new Atherosclerotic CVD (ASCVD) Risk Estimator.[33] This estimator is intended to improve on previous CVD risk estimators, including the Framingham[34] and Adult Treatment Panel III[35] risk algorithms. It was derived from several longitudinal epidemiologic cohort studies of non-Hispanic whites and blacks, and was validated externally in 2 cohort studies with similar populations (MESA and REGARDS),[36] as well as in contemporary samples of the derivation cohorts. However, studies among other race/ethnic minority groups are lacking. The ACC/AHA Work Group, which developed the algorithm for the ASCVD Risk Estimator, acknowledges that it should be used only in men and women of non-Hispanic white or non-Hispanic black decent, and that it may not accurately predict risk in other racial/ethnic groups.[37] Specifically, there is concern of overestimation of risk in Mexican Americans and East Asians and underestimation of risk in other groups, such as Puerto Ricans and South Asians.[37,38] Other countries with diverse racial/ethnic minority populations, such as the United Kingdom, have validated algorithms predicting risk for more than 9 specific racial/ethnic subpopulations (available at: http://qrisk.org/).[39]

### Race/Ethnic Differences in Statin Response

#### Statin metabolism and drug sensitivity

Much of the data on race/ethnic differences in statin metabolism have shown that some Asian subgroups are slower to metabolize statins compared with non-Hispanic whites, which leads to higher systemic drug concentrations. Pharmacokinetic studies indicate rosuvastatin plasma concentrations are 2-fold higher in Japanese relative to non-Hispanic white individuals. Rosuvastatin plasma concentrations have been shown to be elevated similarly in other Asian subgroups; these included Chinese, Malay, and Asian Indians, whose rosuvastatin concentrations were approximately 2 times higher relative to Caucasians.[40]

There are several genetic variants associated with altered statin metabolism. Such variants include, but are not limited to, single nucleotide polymorphisms in the genes that encode the organic anion-transporting polypeptide (OATP) 1B1 (521T> C), which regulates hepatic uptake of statins, and the adenosine triphosphate-binding cassette G2 (ABCG2) transporter (421C> A), which regulates hepatic efflux.[41,42] Variants of both genes are associated with increased statin plasma concentrations within multiple race/ethnic groups.[41–44] 421C> A has been found to be a single nucleotide polymorphism candidate to explain the observed racial differences in statin metabolism: the allelic frequency of 421C> A in ABCG2 is higher in Chinese (~35%) relative to Caucasians (9%–14%).[43,45]

Higher plasma levels of statins in Asians compared with non-Hispanic whites has led to concern about increased risk for statin-induced side effects in this population. Such concerns have led to a revised package insert recommending lower starting doses of rosuvastatin in this population (5 vs 10 mg for non-Hispanic whites).[46] Notably, in Japan, starting doses for most statins are one-half of what is recommended in the United States.[47]

There is less information on statin metabolism in other racial/ethnic minority groups. We are aware of 1 study that evaluated the pharmacokinetics of single-dose pravastatin in non-Hispanic blacks versus European Americans.[44] In this study, the OATP1B1 521T> C polymorphism was associated significantly with higher statin plasma concentrations in subjects of European versus African ancestry.[44] This may be explained by the low allelic frequency of OATP1B1 521T> C in non-Hispanic blacks (~1%)[44] relative to non-Hispanic whites. To our knowledge, no studies have been published on the pharmacokinetics of statins in Hispanics.

Myalgia (muscle pain) is one of the most commonly observed side effects associated with statins, but has been reported to occur at varying frequencies (5%–20%) in randomized controlled trials (RCT) and observational studies.[48–50] More severe but rare muscle side effects have also been reported, including myopathy (0.01%–0.3%) and rhabdomyolysis (0.003%–0.01%).[51] To date, high-dose simvastatin (80 mg) is the only statin to receive a US FDA warning for increased risk of muscle damage.[52] The use of statins in combination with other drugs has also been shown to increase the risk of adverse events.[53,54] In HPS2-THRIVE, which included 25,673 adults from Europe and China on simvastatin 40 mg/d, a higher risk of adverse events, including myopathy, were reported in patients randomized to niacin–laropiprant relative to placebo.[55] Furthermore, the relative risk of musculoskeletal events (mostly myopathy) in the niacin–laropiprant versus placebo group was markedly higher among Chinese participants than European participants.[55] To our knowledge no safety concerns have been raised for statins alone or in combination with agents in non-Hispanic blacks or Hispanics.

#### Statin efficacy in Asian populations

Studies conducted in Asian countries have documented that lower statin doses can achieve similar therapeutic effects in Asian populations.

- In an open-label study of Japanese patients receiving simvastatin (initial dose 5 mg/d), LDL-C decreased by 26% over 6 months, an effect that corresponds with simvastatin 20 mg/d in Western studies[56]
- In a multicenter, double-blind, RCT in 6 Asian countries, patients randomized to receive 10 mg simvastatin or atorvastatin daily over 8 weeks had an average LDL-C reduction of 35% and 43%, respectively, with more than 80% of patients achieving a National Cholesterol Education Program LDL-C target.[57] To see similar effects in non-Hispanic whites would generally require at least double this dose of simvastatin.

- In a prospective RCT of the primary prevention of CVD in Japan, pravastatin 10 to 20 mg/d reduced LDL-C by only 18% but reduced CHD by 33% relative to diet alone[58]; this level of risk reduction in CVD is similar to trials of predominantly non-Hispanic white populations taking higher daily doses of pravastatin (40 mg)[59] or a higher potency statin (atorvastatin 10 mg/d).[60]

It is tempting to speculate that the apparently increased effect of statins in Asians relative to non-Hispanic whites is owing to genetic differences in statin metabolism; however, because comparisons in these studies were indirect and were conducted on ethnic populations outside of the United States or Europe, underlying cultural differences in diet and lifestyle cannot be ruled out as a causal factor.

In addition, other studies have failed to demonstrate differences in response to statins in Asian and non-Hispanic white populations.

- In a combined analysis of 2 small multicenter open-label studies, GOALLS (included non-Asian and Asian participants) and STATT (included Asians only), the authors compared cholesterol outcomes among patients with CHD treated with simvastatin for 14 weeks.[61] There were no differences in changes in LDL-C among Asians in the STATT study (n = 133; −45.4 mg/dL) relative to Asians (n = 15) or non-Asians (n = 183) in the GOALLS study (−41.1 and −41.2 mg/dL, respectively)[61]
- In an observational, prospective study in Canada, no difference in the magnitude of LDL-C lowering was observed among non-Hispanic whites and South Asians (−41% vs −43%, respectively; $P = .40$), taking atorvastatin or simvastatin (20 mg median dose for each) for more than 3 years in the secondary prevention of CVD[62]
- Using data from an RCT evaluating atorvastatin versus placebo in a multiethnic population in the UK, Chapman and colleagues[63] matched White (n = 198) and South Asian (n = 76) cohorts receiving atorvastatin to evaluate the effects of statins across race/ethnic groups. The authors again found no difference in the percent reduction in LDL-C among whites and South Asians (−40% vs −39%; $P = .92$)[63]

To our best knowledge, no existing studies have shown differences in statin efficacy in non-Hispanic blacks, Hispanics, and non-Hispanic whites.[63–65]

## Lifestyle Modification in Special Racial/Ethnic Groups

Lifestyle modification has been recommended to treat dyslipidemia and to reduce ASCVD risk, both before and in addition to the use of lipid-lowering agents.[1] These lifestyle risk factors include unhealthy diet, overweight and obesity, and physical inactivity. The AHA has the following specific recommendations for individuals with dyslipidemia[66]:

- Diet: increase the intake of vegetables, fruits, and whole grains and limit intake of sweets; reduce the intake of saturated fat and trans fat.
- Physical activity: engage in aerobic physical activity; three to four 40-minute sessions per week; moderate-to-vigorous intensity physical activity.

Racial/ethnic disparities also exist in these lifestyle risk factors. According to data from the Behavioral Risk Factor Surveillance System in 2002, non-Hispanic whites had more fruits and vegetables in their diet compared with Hispanics and non-Hispanic blacks.[6,67] According to the National Health Interview Survey for 2008 through 2010, 71% of Hispanics were overweight or obese, followed by non-Hispanic blacks (70%), non-Hispanic whites (62%), and Asian Americans (42%). In addition, National Health Interview Survey for 2008 through 2010 also found that, compared with non-Hispanic whites (20%), non-Hispanic black (17%), Asian American (16%), and Hispanic (13%) adults were less likely to meet the 2008 guidelines for aerobic and muscle strengthening through leisure time activity.[68] All these data indicate that both non-Hispanic blacks and Hispanics are at higher risk for having both diet and lifestyle risk factors, and Asian Americans are more likely to be physically inactive.

A recent systematic review included nutrition and physical activity intervention studies in adult African Americans, from 2000 to 2011.[69] This study found both diet and physical activity interventions for weight loss improved cholesterol clinical outcomes among African Americans.[69] In particular, it provided evidence to support interventions in community-based settings among African Americans. A 2011 systematic review included intervention studies that promote physical activity in Hispanic adults published between 1988 and 2011.[70] This study concluded that physical activity interventions in Hispanics should include community-based settings, social support strategy, culturally sensitive intervention design, and staff from the same ethnic group. A systemic review of RCTs of lifestyle interventions for Asian Americans published between 1995 and 2013 concluded that lifestyle interventions improved physical activity, healthy diet, and weight control in Asian Americans.[71] However, the studies included in this review were limited in cultural appropriateness. In particular, Asian subgroups were aggregated together although they have different cultures and health behavior patterns. Other recommendations include individual tailoring, education and modeling of lifestyle behaviors, and providing support during a maintenance phase.

Immigration and acculturation have a profound impact on lifestyle in both Hispanics and Asians in the United States. For example, traditional Hispanic diets contain high levels of fiber. However, studies found US-born Hispanics had a hard time retaining traditional diets and consumed more fat and sugar compared with their counterparts in their home countries.[72,73] They have less access to high nutritional quality foods and are at risk for overweight/obesity.[72,74] Similarly, traditional East Asian diets contain less total and saturated fat but more sodium intake compared with Western diets and Asian Indian diets.[75,76] However, Chinese immigrants who have lived in the United States for longer than 10 years had a more unhealthy diet and less physical activity compared with recent immigrants.[30] In contrast, higher acculturation levels were associated with more physical activity among Korean Americans.[77] Future studies should consider providing culturally tailored, ethnic-specific interventions to these diverse immigrant populations.

## SUMMARY

There are significant racial/ethnic differences in dyslipidemia prevalence, dyslipidemia-related mortality rates, and response to lipid-lowering agents. Among all racial/ethnic groups, Asian Indians, Filipinos and Hispanics are at most elevated risk for dyslipidemia, which is consistent with the higher CHD mortality rates in these groups. More attention should be paid to these at-risk groups for screening and treatment purposes. Compared with other racial/ethnic groups, statins may have a higher efficacy for Asians, which may potentially be explained by genetic differences in statin metabolism, but overall the data are mixed. At present it may be wise to start with a lower statin dose in an individual with Asian ancestry until the treatment and adverse effects can be determined. In addition, racial/ethnic differences in health behavior patterns should be taken into consideration when promoting lifestyle modification among individuals with dyslipidemia. In particular,

Hispanic subgroups (Mexican, Puerto Rican, etc) and Asian (Chinese, South Asian, etc) subgroups should be disaggregated in lifestyle interventions. Further studies are needed to better understand racial/ethnic-specific risk factors contributing to the observed differences in dyslipidemia, CHD, and stroke. Culturally tailored prevention and intervention should be provided to the minority populations with elevated risk for dyslipidemia and considerably more research is needed to determine the best approaches to helping specific subgroups.

## REFERENCES

1. Stone NJ, Robinson J, Lichtenstein AH, et al. 2013 ACC/AHA guideline on the treatment of blood cholesterol to reduce atherosclerotic cardiovascular risk in adults: a report of the American College of Cardiology/American Heart Association task force on practice guidelines. Circulation 2014;129:S1–45.

2. Toth PP, Potter D, Ming EE. Prevalence of lipid abnormalities in the United States: the National Health and Nutrition Examination Survey 2003-2006. J Clin Lipidol 2012;6(4):325–30.

3. Frank AT, Zhao B, Jose PO, et al. Racial/ethnic differences in dyslipidemia patterns. Circulation 2014; 129(5):570–9.

4. Holland AT, Palaniappan LP. Problems with the collection and interpretation of Asian-American health data: omission, aggregation, and extrapolation. Ann Epidemiol 2012;22(6):397–405.

5. Statistical fact sheet 2013 update: high blood cholesterol & other lipids. 2013. Available at: http://www.heart.org/idc/groups/heart-public/@wcm/@sop/@smd/documents/downloadable/ucm_319586.pdf. Accessed November 15, 2014.

6. Rodriguez CJ, Allison M, Daviglus ML, et al. Status of cardiovascular disease and stroke in Hispanics/Latinos in the United States: a science advisory from the American Heart Association. Circulation 2014;130:593–625 (1524–4539 [Electronic]).

7. Anand SS, Yusuf S, Vuksan V, et al. Differences in risk factors, atherosclerosis and cardiovascular disease between ethnic groups in Canada: the Study of Health Assessment and Risk in Ethnic groups (SHARE). Indian Heart J 2000;52(7 Suppl):S35–43.

8. Aoki Y, Yoon SS, Chong Y, et al. Hypertension, abnormal cholesterol, and high body mass index among non-Hispanic Asian adults: United States, 2011-2012. NCHS Data Brief 2014;(140):1–8.

9. Miller M, Stone NJ, Ballantyne C, et al. Triglycerides and cardiovascular disease: a scientific statement from the American Heart Association. Circulation 2011;123(20):2292–333.

10. Goff DC Jr, Bertoni AG, Kramer H, et al. Dyslipidemia prevalence, treatment, and control in the Multi-Ethnic Study of Atherosclerosis (MESA): gender,

11. Huang MH, Schocken M, Block G, et al. Variation in nutrient intakes by ethnicity: results from the Study of Women's Health Across the Nation (SWAN). Menopause 2002;9(5):309–19.

12. McKeigue PM, Miller GJ, Marmot MG. Coronary heart disease in South Asians overseas: a review. J Clin Epidemiol 1989;42(7):597–609.

13. Chambers JC, Kooner JS. Diabetes, insulin resistance and vascular disease among Indian Asians and Europeans. Semin Vasc Med 2002; 2(2):199–214.

14. Radhika G, Ganesan A, Sathya RM, et al. Dietary carbohydrates, glycemic load and serum high-density lipoprotein cholesterol concentrations among South Indian adults. Eur J Clin Nutr 2009; 63(3):413–20.

15. Enas EA. Clinical implications: dyslipidemia in the Asian Indian population. 2002. Available at: https:// southasianheartcenter.org/docs/AAPImonograph.pdf. Accessed November 15, 2014.

16. Roger VL, Go AS, Lloyd-Jones DM, et al. Heart disease and stroke statistics—2011 update: a report from the American Heart Association. Circulation 2011;123(4):e18–209.

17. Jose PO, Frank AT, Kapphahn KI, et al. Cardiovascular disease mortality in Asian Americans (2003 to 2010). J Am Coll Cardiol 2014;64(23):2486–94.

18. Palaniappan L, Wang Y, Fortmann SP. Coronary heart disease mortality for six ethnic groups in California, 1990-2000. Ann Epidemiol 2004;14(7): 499–506.

19. Keppel KG, Pearcy JN, Heron MP. Is there progress toward eliminating racial/ethnic disparities in the leading causes of death? Public Health Rep 2010; 125(5):689–97.

20. Farnier M, Chen E, Johnson-Levonas AO, et al. Effects of extended-release niacin/laropiprant, simvastatin, and the combination on correlations between apolipoprotein B, LDL cholesterol, and non-HDL cholesterol in patients with dyslipidemia. Vasc Health Risk Manag 2014;10:279–90.

21. Enas E, Yusuf S, Mehta J. Meeting of international working group on coronary artery disease in South Asians. Indian Heart J 1996;48:727–32.

22. Hoyert DL. 75 years of mortality in the United States, 1935-2010. NCHS Data Brief 2012;(88):1–8.

23. Ye J, Rust G, Baltrus P, et al. Cardiovascular risk factors among Asian Americans: results from a national health survey. Ann Epidemiol 2009;19(10):718–23.

24. Klatsky AL, Tekawa IS, Armstrong MA. Cardiovascular risk factors among Asian Americans. Public Health Rep 1996;111(Suppl 2):62–4.

25. Marmot MG, Syme SL, Kagan A, et al. Epidemiologic studies of coronary heart disease and stroke in Japanese men living in Japan, Hawaii and California: prevalence of coronary and hypertensive heart disease and associated risk factors. Am J Epidemiol 1975;102(6):514–25.

26. Balarajan R. Ethnic differences in mortality from ischaemic heart disease and cerebrovascular disease in England and Wales. BMJ 1991;302(6776): 560–4.

27. Enas EA, Garg A, Davidson MA, et al. Coronary heart disease and its risk factors in first-generation immigrant Asian Indians to the United States of America. Indian Heart J 1996;48(4):343–53.

28. Karthikeyan G, Teo KK, Islam S, et al. Lipid profile, plasma apolipoproteins, and risk of a first myocardial infarction among Asians: an analysis from the INTERHEART Study. J Am Coll Cardiol 2009;53(3): 244–53.

29. Marmot MG, Syme SL. Acculturation and coronary heart disease in Japanese-Americans. Am J Epidemiol 1976;104(3):225–47.

30. Taylor VM, Yasui Y, Tu SP, et al. Heart disease prevention among Chinese immigrants. J Community Health 2007;32(5):299–310.

31. Gupta M, Brister S. Is South Asian ethnicity an independent cardiovascular risk factor? Can J Cardiol 2006;22(3):193–7.

32. Bartholow M. Rx focus: top 200 drugs of 2012. Pharm Times 2012.

33. Pencina MJ, Navar-Boggan AM, D'Agostino RB Sr, et al. Application of new cholesterol guidelines to a population-based sample. N Engl J Med 2014; 370(15):1422–31.

34. D'Agostino RB Sr, Vasan RS, Pencina MJ, et al. General cardiovascular risk profile for use in primary care: the Framingham heart study. Circulation 2008;117(6):743–53.

35. National Cholesterol Education Program (NCEP) Expert Panel on Detection, Evaluation, and Treatment of High Blood Cholesterol in Adults (Adult Treatment Panel III). Third report of the national cholesterol education program (NCEP) expert panel on detection, evaluation, and treatment of high blood cholesterol in adults (Adult treatment panel III) final report. Circulation 2002;106(25):3143–421.

36. Goff DC Jr, Lloyd-Jones DM, Bennett G, et al. 2013 ACC/AHA guideline on the assessment of cardiovascular risk: a report of the American College of Cardiology/American Heart Association Task Force on Practice Guidelines. J Am Coll Cardiol 2014; 63(25 Pt B):2935–59.

37. Goff DC Jr, Lloyd-Jones DM. 2013 Report on the assessment of cardiovascular risk: full work group report supplement. 2013. Available at: http://jaccjacc. cardiosource.com/acc_documents/2013_FPR_S5_ Risk_Assesment.pdf. Accessed May 22, 2014.

38. Stone NJ, Robinson JG, Lichtenstein AH. 2013 Report on the treatment of blood cholesterol to reduce atherosclerotic cardiovascular disease in

The following references appear at the top of the first column and continue the list:

ethnicity, and coronary artery calcium. Circulation 2006;113(5):647–56.

adults: full panel report supplement. 2013. Available at: http://www.kcumb.edu/uploadedFiles/Content/Academics/_Assets/CME_Presentations/Moriarty12_5_full.pdf. Accessed May 23, 2014.

39. Hippisley-Cox J, Coupland C, Vinogradova Y, et al. Predicting cardiovascular risk in England and Wales: prospective derivation and validation of QRISK2. BMJ 2008;336(7659):1475–82.

40. Lee E, Ryan S, Birmingham B, et al. Rosuvastatin pharmacokinetics and pharmacogenetics in white and Asian subjects residing in the same environment. Clin Pharmacol Ther 2005;78(4):330–41.

41. Nishizato Y, Ieiri I, Suzuki H, et al. Polymorphisms of OATP-C (SLC21A6) and OAT3 (SLC22A8) genes: consequences for pravastatin pharmacokinetics. Clin Pharmacol Ther 2003;73(6):554–65.

42. Niemi M. Transporter pharmacogenetics and statin toxicity. Clin Pharmacol Ther 2010;87(1):130–3.

43. Zhang W, Yu BN, He YJ, et al. Role of BCRP 421C>A polymorphism on rosuvastatin pharmacokinetics in healthy Chinese males. Clin Chim Acta 2006; 373(1–2):99–103.

44. Ho RH, Choi L, Lee W, et al. Effect of drug transporter genotypes on pravastatin disposition in European- and African-American participants. Pharmacogenet Genomics 2007;17(8):647–56.

45. Keskitalo JE, Zolk O, Fromm MF, et al. ABCG2 polymorphism markedly affects the pharmacokinetics of atorvastatin and rosuvastatin. Clin Pharmacol Ther 2009;86(2):197–203.

46. AstraZeneca. CRESTOR (rosuvastatin) prescribing information. 2014. Available at: http://www1.astrazeneca-us.com/pi/crestor.pdf. Accessed November 12, 2014.

47. Liao JK. Safety and efficacy of statins in Asians. Am J Cardiol 2007;99(3):410–4.

48. Bruckert E, Hayem G, Dejager S, et al. Mild to moderate muscular symptoms with high-dosage statin therapy in hyperlipidemic patients–the PRIMO study. Cardiovasc Drugs Ther 2005;19(6):403–14.

49. Stewart A. SLCO1B1 polymorphisms and statin-induced myopathy. PLOS Currents Evidence on Genomic Tests. December 4, 2013. Edition 1. http://dx.doi.org/10.1371/currents.eogt.d21e7f0c58463571bb0d9d3a19b82203.

50. Fung EC, Crook MA. Statin myopathy: a lipid clinic experience on the tolerability of statin rechallenge. Cardiovasc Ther 2012;30(5):e212–8.

51. Law M, Rudnicka AR. Statin safety: a systematic review. Am J Cardiol 2006;97(8A):52C–60C.

52. FDA drug safety communication: new restrictions, contraindications, and dose limitations for Zocor (simvastatin) to reduce the risk of muscle injury. 2011. Available at: http://www.fda.gov/Drugs/DrugSafety/ucm256581.htm. Accessed November 15, 2014.

53. Thompson PD, Clarkson P, Karas RH. Statin-associated myopathy. JAMA 2003;289(13):1681–90.

54. Pasternak RC, Smith SC Jr, Bairey-Merz CN, et al. ACC/AHA/NHLBI clinical advisory on the use and safety of statins. J Am Coll Cardiol 2002;40(3):567–72.

55. Group HT, Landray MJ, Haynes R, et al. Effects of extended-release niacin with laropiprant in high-risk patients. N Engl J Med 2014;371(3):203–12.

56. Matsuzawa Y, Kita T, Mabuchi H, et al. Sustained reduction of serum cholesterol in low-dose 6-year simvastatin treatment with minimum side effects in 51,321 Japanese hypercholesterolemic patients. Circ J 2003;67(4):287–94.

57. Wu CC, Sy R, Tanphaichitr V, et al. Comparing the efficacy and safety of atorvastatin and simvastatin in Asians with elevated low-density lipoprotein-cholesterol–a multinational, multicenter, double-blind study. J Formos Med Assoc 2002;101(7):478–87.

58. Nakamura H, Arakawa K, Itakura H, et al. Primary prevention of cardiovascular disease with pravastatin in Japan (MEGA Study): a prospective randomised controlled trial. Lancet 2006;368(9542):1155–63.

59. Shepherd J, Cobbe SM, Ford I, et al. Prevention of coronary heart disease with pravastatin in men with hypercholesterolemia. West of Scotland coronary prevention study group. N Engl J Med 1995;333(20):1301–7.

60. Colhoun HM, Betteridge DJ, Durrington PN, et al. Primary prevention of cardiovascular disease with atorvastatin in type 2 diabetes in the Collaborative Atorvastatin Diabetes Study (CARDS): multicentre randomised placebo-controlled trial. Lancet 2004;364(9435):685–96.

61. Morales D, Chung N, Zhu JR, et al. Efficacy and safety of simvastatin in Asian and non-Asian coronary heart disease patients: a comparison of the GOALLS and STATT studies. Curr Med Res Opin 2004;20(8):1235–43.

62. Gupta M, Braga MF, Teoh H, et al. Statin effects on LDL and HDL cholesterol in South Asian and white populations. J Clin Pharmacol 2009;49(7):831–7.

63. Chapman N, Chang CL, Caulfield M, et al. Ethnic variations in lipid-lowering in response to a statin (EVIREST): a substudy of the Anglo-Scandinavian Cardiac Outcomes Trial (ASCOT). Ethn Dis 2011; 21(2):150–7.

64. Albert MA, Glynn RJ, Fonseca FA, et al. Race, ethnicity, and the efficacy of rosuvastatin in primary prevention: the justification for the use of statins in prevention: an intervention trial evaluating rosuvastatin (JUPITER) trial. Am Heart J 2011;162(1):106–14.e102.

65. Lipworth L, Fazio S, Kabagambe EK, et al. A prospective study of statin use and mortality among 67,385 blacks and whites in the Southeastern United States. Clin Epidemiol 2014;6:15–25.

66. Eckel RH, Jakicic JM, Ard JD, et al. 2013 AHA/ACC guideline on lifestyle management to reduce cardiovascular risk: a report of the American College of Cardiology/AMERICAN HEART ASSOCIATION Task Force on Practice Guidelines. J Am Coll Cardiol 2014;63:2960–84 (1524–4539 (Electronic)).

67. Behavioral risk factor surveillance system: BRFSS 2002 survey data and documentation. Available at: http://www.cdc.gov/brfss/annual_data/annual_2002.htm. Accessed November 15, 2014.

68. Schoenborn CA, Adams PF, Peregoy JA. Health behaviors of adults: United States, 2008-2010. Vital Health Stat 10 2013;(257):1–184.

69. Lemacks J, Wells BA, Ilich JZ, et al. Interventions for improving nutrition and physical activity behaviors in adult African American populations: a systematic review, January 2000 through December 2011. Prev Chronic Dis 2013;10:E99.

70. Ickes MJ, Sharma M. A systematic review of physical activity interventions in Hispanic adults. J Environ Public Health 2012;2012:156435.

71. Bender MS, Choi J, Won GY, et al. Randomized controlled trial lifestyle interventions for Asian Americans: a systematic review. Prev Med 2014;67:171–81.

72. Dhokarh R, Himmelgreen DA, Peng YK, et al. Food insecurity is associated with acculturation and social networks in Puerto Rican households. J Nutr Educ Behav 2011;43:288–94 (1878–2620 [Electronic]).

73. Mainous AG 3rd, Diaz VA, Geesey ME. Acculturation and healthy lifestyle among Latinos with diabetes. Ann Fam Med 2008;6:131–7 (1544–1717 [Electronic]).

74. Lin H, Bermudez OI, Tucker KL. Dietary patterns of Hispanic elders are associated with acculturation and obesity. J Nutr 2003;133:3651–7 (0022–3166 [Print]).

75. Palaniappan LP, Araneta MR, Assimes TL, et al. Call to action: cardiovascular disease in Asian Americans: a science advisory from the American Heart Association. Circulation 2010;122(12):1242–52.

76. Zhou BF, Stamler J, Dennis B, et al. Nutrient intakes of middle-aged men and women in China, Japan, United Kingdom, and United States in the late 1990s: the INTERMAP study. J Hum Hypertens 2003;17:623–30 (0950–9240 [Print]).

77. Song YJ, Hofstetter CR, Hovell MF, et al. Acculturation and health risk behaviors among Californians of Korean descent. Prev Med 2004;39:147–56 (0091–7435 [Print]).

# Index

*Note:* Page numbers of article titles are in **boldface** type.

## A

ACC/AHA. *See* American College of Cardiology/
American Heart Association (ACC/AHA)
ACE inhibitors. *See* Angiotensin-converting enzyme
(ACE) inhibitors
American College of Cardiology/American Heart
Association (ACC/AHA)
2013 cholesterol guidelines of, 182–186. *See also*
2013 American College of Cardiology/
American Heart Association (ACC/AHA)
cholesterol guidelines
Angiotensin-converting enzyme (ACE) inhibitors
in residual risk management after MI among
LDL–C persons, 302
Antiplatelet therapy
in residual risk management after MI among
LDL–C persons, 301–302
Antiretroviral therapy (ART)
in dyslipidemia management in HIV patients
statin interactions with, 286
switching drugs in, 293
in HIV management, 279
Apheresis
LDL
in FH management, 174–175
lipoprotein, **197–208**. *See also* Lipoprotein
apheresis (LA)
Apolipoprotein(s)
alteration by LA, 201–203
ART. *See* Antiretroviral therapy (ART)
ASCVD. *See* Atherosclerotic cardiovascular disease
(ASCVD)
Atherogenesis
accelerated
in hypertriglyceridemia
mechanisms of, 311–312
Atherogenic cholesterol
in patient-centered management of dyslipidemia,
186–187
Atherogenic dyslipidemia, 312–313
Atherosclerotic cardiovascular disease (ASCVD)
assessment of
in patient-centered management of
dyslipidemia, 187–188
hypertriglyceridemia *vs.*
association and causation, 311–313
management of
new cholesterol guidelines in, **181–196**

ACC/AHA, 182–186. *See also* 2013
American College of Cardiology/
American Heart Association (ACC/AHA)
cholesterol guidelines
prevention of
hypertriglyceridemia management in, **309–323**.
*See also* Hypertriglyceridemia,
management of, in ASCVD prevention
risk assessment for, 192–193

## B

β-blockers
in residual risk management after MI among
LDL–C persons, 302–303
Bile acid sequestrants
in dyslipidemia management in HIV patients,
291
Breastfeeding
dyslipidemia in women who are
recommendations for, 222

## C

Cardiac rehabilitation
in residual risk management after MI among
LDL–C persons, 301
Cardiovascular disease (CVD)
atherosclerotic
management of
new cholesterol guidelines in, **181–196**. *See
also* Atherosclerotic cardiovascular
disease (ASCVD)
HCV and, 278–279
risk factors for
in pregnancy, 210–211
Cholestatic liver disease
statin use in patients with, 261–262
Cholesterol
atherogenic
in patient-centered management of
dyslipidemia, 186–187
fetal development effects of, 209–210
HDL. *See* High-density lipoprotein cholesterol
(HDL–C)
LDL. *See* Low-density lipoprotein cholesterol
(LDL–C)
management of

cardiology.theclinics.com

# Moving?

## Make sure your subscription moves with you!

To notify us of your new address, find your **Clinics Account Number** (located on your mailing label above your name), and contact customer service at:

**Email: journalscustomerservice-usa@elsevier.com**

**800-654-2452** (subscribers in the U.S. & Canada)
**314-447-8871** (subscribers outside of the U.S. & Canada)

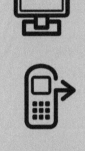

**Fax number: 314-447-8029**

**Elsevier Health Sciences Division**
**Subscription Customer Service**
**3251 Riverport Lane**
**Maryland Heights, MO 63043**